# Millets and Other Potential Crops

## Ensuring Climate Resilience and Nutritional Security

# Millets and Other Potential Crops

## Ensuring Climate Resilience & Nutritional Security


*Editors :*

**Dr. Jyostnarani Pradhan**
Department of Botany, Plant Physiology and Biochemistry
College of Basic Sciences and Humanities, Dr. Rajendra Prasad
Central Agricultural University, Pusa, Samastipur - 848125, Bihar

**Dr. Jyoti Prakash Sahoo**
Department of Agriculture and Allied Sciences
C. V. Raman Global University, Bhubaneswar - 752054, Odisha

**Prof. Kailash Chandra Samal**
College of Horticulture, Odisha University of Agriculture and Technology
Chiplima - 768025, Odisha

**Dr. Manasi Dash**
Department of Genetics and Plant Breeding
College of Agriculture, Odisha University of Agriculture and Technology,
Bhubaneswar - 751003, Odisha



**NARENDRA PUBLISHING HOUSE**
New Delhi-110 085

CRC Press
Taylor & Francis Group
Boca Raton London New York

CRC Press is an imprint of the
Taylor & Francis Group, an **informa** business

First published 2025
by CRC Press
2 Park Square, Milton Park, Abingdon, Oxon OX14 4RN

and by CRC Press
6000 Broken Sound Parkway NW, Suite 300, Boca Raton, FL 33487-2742

*CRC Press is an imprint of Informa UK Limited*



*British Library Cataloguing-in-Publication Data*
A catalogue record for this book is available from the British Library

Print edition not for sale in South Asia (India, Sri Lanka, Nepal, Bangladesh, Pakistan or Bhutan)

ISBN: 9781032873008 (hbk)
ISBN: 9781032873022 (pbk)
ISBN: 9781003531937 (ebk)

DOI: 10.1201/9781003531937

Typeset in Times New Roman

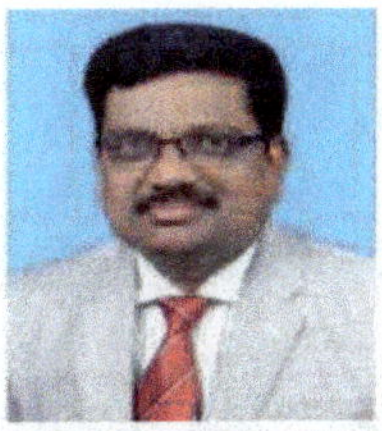


ପ୍ରଫେସର ପ୍ରଭାତ କୁମାର
ରାଉଳ
କୁଳପତି
**Prof. Pravat Kumar Roul**
Vice-Chancellor



**ଓଡ଼ିଶା କୃଷି ଓ ବୈଷୟିକ ବିଶ୍ୱ ବିଦ୍ୟାଳୟ,**
**ଭୁବନେଶ୍ୱର**
**ODISHA UNIVERSITY OF AGRICULTURE AND TECHNOLOGY**
**BHUBANESWAR – 751003**


**Dated the 6th June, 2023**

## MESSAGE

Millets include a diverse group of crops such as finger millet, pearl millet, foxtail millet, proso millet, barnyard millet, little millet, etc. Millets are grown in India since ancient time and occupy a conspicuous place in our culture heritage. These crops provide reasonable options for nutritional security in global agri-food system.

I am glad to know that a book entitled “Millets and other potential crops: ensuring climate resilience and nutritional security” is being published with efforts of some of our faculty members. I hope, the book will throw insight into technology innovations of millet crops for the benefit of students, academicians, researchers, farmers and others interested in millet cultivation.

I congratulate the authors and wish this endeavour all success.

**(P. K. Roul)**


**Visit us at www.ouat.nic.in**
Tel: 0674-2397700 (O) Fax-0674-2397780
E-mail: vc@ouat.nic.in/ vouat@gmail.com

C. V. RAMAN GLOBAL UNIVERSITY
**Department of Agriculture and Allied Sciences**
**PO-Mahura, Pin-752 054, Dist. Khorda, Odisha, India**
Email: deanagriculture@cgu-odisha.ac.in

**Dr. Dilip Kumar Dash**
M. Sc. (Hort), Ph.D.
Dean, Department of Agriculture and Allied Sciences

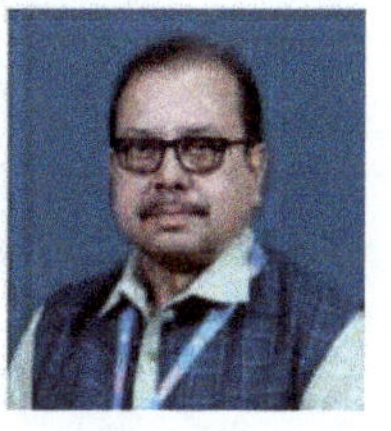

## MESSAGE

Millets are resilient cereals that can provide an affordable and nutritious option towards food security. These are among the first plants to be domesticated and are considered "nutri-cereals" due to their high nutritional content. However, other potential crops mentioned in this book can also provide nutritional security during changing climatic condition.

I appreciate the publication of this book entitled "Millets and Other Potential Crops: Ensuring Climate Resilience and Nutritional Security" composed by Dr. Jyostnarani Pradhan, Dr. Jyoti Prakash Sahoo, Dr. Kailash Chandra Samal, and Dr. Manasi Dash, which plays an important role in enriching teaching courses and research related to millets and other potential crops towards climate resilience and nutritional security.

The major goal of this book is to promote the sustainable cultivation of millets and other potential crops, under changing climatic conditions for improving their quality, highlighting their potential to provide new sustainable market opportunities for producers and consumers.

I express my best wishes to the editors and contributors for the grand success of the book.

With best compliments.

22.05.2023

(D K Dash)

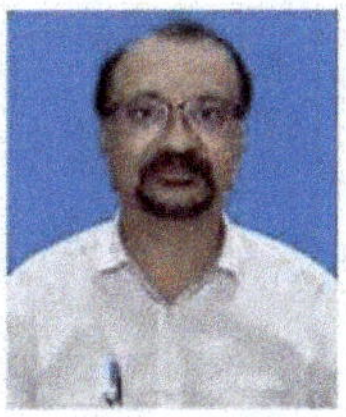

APEX PROFESSIONAL UNIVERSITY

Established by Government of Arunachal Pradesh

**Dr. Somnath Roy Chowdhury**
**Pro-Vice Chancellor**

**Apex Professional University, NH – 52, Pasighat Smart City, District East Siang – 791102, Arunachal Pradesh – India**

## MESSAGE

*"Knowledge shared is knowledge squared."*

It is heartening to note that in this International year of Millets, 2023 such a book on millets and other under exploited crops is being brought out. It is an appreciable contribution to the agriculture, health and well-being sector. Sincere effort has been made to make reader(s) aware about the millets (super food) and other potential under-exploited crops and strategise for food and nutritional security. Millets are known for their better resilience against harsh weather like heat, drought etc. compared to other conventional cereals and can provide affordable food and nutritional security. The information provided in this book is regarding importance, scope for its improvement, utilisation and packages of practices for cultivation of millets and other underutilised crops.

I express my best wishes to the editors and contributors for their appreciable effort to bring out this book in appropriate time when nation has pledged to provide food and nutritional security to our citizen.

With best compliments

(S. Roy Chowdhury)

Visit our website @ www.apexuniversity.edu.in

# Contents

# Preface

The first edition is an attempt to provide a true "Millets and Other Potential Crops: Ensuring Climate Resilience and Nutritional Security" text that is up-to-date, readable, and challenging. The major goal is to promote the sustainable cultivation of millets, also under adverse and changing climatic conditions and improving their quality, highlighting their potential to provide new sustainable market opportunities for producers and consumers. Millets are resilient cereals that can provide an affordable and nutritious option and help guarantee food security. They are also deeply rooted in Indigenous Peoples' culture and traditions. Millets are among the first plants to be domesticated and are considered "nutri-cereals" due to their high nutritional content. Millets are incredible ancestral crops with high nutritional value. Millets can play an important role and contribute to our collective efforts to empower smallholder farmers, achieve sustainable development, eliminate hunger, adapt to climate change, promote biodiversity, and transform agri-food systems. According to The International Crop Research Institute for the Semi-Arid Tropics (ICRISAT), more than 90 million people in Africa and Asia depend on millets in their diet. Although the global millet consumption has declined at a rate of 9 percent, the Millet Market forecast for 2022-27 shows promising trends. India dominates the global production at 41 percent, whereas the consumption has been receding over the years. On the other hand, Africa has become the largest consumer of millets at 40 percent.

The United Nations General Assembly at its 75th session in March 2021 declared 2023 the International Year of Millets (IYM 2023) with the Food and Agriculture Organization of the United Nations (FAO) as the lead agency. The International Year of Millets 2023 will focus on raising awareness of the nutritional and health benefits of millets and promoting millets as a key component of the food basket, raising awareness of the contribution of millets to food security and their important role in keeping a check on food wastage, promoting the sustainable cultivation of millets, also under adverse and changing climatic conditions and improving their quality, highlighting their potential to provide new sustainable market opportunities for producers and consumers, promoting a better utilization of crop rotations, and enhancing investment in research and development.

As the global agrifood systems face challenges to feed an ever-growing global population, resilient cereals like millets provide an affordable and nutritious option, and efforts need to be scaled-up to promote their cultivation. The authors believe that, this edition presents the basic principles and practices of Millets and other potential crops towards climate resilience and nutritional security in a clear and logical sequence. This edition begins with a introductory Chapter-1 that attempts to convey some important facts and figures of International Year of Millets. Chapter 2 describes the millets as super food for nutrition security and livelihood improvement. Meanwhile, a detailed study of climate change and its impact on millets is described in Chapter 3. Chapter 4 highlights the vital role of millets in sustainable agriculture. Chapter 5 describes the role of small millets in the context of climate change and genomic resources. Organic agriculture is a holistic production management system which promotes and enhances agro-ecosystem health, including biodiversity, biological cycles, and soil biological activity. Meanwhile, Chapter 6 covers the cultivation practices of millets in organic agriculture system. The breeding and biotechnological aspects of millets genetic improvement are described in Chapter 7 and Chapter 8 respectively. Chapter 9, 10 and 11 describe the sustainable approach for nutritional security and biofortification of finger millets, origin, production, nutritional benefits and medicinal use of foxtail millet and nutritional composition, health benefits and food product developments of kodo millet. Chapter 12, 13, 14 and 15 dissect the economic important of major disease and pest of millets and their integrated management strategies.

As this edition also focuses on other potential crops, Chapter 16 describes some exotic fruits in India, their production, nutritional benefits, and medicinal properties. However, Chapter 17 and 18 deal with the climate resilient fruit and vegetable crops to ensure global food and nutritional security. However, there are many Unani medications with antihyperlipidemic properties, and one of them is Jamun. It is a suitable source of iron and ascorbic acid, and it can even help with heart and liver problems. The dried and powdered seed of the Jamun is frequently used in India to manage diabetes. In this context, Chapter 19 deals with the bioactive compounds in Jamun maintaining nutritive sanctuary. Meanwhile, Chapter 20 helps to meet the incredible, the unsung heroes of crops in alleviating iron deficiency anemia. Chapter 21 describes the importance of millets for enhancement of calcium content and thickness in eggshell of granivorous birds, while Chapter 22 describes the climate change resilient through modern farming in vegetable cultivation.

The authors are thankful to students, teachers and colleagues who have suggested improvements for the book. Authors especially thank Sibasis Mahapatra, Sheetal Das, Akash Kumar Jena and Sonali Behera for their valuable input for this edition. The authors are thankful to all the contributors, who have contributed their chapters for this book. Credits for illustrations and tables from other individuals or publications are given with the individual items.

**Dr. Jyostnarani Pradhan**

**Dr. Jyoti Prakash Sahoo**

**Dr. Kailash Chandra Samal**

**Dr. Manasi Dash**

# About the Editors

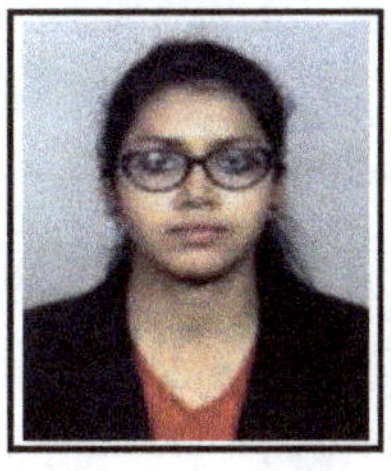

**DR. JYOSTNARANI PRADHAN** is currently working as Assistant Professor in the Department of Botany, Plant Physiology and Biochemistry, College of Basic Sciences and Humanities, Dr. Rajendra Prasad Central Agriculture University, Pusa, Samastipur, Bihar. She pursued her Ph.D. degree in the Department of Plant Physiology, Institute of Agricultural Sciences, Banaras Hindu University with UGC fellowship. She did her bachelor and master degree from Odisha University of Agriculture and Technology (OUAT), Bhubaneswar, India. She worked as research scholar under many national and international scientists during her working period at CSISA project funded by IRRI. She has attended many national and international training programme including IRRI head quarter, Philippines and ICRISAT, Hyderabad. She has been awarded with award of excellence and gold medal for her performance during masters. Her several research papers and articles have been published in national and international journals. She has also published several of books and book chapters. She has contributed in many research projects as P.I. and Co-I. So far she has guided 5 M.Sc.(Plant Physiology) students as Major Advisor. Apart from academic works she is contributing in many administrative works. Presently she is working on stress physiology, secondary metabolites and seed physiology in varoius crops.

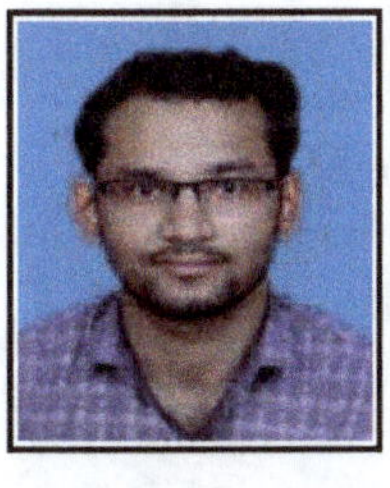

**DR. JYOTI PRAKASH SAHOO** is currently working as Assistant Professor in the Department of Agriculture and Allied Sciences, C. V. Raman Global University, Bhubaneswar, India. He pursued his Ph.D. degree in Agricultural Biotechnology from the Department of Agricultural Biotechnology, College of Agriculture, Odisha University of Agriculture and Technology (OUAT), Bhubaneswar, India, under the guidance of Prof. Kailash Chandra Samal. He authored numerous research and review articles that were published in nationally and internationally reputed agricultural and biological science journals indexed in Scopus, UGC Care List, and Clarivate analytics group and also contributed various book chapters in multitudinous bestseller books related to agricultural biotechnology. He bagged one best article award from "Agriculture Letters – A monthly peer-reviewed newsletter in agriculture and allied sector" for the article entitled "Biotech crop and its consequences in augmenting the soil health status" and two best article awards from "Agriculture and Food e-Newsletter" for the essays entitled "RNA Interference – A Key Tool For Crop Improvement" and "Plant Growth Regulators and Their Mode of Action." He was also awarded with the most Impactful article award (June – 2021) for the article entitled "Covid-19 Mutants Carrying the Global Pandemic towards the Worst" published in "Vigyan Varta – An International E-Magazine for Science Enthusiasts." He is a life member of the "Society of Biotechnology and Bioinformatics, Bhubaneswar, India". He is also working as a potential editorial board member in the journal of Universa Medicina (An official publication of Faculty of Medicine, Trisakti University, Indonesia) and various international journals and newsletters. He is a passionate author who would love to share his knowledge with the world, finding peace by sewing words of hope and trust about life. He is a diligent and persistent individual, his conceptual understanding of agriculture and biotechnology is outstanding. Thou young at age, his contributions to the field of research in agricultural biotechnology and writings is honoured by various prestigious awards such as best oral presenter awards in "National Seminar on Recent Trends in Microbiology and Biotechnology" in the year 2018, young scientist award in the "International Conference on New Paradigms for Agriculture, Food and Sustainability Concerns" in the year 2021 and he is honoured with "Foxcules India prime quality education award - 2021" for the enduring commitments to exceptional contribution towards the education. Dr. Jyoti Prakash Sahoo has an aura of positivity that radiates warmth, smiles to other lives. He is an inspiration for many teenagers and young people out there.

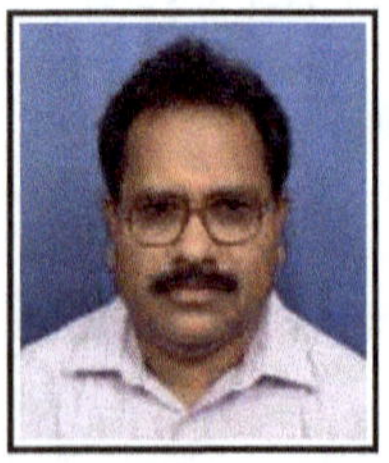

**PROF. KAILASH CHANDRA SAMAL** obtained his M.Sc. degree in Agriculture Biotechnology in the year 1991 from Tamil Nadu Agriculture University, Coimbatore and got his doctoral degree in Biotechnology from Utkal University, Bhubaneswar in the year 2011. He served at Odisha University of Agriculture and Technology (OUAT), Bhubaneswar in different positions for 30 years as a teacher for UG, PG and PhD students and a research scientist. Currently, his areas of specialisation are Plant Molecular Biology, Plant Tissue culture, Microbial technology, DNA fingerprinting, Computational Biology and Bioinformatics,. He has also developed cost-efficient protocols for large-scale micropropagation of several plant species, including banana, ginger, turmeric, sugarcane, stevia and sarpagnadha etc. He has also developed molecular marker based techniques for testing of clonal fidelity (true-to-type nature) of the micropropagated plants. He has also developed a DNA fingerprint database of promising rice varieties in Odisha using microsatellite DNA markers. He has also studied the phenotypic, biochemical and molecular fingerprints of indigenous aromatic rice varieties of Odisha. Molecular fingerprints of different crops such as ragi, wheat, rape seed, and sesamum, blackgram, greengram, eggplant, tomato, etc. So far he has guided 40 M.Sc. (Ag) and PhD students, who did their research on Molecular Biology and Biotechnology. He has 10 externally funded schemes from DBT, RKVY and Ministry of Agriculture, New Delhi. Further, he is a member of several professional bodies of the government and universities. He has isolated and characterised several abiotic stress related genes like DREB etc and deposited them in the GenBank, NCBI, USA. He has published 10 books and more than 128 international and national-level research papers. He currently holds the positions of Professor and Head, Department of Molecular Biology and Biotechnology, Odisha University of Agriculture and Technology, Bhubaneswar, India.

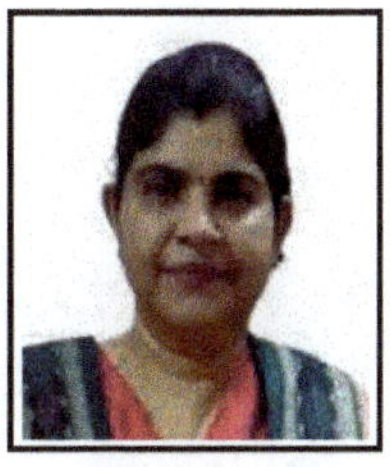

**DR. MANASI DASH,** currently positioned as Faculty in the Department of Genetics and Plant Breeding, obtained her Master's and Ph.D. in Plant Breeding and Genetics from OUAT in the year 1996 and 2005 respectively. She also completed 'Masters in Intellectual Property Law'from IGNOU in the year 2012. She has teaching and research experience of about 18 years in the subject related to Genomics, Plant biotechnology, Molecular Biology, Cell Biology, Plant Breeding and Genetics. She has the credit of releasing one Sesame variety "Kalinga Sesame-3-1". She has been instrumental in carrying out externally funded project from DBT Bio-Care, Govt. of India and RKVY, Govt. of Odisha. She has published several research papers in National and Inter-National journals and also authored many popular science articles. She has edited one book "A Glossary of Biotechnology & Allied Sciences" and is in the Editorial Board of several journals. Her expertise is also commanded by many international journals as a peer reviewer. Further she is a life member in seven international societies. She has successfully guided 17 M.Sc. (Ag.) and Ph.D. students, for their research on transcriptomics, heterosis breeding, anther culture, marker assisted breeding, biotic and abiotic stress resistance. Presently she is working on seed shattering and biofuel traits in varoius crops.

# 1

# International Year of Millets - Unleashing its Potential in Making a Sustainable World

Mamata Mohapatra[1*], Sibasis Mahapatra[2], Sheetal Das[2], Akash Kumar Jena[2], Manaswini Mahapatra[2], Jyoti Prakash Sahoo[2*]

[1] Department of Agricultural Biotechnology, College of Agriculture, Odisha University of Agriculture and Technology, Bhubaneswar - 751003, India

[2] Department of Agriculture and Allied Sciences, C. V. Raman Global University, Bhubaneswar – 752054, India

## ABSTRACT

As the global agrifood systems face challenges to feed an ever-growing global population, resilient cereals like millets provide an affordable and nutritious option, and efforts need to be scaled-up to promote their cultivation. This was the message at the opening ceremony of the International Year of Millets 2023 (IYM) at the headquarters of the Food and Agriculture Organization (FAO) of United Nations. Millets encompass a diverse group of cereals including pearl, proso, foxtail, barnyard, little, kodo, browntop, finger and Guinea millets, as well as fonio, sorghum (or great millet) and teff. They are an important source of nourishment for millions of people in sub-Saharan Africa and Asia. They are deeply rooted in Indigenous Peoples' culture and traditions and also help towards food security in areas where they are culturally relevant. Greater millet production can support the livelihoods of smallholder farmers and can provide decent jobs for women and youth. The revenue created can boost economic growth. With the possibility of a health cereal alternative with millets, the risks associated with production shocks can be mitigated. The IYM 2023 and the push towards increasing millet production will contribute to the 2030 Agenda for Sustainable Development. IYM 2023 hopes to galvanise interest in millets among various stakeholders like farmers, the youth and civil society and push governments and policy makers to priorities the production and trade in these cereals.

*Keywords*: International Year of Millets 2023, Food security, crop prospects, climate change, sustainability

## Introduction

With a request from India, the United Nations has declared 2023 the "International Year of Millets." Declaring 2023 the International Year of Millets has three main

* Corresponding author.

goals: to educate the public about the importance of millets to food security and nutrition; to motivate stakeholders to work toward more sustainable millet production and quality; and to highlight the need for increased investment in research, development, and extension services (FAO, 2023). The resolution designating 2023 as the International Year of Millets urges everyone involved to "support activities aimed at raising awareness of and directing policy attention to the nutritional and health benefits of millet consumption, and their suitability for cultivation under adverse and changing climatic conditions, while also directing policy attention for improving value chain efficiencies."

While FAO strives to create a society where everyone has access to healthy food, one of the greatest challenges is feeding a growing population without depleting arable land. By assisting the revival of millets, scientists are contributing to the attainment of the sustainable development goals (SDGs), especially SDG 2 (zero hunger), SDG3 (excellent health and well-being), SDG 12 (sustainable consumption and production), and SDG 13 (climate action). Millets are cereal grasses that grow annually in warm climates and have small grains. Although the majority of millets are members of the Paniceae tribe, there are a number of other taxa that share the common name. 97% of the world's millet is grown in developing countries, where it serves as an important crop in the semiarid tropics of Asia and Africa (especially in South India, Mali, Nigeria, and Niger). Many regions of the world rely on millet as a staple crop due to its adaptability, versatility, and widespread distribution. Sorghum and pearl millets are two of the most common millets grown, and both are significant in India and other parts of Africa. Other useful plant species include millet varieties such as finger millet, proso millet, and foxtail millet. It's possible that humans have been eating millets for the past seven thousand years, and that it was this crop that paved the way for the development of diversified farming and permanent settlements (Innovate India, 2023).

## Millets

Millets encompass a diverse group of small-grained, dryland cereals including foxtail, barnyard and fonio, among others. As whole grains, millets are a good source of essential nutrients. Millets are primarily grown in Asia and Africa, with India being the top producer followed by Nigeria, Niger and China. They were among the first plants to be domesticated and still serve as a traditional staple crop in parts of Sub-Saharan Africa and Asia. These crops, rooted in ancient cultures and ancestral traditions, have long survived harsh growing conditions. Their climate resilience and adaptability offer opportunities for strengthening food security and bolstering economic growth. In celebration of the International Year of Millets 2023, FAO is collaborating with partners to unlock the great potential of millets as affordable foods that can contribute to healthy diets and a healthy environment (Innovate India, 2023).

## Reasons to bring millets to the market

Millets are a sustainable, nutritious and under-valued food source. Here are six key reasons why millets deserve our attention and a place on our tables.

### Millets are there when others are not.

There is an ever-growing global population that needs sufficient and healthy food amidst climate emergencies and depleting natural resources. Millets can be part of the solution. These grains can survive harsh climate conditions, offering solutions to food scarcity. Because they are often the only crops that can be harvested in dry seasons, millets can be a vital food source for populations vulnerable to food insecurity (Mygov, 2023).

### Millets can contribute to a healthy diet.

Millets provide antioxidants, minerals and protein. As whole grains, each millet variety also offers different types and amounts of fibre, which play a role in regulating bowel function, blood sugar and lipids. Furthermore, millets are gluten-free with a low-glycaemic index making them a great food option for those with celiac disease or gluten intolerance, high-blood sugar or diabetes. They can also be a cost-effective source of iron. Incorporating millets in our diets can provide us with nutritious and healthy alternatives to the usual refined grains in the global market. Start exploring some millet recipes, such as this finger millet pancakes option, to revamp your diet (Mygov, 2023).

### Millets are climate-resilient.

Millets are resistant to drought and tolerant to crop diseases and pests, allowing them to survive in adverse climatic conditions. Because millets can be grown with minimal inputs and maintenance and can adapt to climate shocks, expanding production of millets can transform local agrifood systems to be more efficient, resilient and inclusive. The ability of millets to grow in poor, degraded soils can also provide land cover in arid areas, reducing soil degradation and supporting biodiversity (Mygov, 2023).

### Millets offer promising livelihood opportunities for small-scale farmers.

As other cereals have become widespread, dietary preferences have shifted and led to a decline in the production and demand for millets. By encouraging the consumption and production of these underutilized crops, we can help millets regain market share and create additional opportunities for small-scale farmers (Mygov, 2023).

### Millets' trade can improve the diversity of the global food system.

Currently, millets account for less than three percent of the global grains trade. When sudden shocks affect the foodgrain market, millets can provide a valuable alternative to typically traded grains. This added diversity can improve the resilience of the global trade markets and mitigate our reliance on other grains.

### Millets can be used in many innovative ways.

The genetic diversity of millets lends itself to many diverse and innovate applications of millets in areas such as therapeutics and pharmaceuticals. Used innovatively, millets offer even greater market opportunities for regional and international trade (Mygov, 2023).

## International Year of Millets

Millet is a staple food in many parts of the world, but its origins are in Asia and Africa. Cultivation sites have been discovered in Asia dating back to between 10,300 and 8,700 years ago. Therefore, it predated rice in Asia. It is believed to be the oldest cultivated dry crop in East Asia. In 2005, archaeologists in northwest China unearthed a bowl containing foxtail millet noodle remnants dating back 4000 years. The Old Testament and an ancient Indian text called the Yajurveda both make reference to millet as a common crop. However, its popularity waned with the rise of refined flours and packaged foods, as is the case with all whole grains.

Millets are primarily grown in India during the kharif season, requiring less water and agricultural inputs. Millets are significant because of their enormous ability to support human life, raise farmers' incomes, and guarantee global food and nutritional security. The Government of India has made millets a top priority because of their huge potential and the fact that they are in line with numerous UN Sustainable Development Goals (SDGs). In order to generate more interest in and demand for millets, it is rebranded as "Nutri Cereals" in April 2018 and designated 2018 the National Year of Millets (Mygov, 2023).

While both rice and wheat are good providers of carbs, millets, which were traditionally known as coarse cereals, offer more protein, fiber, iron, and calcium. Research has shown that millets are an excellent defense against diabetes and obesity, as well as a rich source of minerals and gluten-free alternative, according to an official statement released in 2018. Because of their low glycemic index, millets have less of an impact on blood glucose levels than other foods. The government has rebranded millets as "Nutri cereals" to make the product more accessible to consumers. Millets are especially useful for providing dietary stability and protecting against nutritional deficiencies for children and women. Owing to its high iron content, it can aid in the prevention of anaemia, a condition that is surprisingly common among pregnant Indian women and babies. In terms of crude fiber content, barnyard millet has an average of 12.8 g/100 g, making it the richest source.

Little millet (*Panicum sumatrense*) and kodo millet (*Paspalum scrobiculatum*) have been found to have the greatest fiber content, at 38% and 37%, respectively. Methionine, valine, and lysine are just a few examples of the necessary amino acids found in abundance in finger millet protein; in fact, 44.7% of the total amino acids found in finger millet protein are essential amino acids. This amount exceeds the 33.9% threshold established by the FAO as the minimum for essential amino acids in reference protein. Based on the average protein content reported across studies, proso millet stands out as the millet with the highest protein content. Proso millet has a protein content similar to wheat, but it contains more essential amino acids like leucine, isoleucine, and thiamine. Finger millet has a calcium content about eight times higher than wheat and can prevent osteoporosis because it is the richest source of calcium (348 mg/100 g). Pregnant women with anaemia can meet their iron needs through the consumption of barnyard millet and pearl millet. Barnyard millet has an iron level of 17.47 mg/100 g. Foxtail millet has the highest zinc content (4.1 mg/100 g) and is a good source of iron (2.7 mg/100 g) among all millets. Zinc and iron are two minerals that have been shown to boost immunity. Moreover, a number of B vitamins, including riboflavin, niacin, and folic acid, may be found in millets. Millets have a similar thiamine and niacin level to both rice and wheat. Foxtail millet, with 0.60 mg/100 g, has the highest thiamine concentration among millets. Barnyard millet (4.20 mg/100 g), foxtail millet (1.65 mg/100 g), and pearl millet (1.48 mg/100 g) all have significantly higher riboflavin contents than common cereals (Innovate India, 2023).

Millets are an excellent crop since they do not require a certain photoperiod to blossom and they are resistant to climate change. Millets may even grow in very poor soils with very little help from outside sources. Millets are able to thrive in arid climates without irrigation, and they may be harvested even during extended periods of low precipitation. Millets require half the time and energy to cultivate as wheat while using a whopping 70% less water. These are hardy plants that can survive under scorching conditions. Cultivating millets may also encourage a transition towards sustainable agriculture by diversifying crop rotations and preventing the promotion of mono-cropping systems, both of which contribute to greater sustainability. Crop residues, due to their high carbon content, play an essential role in preserving and enhancing soil carbon levels, which is crucial for the success of sustainable farming systems and, in certain cases, in supplying feed for animals (Innovate India, 2023).

Millets have a smaller impact on water resources than more well-known cereals like wheat, rice, and maize because they can thrive on dry, non-irrigated soil with little rainfall. With a predicted worldwide population of 8.5 billion in 2030 and a whopping 9.7 billion by 2050, more food production is essential. As the climate crisis worsens and environmental challenges multiply, it becomes increasingly important to diversify food production by encouraging the growth of crops that can thrive under extreme conditions. Specifically, the UN resolution recognizes the "urgent need to raise awareness of the climate-resilience and nutritional advantages of millets and to advocate for diverse, balanced, and nutritious diets through the increasing sustainable production and consumption of millets (PIB, 2023)."

As millets can thrive in a wide range of soil conditions, from the very acidic (pH 4.5) to the very basic (pH 8.0), their cultivation may provide a solution. In acidic soils, millets can be a viable wheat substitute. Soil salinity of 11–12 dS/m is suitable for growing millets such as pearl millet (*Pennisetum glaucum*) and finger millet. Millets have a short growing season and require little water during their development. Some millets, such as pearl millet and proso millet (*Panicum miliaceum*), only need 20 cm of rain, significantly less than the 120-140 cm needed by rice. Most millets are ready for harvest 60-90 days after sowing and require very little irrigation. In comparison to rice (120-140 days), the barnyard millet (Echinochloa frumentacea) only takes 45-70 days to mature. Millets are classified as a $C_4$ cereal. $C_4$ cereals are better for the environment because they capture more carbon dioxide, transform it into oxygen, use water efficiently, and use less resources to grow. As a result, millets can aid in eradicating climatic uncertainties, cutting down on carbon dioxide in the atmosphere, and helping to slow the progression of climate change (Innovate India, 2023).

Yet, there are certain barriers to the widespread adoption of millet as a food source. For example, the selling price of millet was low but is currently reducing. For farmers, the national average of about 1 tonne for jowar, 1.5 tonne for bajra, and 1.7 tonne for ragi, as opposed to 3.5 tonne for wheat, and 4 tonne for rice, are a disincentive. By spreading the word, we can increase demand for this nutritious grain. The latest official data for 2021-22 shows that there are 26.52 crore children in India attending pre-primary through higher-level education at 14.89 lakh schools. Millets could be served as ready-to-eat foods such as cookies, laddu, murukku, nutrition bars, and extruded snacks (healthier versions of Maggi, Kurkure, or Cheetos). In addition, 13.91 million anganwadi care centres provide supplementary nutrition to 7.71 crore children and 1.80 crore pregnant and lactating women (PIB, 2023). Millets could be incorporated into children's diets as a means of reducing micronutrient malnutrition, particularly iron and zinc deficiency, which are major causes of anaemia and stunting, respectively, and which also contribute to diminished cognitive performance and susceptibility to diarrhoea.

School children and those who benefit from anganwadis can each get one hot meal each day consisting of bajra, jowar, ragi, kodo, or kutki, as well as a glass of milk and an egg. The Centre already has two schemes, Pradhan Mantri Poshan Shakti Nirman and Saksham Anganwadi & Poshan 2.0, with a combined budget of Rs 30,496.82 crore in 2022-23, which will help combat hidden hunger while also giving a boost to crop diversification by creating demand for millions of small millet, dairy, and poultry farmers. One way to maximize the impact of these programs is to shift their focus to millets. The federal government might provide funding to any state that is interested in acquiring regionally appropriate millets for distribution in schools and nutrition centers. In 2021-22, Odisha's millet mission planned to purchase 32,302 metric tons of millet, mostly ragi, for a total of Rs 109.08 crore (PIB, 2023) (Figure 1).

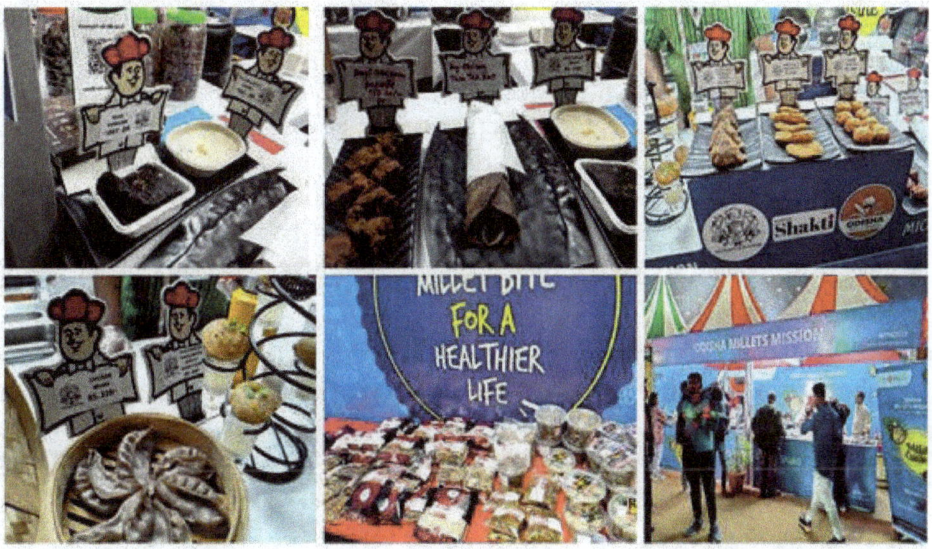


**Figure 1 :** Odisha Millets Mission to promote millets through urban campaigns and promotional events to create awareness on nutritional aspects and health benefits of millets

A combination of central funding with decentralized procurement linked to nutrition goals — specifically the eradication of hidden hunger among school-age children — can do for millets what the Food Corporation of India did with rice and wheat. This could include Rajasthan, Uttar Pradesh, and Haryana for bajra, Maharashtra for jowar, Karnataka for ragi, and Madhya Pradesh for kodo/kutki. The government has taken several steps, including the Programme for the Intensified Promotion of Millet for Nutritional Security(INSIMP), to increase the consumption of millets. To provide farmers a financial boost, the government raised the minimum support price (MSP) for millets. The government has placed millets in the public distribution system to guarantee a consistent demand for the product.

Farmers have been receiving seed kits and other inputs from the government, and value chains have been established through Farmer Producer Associations. The Indian Institute of Millets Research in Hyderabad was designated by the government as an Institution of Excellence in the most recent budget (2023–2024) to further study and advocacy for millets (PIB, 2023).

A whole month has been set aside for IYM to be promoted by the federal government, state governments, and Indian embassies abroad. The sports ministry has planned 15 such events, such as involving sports people, nutritionists, and fitness experts through video messages, organizing webinars on millets with leading nutritionists, dietitians, and elite athletes, and amplifying through the Fit India App.The Food Processing Industries will host millet fair-cum-exhibitions in Punjab, Kerala, and Tamil Nadu and Food Safety and Standards Authority of Indiais hosting "Eat Right Melas". Chhattisgarh, Mizoram, and Rajasthan will host mahotsav or melas, food festivals, training of farmers, awareness campaigns, workshops, seminars, placement of hoardings.The Indian embassy in Azerbaijan and Belarus has invited local chambers of commerce, food bloggers, importers of food goods, and restaurants to participate in business-to-business meetings. To solve these issues and develop new methods to position millets as alternative staples around the world, the "Start-up Innovation Challenge" is a program to foster young people's creative thinking and innovative initiatives in the millet industry (PIB, 2023).

Several wild types of millets may even survive in permanently wet environments, proving their resilience in the face of a wide range of environmental stresses. They are high in protein and minerals (such calcium, iron, copper, magnesium, etc.), as well as B vitamins and antioxidants, and they have a low glycemic index. These exceptional qualities allow these plants to adapt to changing climates while still providing a healthy diet. Farmers may profit from these, and they also have the potential to boost community health. Scientific interventions have the potential to remove pre-existing constraints, such as the existence of anti-nutritional components and the low sensory acceptance of millet-based goods. Cooking, roasting, germination, and fermentation are only some of the ways that the anti-nutritional elements can be neutralized. By combining millet flours with other flours of high acceptance and making composite meals, the sensory acceptability of millet-based goods can be increased. Farmers will be energized by the new doors that will open to them thanks to the usage of millets in commercial/packaged meals. The current dietary deficits of protein, calcium, and iron in poor nations can be overcome with the inclusion of millet-based meals in international, national, and state-level feeding programs (Firstpost, 2023).

## Conclusion

The United Nations General Assembly at its 75th session in March 2021 declared 2023 the International Year of Millets (IYM 2023). FAO is the lead agency for celebrating the Year in collaboration with other relevant stakeholders. Millets can grow on arid lands with minimal inputs and are resilient to changes in climate. They are therefore an ideal solution for countries to increase self-sufficiency and reduce reliance on imported cereal grains. IYM 2023 will be an opportunity to raise awareness of, and direct policy attention to the nutritional and health benefits of millets and their suitability for cultivation under adverse and changing climatic conditions. The Year will also promote the sustainable production of millets, while highlighting their potential to provide new sustainable market opportunities for producers and consumers. The development and release of high-yielding varieties of millets across the world may be attributed to scientific interventions such as the use of molecular biomarkers, sequence information, the generation of mapping populations, and the introduction of mutants. Hybrids created recently have higher yields per hectare and more disease resistance than their parent kinds. Moreover, the benefits derived from millets can give them the title of being a future food security of the world.

## References

FAO 2023. Six reasons to bring millets to the market! Available at: https://www.fao.org/fao-stories/article/en/c/1628815/. Accessed on: 15th April 2023.

Firstpost 2023. Millets are the New Yoga: India's big plan to make the cereals its biggest export in 2023. Available at: https://www.firstpost.com/explainers/millets-are-the-new-yoga-indias-big-plan-to-make-the-cereals-its-biggest-export-in-2023-11914572.html. Accessed on: 15th April 2023.

Innovate India 2023. Start-up Innovation Challenge. Available at: https://innovateindia.mygov.in/millet-year-startup-challenge/. Accessed on: 15th April 2023.

Mygov 2023. Millets 2023. Available at: https://www.mygov.in/campaigns/millets/. Accessed on: 15th April 2023.

PIB 2023. International Year of Millets (IYM) 2023 kick starts with Focussed Activities being undertaken by Central Ministries, State Governments and Indian Embassies. Available at: https://pib.gov.in/PressReleasePage.aspx?PRID=1887847. Accessed on: 15th April 2023.

# 2

# Millets: Super Food for Nutrition Security and Livelihood Improvement

Subrat Pattanaik[1, 2*] and Arati Priyadarshini[1, 2]

[1] Department of Agriculture and Allied Sciences, C. V. Raman Global University, Bhubaneswar - 752054, India

[2] College of Agriculture, Odisha University of Agriculture and Technology, Bhubaneswar - 751003, India

**ABSTRACT**

India possesses one of the world's fastest emerging economies. Despite India's astounding economic growth, there are still concerns regarding hunger and malnutrition. Significant issues have evolved around the world such as food security, livelihood security, as well as natural resources conservation. As per the Global Hunger Index Report 2022, India secured the rank of 107 out of 121 countries scoring 29.1 coming under 'serious' category. One of the main causes of the prevalence of malnutrition is the lack of a diverse diet. The Government of India is encouraging and promoting the production of millets in order to raise consumer level of knowledge on nutrition and enhance farmers' income in the nation. In 2020, India accounted for over 41% of the world's millets production. The United Nations General Assembly (UNGA) also declared 2023 as the International Year of Millets. Millets are regarded as store house of nutrition and are widely consumed by vegans. Millets are by far more superior as compared to rice and wheat in terms of nutritional parameters. Millets have a number of health advantages, including the ability to improve digestive system, lower the risk of cancer, improve respiratory health, strengthen the immune system etc. Apart from nutrition, Millets are dry crop which consume 2.5% less water than other major cereal crops. The Government of India is taking necessary steps such as implementing schemes like POSHAN Abhiyan, Nutri-Sensitive Agriculture, Millet Mission etc to boost and strengthen the supply chain. Diversification of crop in favour of millets and increasing MSP for millets can encourage the farmers.

*Keywords*: Millets, Super Food, Nutrition Security, Livelihood Improvement

## Introduction

India's economy has grown significantly over the past several years and is now expanding at one of the fastest rates in the world. Despite great achievements,

* Corresponding author.

the problems of hunger and malnutrition still exist. In the Global Hunger Index (GHI) 2022, India dropped six positions to settle at position 107 out of 121 nations. Major issues such as food security, livelihood security, as well as natural resources conservation and environmental protection have emerged across the globe. One of the main causes of malnutrition and the prevalence of non-communicable diseases like diabetes in India is a lack of nutritional diversification. Because of their numerous advantages, millets can be cultivated in addition to other crops to help provide a solution. Millets are considered a climate-resilient cereal globally. The diverse production of different varieties of millets can be the alternate option for the small and marginal farmers to sustain their livelihood and maintain nutrition security for themselves as well as increasing population in this era of global climate change. Particularly in Asia and Africa, millets serve as one of the major sources and fodder crops.

Millets are a crop that is exceptionally nutrient-dense and contain significant levels of vitamins and minerals. They are otherwise referred as "super-food" and its production can address the issues related nutrition security and farmer's livelihood. Millets are one of the oldest foods which are small seeded cereal grass that can be cultivated in low fertile, mountainous and arid or rain-fed areas. Millets are a great source of energy, dietary fibre, slowly digestible starch, and resistant starch, which results in a prolonged release of glucose and satiety. Millets are exceptionally nutritious, non-glutinous, and acid-free meals. As a result, they are relaxing and very easily digestible, contain a lot of lecithin, and are beneficial for stimulating the neurological system (Michaelraj and Shanmugam, 2013). Before consumption, millets are typically treated to eliminate the undesirable parts, enhance their shelf life, and enrich their nutritional and sensory characteristics. Millets provide vital micro nutrients like vitamin B, Calcium, Iron Folic acid and Sulphur, as well as dietary fiber making them a valuable tool in the fight against nutrition.

As per the fourth advance estimate, More than 50.9 million tonnes of millet were produced in India, accounting for 20% of global production and 80% of that in Asia. India has a greater average yield than the rest of the world, at 1239 kg/ha compared to 1229 kg/ha globally. In 2020, India accounted for over 41% of the entire world production of millets. (FAO, 2018 and APEDA, 2020). 97% of the millet produced and the seed required globally are produced in developing countries. Compared to USD 28.5 million in 2019–20, India exported millets valued USD 26.97 million in 2020–21. Sorghum, Pearl millet and finger millet are the most commonly grown millets varieties in India. Millets are grown in about 21 States out of which Rajasthan, Andhra Pradesh and Telangana are regarded as the major state producer of millets among all other states. India is leading the way in promoting millets; the substantial increase in MSP over the past five years has contributed to higher millet output and increase farmers ' incomes in the country.

The Government of India declared 2018 as the Year of Millets in order to facilitate and promote mass production of millets. The United Nations General Assembly declared 2023 as the "International Year of Millets" during its 75th Session in March 2021 in order to encourage local and international demand and supply healthy and nutritious food for the expanding population.

## Millets in India: Facts and Figures

Globally, India is the largest producer with 41.04% market share and the fifth largest exporter of millets. (Rao *et al,* 2021) The consumption and the area under production was significantly decreased over the years due to adoption of commercial crops which were supported by several other policies such as subsidized inputs and incentivized procurement. In recent times, the Government of India declared millets to be "Nutri-cereals" in April, 2018, after realising the significance of millets in ensuring the nation's nutritional security. As per the 4th Advance estimate 2021-22, Pearl millet (60%) followed by Sorghum (27%), Finger millet (11%) are the three major millets produced in India with a 27% increase in total millet output over the previous year. Rajasthan (39%), Uttar Pradesh (20%), Haryana (12%), Gujarat (11%), and Madhya Pradesh (9%) are the top five major millet producing states followed by Maharashtra, Karnataka, Tamil Nadu, Andhra Pradesh and Telangana. India's millets exports have risen steadily during the past five years, from 2010 to 2020, at a CAGR of about 3%.

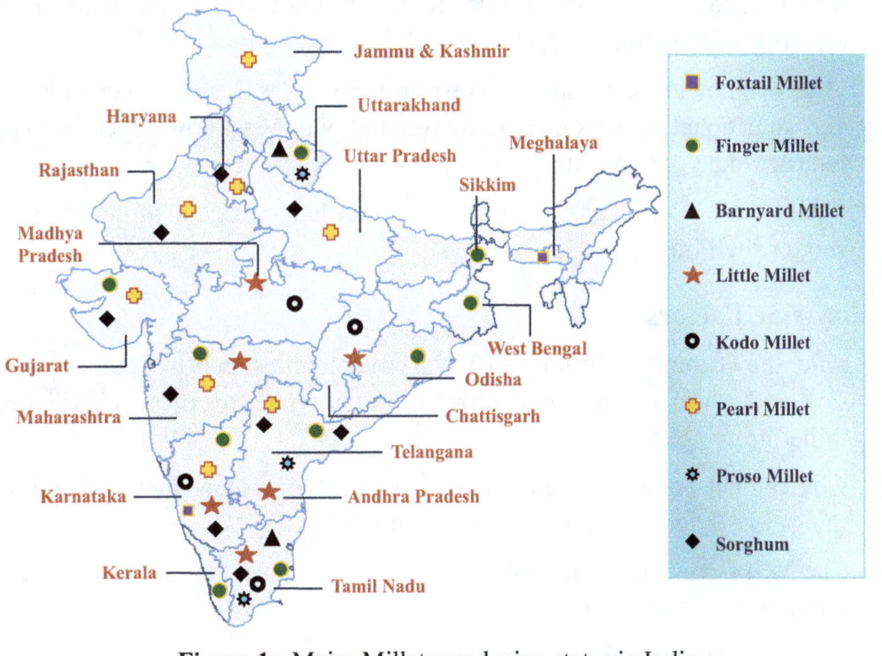


**Figure 1 :** Major Millets producing states in India

## Challenges in Millet Production

### Supply Side Factors

1. Lack of appropriate post-harvest processing technologies: The processing is usually done to make it fit for consumption but significant amount of nutrients are lost due to processing which involves polishing and milling, fermenting, parboiling, baking etc.
2. Consistent supply of raw material: Marginalised agriculture is expanding and incentives for millet production are woefully inadequate.
3. FPOs/ Cooperatives/ SHGs focusing on millet production are still few.
4. Lower yields supported by less remunerative farming leading to lack of commercialization and reduced profits.

### Demand-side Factors

1. Shifting consumer preferences & tastes: Consumer preferences have changed over the years to embrace tastier and more convenient foods, either as a result of the influence of western culture or due to the "indigenous misperception on millets as poor man's foods."
2. Rapid urbanization, increasing population and changing life style have increased the demand for healthy foods but the marginalized cultivation of millets is contributing to decline in millets consumption in India
3. Lack of knowledge of millets' nutritional benefits: Despite other causes, the very nutritional benefits of millets were not widely acknowledged by people, industry and governments.
4. Shelf Life: Millets after processed such as milled grains and millets flour have shorter shelf life.

### Policy-side Factors

1. After the Green Revolution of 1970's, government support of policies mainly favoured wheat and rice in contrast to millet which resulted in shrinking of millet-growing area.
2. Government policy favours irrigated crops by providing input subsidies for things like irrigation, fertilisers, and other things.
3. The MSPs granted by the policymakers are the ones that are driving millets farming.
4. Lack of public procurement and marketing support

## Importance of Millets

Millets can contribute to several Sustainable Development Goals such as it can contribute towards food security and nutrition (SDG 2; End Hunger), it is an important healthy diet providing high quality nutritional benefits (SDG 3; Good Health and Well-Being) and it can avail opportunities to small and marginal farmers to improve their livelihoods (SDG 8; Decent Work and Economic Growth). It can fetch higher price in contrast to other major cereal crops (rice & wheat). Unlike other crops, millets are ecologically sustainable which means it is not dependent on chemical fertilizers and are minimally affected by pests and diseases. Cereal crops like Rice which is grown in majority parts of the nation consume around 4,000-5000 litres of water to produce one kilogram of rice. Millets require less water as compared to other cereal crops, thus support climate resilient agriculture (SDG 13; Climate Action and SDG 15; Life on Land). Millets are rich in protein, fibre, and micronutrients and may be used as both a healthy diet for humans and livestock respectively. Farming millets can help in bringing down the carbon footprint. The urban population may readily obtain and take advantage of the benefits of millet-based value-added products in the category of ready to cook and ready to eat foods.

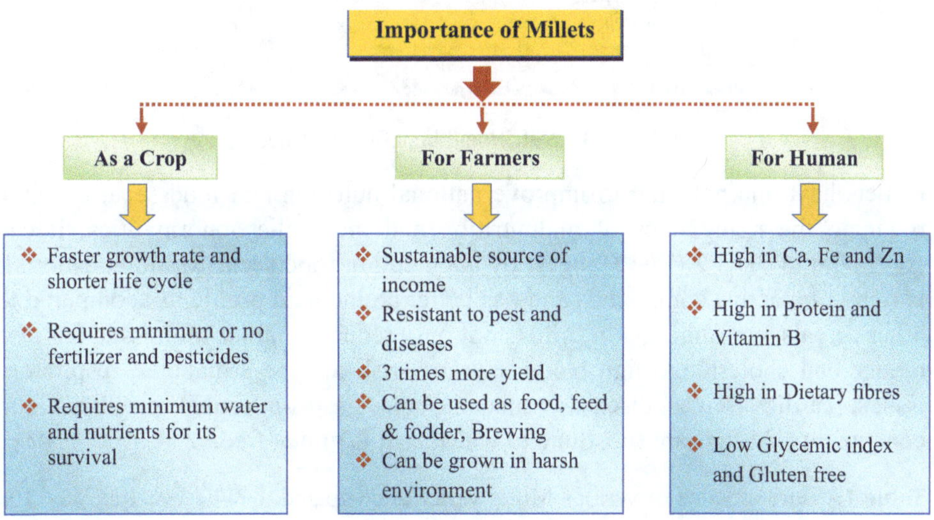


**Figure 2 :** Importance of Millets

## Food and Nutritional Security

Due to increase in global population and changing world climate, people are facing food shortages and malnutrition. India has slipped 6 positions from its previous rank of 101. India scored 29.1 in the recent report which means that the level of hunger is serious. The global score of 18.2 in 2022 which is stagnated in comparison to 2014 is still considered "moderate". Approximately one-third of the malnourished children in the world are reported from India alone. (GHI, 2022 and Nainwal, 2018). Millets was earlier termed as "coarse grains" and nowadays it is regarded as nutri-cereals. Millets are regaining popularity after being neglected for several decades can replace major producing staple foods such as paddy and wheat. Millets are resistant to harsh climatic conditions, pest and diseases unlike other cereal crops.

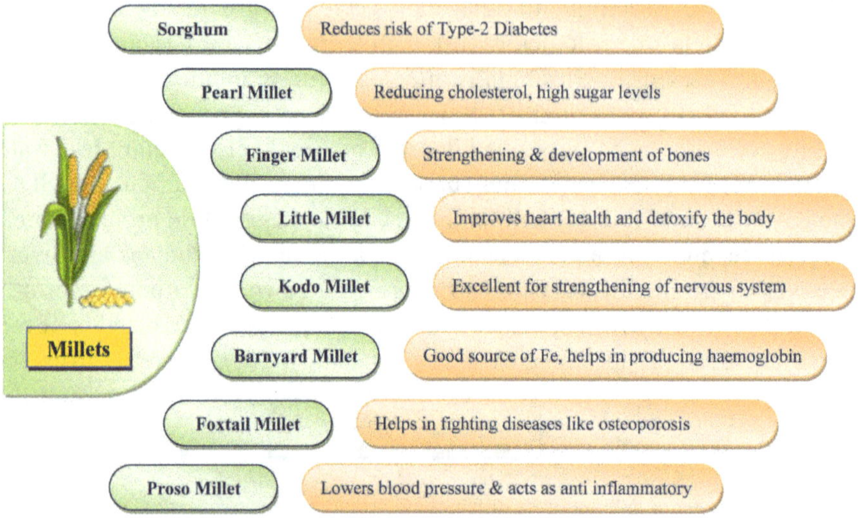


**Figure 3 :** Nutritional benefits of Millets

Millets have the potential to improve national nutrition and food security while reducing the rising rates of malnutrition and metabolic abnormalities. It can contribute to SDG 2 (End Hunger) by augmenting food security and nutrition. It is rich in bioactive compounds and has better amino acid profile. As compared to other cereals, consumption of millets not only reduces malnutrition issue but also reduce bad cholesterol, high blood pressure, risk of type-2 diabetes, respiratory issues, cardiovascular diseases, anaemia and gastro-intestinal problems and constipation. Millets are substitute to wheat as it is gluten free.

**Table 1:** Nutrient value of various Millet varieties compared to Wheat & Rice (for 100 gms)

| **Millet** | **Protein (g)** | **Carbs (g)** | **Fat (g)** | **Minerals (g)** | **Fiber (g)** | **Ca (mg)** | **P (mg)** | **Fe (g)** | **Energy (kcal)** |
|---|---|---|---|---|---|---|---|---|---|
| Finger | 7.3 | 72 | 1.3 | 2.7 | 3.6 | 344 | 283 | 3.9 | 336 |
| Sorghum | 10.4 | 70.7 | 3.1 | 1.2 | 2 | 25 | 222 | 5.4 | 329 |
| Pearl | 11.8 | 67 | 4.8 | 2.2 | 2.3 | 43 | – | 11 | 363 |
| Foxtail | 12.3 | 60.2 | 4.3 | 4 | 6.7 | 31 | 290 | 2.8 | 351 |
| Little | 7.7 | 67 | 4.7 | 1.7 | 7.6 | 17 | 220 | 9.3 | 329 |

| | | | | | | | | | |
|---|---|---|---|---|---|---|---|---|---|
| Kodo | 8.3 | 65.9 | 1.4 | 2.6 | 5.2 | 35 | 188 | 1.7 | 353 |
| Proso | 12.5 | 70.4 | 1.1 | 1.9 | 5.2 | 8 | 206 | 2.9 | 354 |
| Barnyard | 6.2 | 65.5 | 4.8 | 3.7 | 13.6 | 22 | 280 | 18.6 | 300 |
| Paddy | 6.8 | 78.2 | 0.5 | 0.6 | 1 | 33 | 160 | 1.8 | 362 |
| Wheat | 11.8 | 71.2 | 1.5 | 1.5 | 2 | 30 | 306 | 3.5 | 348 |

*Source*: Nutritive value of Indian foods, NIN 2007

## Livelihood Security

- Improved Connectivity & Doubling farmer's Income: Small farmers, who are among the poorest households in rural India, would only produce millets if it yields them high returns. These farmers are typically found in hilly regions, dryland plains, and communities located in the most remote areas. The problem may be resolved by farm diversification, improving transportation infrastructure and including more stakeholders in effective and timely procurement. Millets are more profitable for farming since they may be used for both food and feed.
- Processing and Value-Added Products: Millet-based goods may become more appealing to both traditional and modern consumers by enhancing processing methods and diversifying the supply of value-added millet products. As compared to other cereal crops, millets require very less investment for its production and can lead to higher economic returns through value addition. For e.g., bakery products, snacks, millet flours, semolina, instant mixes etc.
- Availability, Accessibility and Affordability: Promoting and raising awareness through advertising in print media, electronic media (TV Channels, Radio), and social media, about nutrition and health facts. Millets are expensive for low income consumers than other cereal crops. Consumption may be increased by highlighting affordability through government subsidies.
- Branding: Innovative and eye catchy packaging efforts to target and create more demand in urban areas.
- Shifting Perception: By marketing and promotion, the stereotype that millets are poor man's food needs to be put to rest. Creating awareness of nutritional value of millets foods are most important areas to increase the consumption and utilization of millets. Initiatives to replace existing diets with millet based diets in hospitals and in school's mid day meal programme.
- Promoting Entrepreneurship: Fostering entrepreneurship can promote and develop local market. Maximizing millet farming can boost rural economy, increase productivity, alleviate food and nutrition security and stimulate demand among urban masses.
- Private sector food processing Industries: Encourage private sector investment in millets processing and R&D.

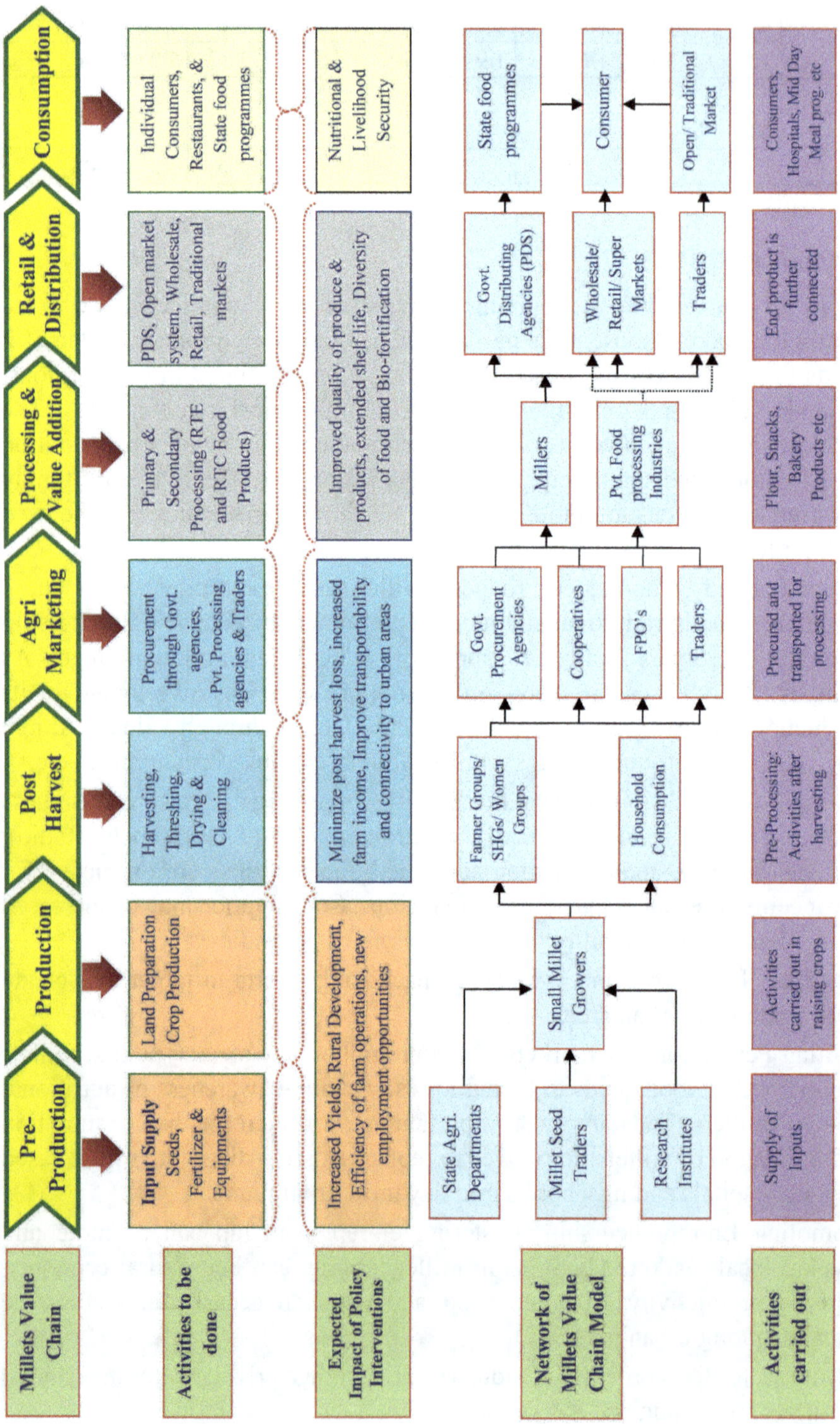


**Figure 4 :** Value Chain Model for Small Millets Growers

## Value Chain Model for Small Millets Growers

The Millet Value Chain is developed to provide maximum benefit to the small millet growers and create awareness among the increasing population for its nutritional benefits and livelihood security. The chain starts form pre-production phase where the role of Research Institutes (Govt. and Private), State Agricultural Departments and traders supply inputs such as good quality seeds, equipments etc to the small millet growers. In production phase, the millet growers grow a wide variety of millets by utilizing improved and sustainable farming practices. The two phase result in increased in yield which in result generate new employment opportunities leading to development in backward rural areas. Once the production is done, the pre-processing or the post harvest stage starts where the Farmer Groups/ SHGs/ Women Groups would directly sell the produce to agri-marketing channels like government procuring agencies/ Cooperatives/ FPOs/ traders after threshing, drying & cleaning. Some of the produce is also kept for household consumption. The two phase result in reduce post harvest losses; enhance transportability and connection to urban demand. Different agencies procure grains; again the produce is transferred or sold to the millers or private food processing Industries for further processing and value addition (RTE and RTC Food Products) such as flour, snacks, bakery products, cookies, millet snacks, namkeen etc. Then the final processed product is distributed through various agencies via Public distribution system which is further connected to the end user i.e., the consumers. The private food processing industries supply the goods through their retail chain market to the consumers. The traders do so in an indirect manner through the traditional/open retail market, which is followed by a series of small shops and outlets before reaching the consumers. The 5th and 6th stage is mainly responsible for improved quality of produce & products, extended shelf life, diversity of food and Bio-fortification which in final stage is responsible for nutritional benefits to the end user through buying from retail markets/ consuming through inclusion of state govt. initiatives like mid day meal schemes/ incorporating millets in their hospital diets.

## Various Policy Implementations in India

### A. Government of India Initiatives

- In 2018, Millets was officially declared as "Nutricereals". As part of the same year's "National Year of Millets" declaration, the GoI also announced the NFSM Sub-mission on Nutri-Cereals with a budget of INR 300.00 crore for the financial year 2018–19.
- In 2018, GoI has proposed the United Nations to designate 2023 as the 'International Year of Millets', the proposal was eventually approved in 2021, and 2023 was subsequently designated as the "International Year of Millets".

### B. State Government Initiatives

- In 2018, the government of Odisha began the Odisha Millet Mission, with the slogan "Reviving millets in farm and on plates" across 15,292 villages over 81 blocks in 15 districts. The mission is largely concentrated on the tribal regions of Odisha where millets are the major crop in order to overcome the significant supply chain and consumer obstacles.
- The Karnataka government introduced the "Karnataka Organic Farming Policy 2017", to encourage the growth of millets and the next stage of development in organic farming.
- The Telangana Millet Mission project was launched on 2nd July, 2018, in an effort to increase the area, production and consumption of millets through improved agricultural techniques, development of processing facilities, rural entrepreneurship and market linkages.
- Maharashtra government is promoting Millets through Project on Climate Resilient Agriculture.
- Andhra Pradesh government has initiated a program on the "Comprehensive Revival of Millets cultivation' by tribals in north Coastal Andhra and sections of Rayalaseema.

### C. Private Sector Initiatives

- Private players like ITC Foods and ITC ABD have introduced products under the brand name Aashirvaad Nature's Super Foods, comprising jowar flour, ragi flour, multi-grain mix flour, and khatta meetha poha, as well as gluten-free flour.
- Under the brand name Nutri Choice, Britannia Industries Ltd. produced Ragi cookies and 5-grain Digestive biscuits for those who suffer from diabetes.
- MTR Foods: A Multi-grain Dosa Mix and Ragi Idli are two of the three new items the company has released under its DeLite brand.
- Big Basket: has over 50 millet-based products available and is always trying to develop new options to fulfil the demands of a wide range of customers who value health and wellness
- Kellogg's India: The Company just introduced Ragi Chocos, a tasty and nutritious breakfast option for growing kids.

## Conclusion

They are the ideal alternative to staple cereal crops because of their exceptional capacity to thrive under adverse conditions. Production and productivity of millets needs to be enhanced by strengthening the procurement process in seed chain. Demand needs to be created through awareness regarding its properties to withstand climate change, farm income and especially on human health. To boost rural or grass root level economies, ensure food, nutritional and livelihood security of the small and marginal farmers, supportive agricultural policies in favour of them needs to modify such as sensitizing farmers and government to change MSP structure in accordance with other cereal crops. Widespread adoption of improved sustainable farming practices and proper science and technology needs to be adopted for increasing the productivity. A number of these issues will be resolved by this strategy, improving agricultural productivity, soil health, and environmental safety.

The key factor preventing millets from becoming widely available and utilized was the lack of equilibrium between the factors affecting their supply and demand. In recent years, Government has taken various commendable initiatives but to achieve broader goals, issues such fall of area under millets such as low remuneration, absence of input subsidies and pricing incentives, subsidized distribution through the public distribution system (PDS) and alterations in consumer preferences and reduced demand need to be strategically addressed. The year 2023 is celebrated as International Year of Millets; it is an opportunity for India to promote Millets which was once regarded as "Poor Person's Food". One of the main goals is to place this super food in the world's 'food map' and positioning India as the 'Global Hub for Millets' with PM Modi's vision of "Vasudaiva Kutumbakam" (The World is One Family). The importance of this event is to generate "Millet Mindfulness" via increasing awareness, production and consumption.

## References

Annor G.A., Tyl C., Marcone M., Ragaee S., Marti A. Why do millets have slower starch and protein digestibility than other cereals? Trends Food Sci. Technol. 2017;66:73–83. doi: 10.1016/j.tifs.2017.05.012. [CrossRef]

APEDA. Ministry Of Commerce & Industry. 2020-21. India Millets Production. https://apeda.gov.in/milletportal/Production.

Ashoka, P.; Gangaiah, B.; Sunitha, N. Millets-foods of twenty first century. Int. J. Curr. Microbiol. Appl. Sci. 2020, 9, 2404–2410. [Google Scholar] [CrossRef]

B. Dayakar Rao, Raj Bhandari, and Tonapi, VA, K. 2021. "White Paper on Millets – A Policy Note on Mainstreaming Millets for Nutrition Security". ICAR-Indian Institute of Millets Research (IIMR), Rajendranagar, Hyderabad-500030

FAO. 2018. FAOSTAT database Rome: Food and Agriculture Organization. http://www.fao.org/faostat/en/#data/.

Global Hunger Index Report; 2022. https://www.globalhungerindex.org/india.html. Accessed 18th February, 2023

Michaelraj Stanly Joseph and Shanmugam. 2013. "A study on Millets based Cultivation and Consumption in India", International Journal of Marketing, Financial Services and Management Research, Vol.2,No.4,pp. 49-50.

NAAS 2022. Promoting Millet Production, Value Addition and Consumption. Policy Paper No. 114, National Academy of Agricultural Sciences, New Delhi: 24 p.

Nainwal, K. Conservation of minor millets for sustaining agricultural biodiversity and nutritional security. J. Pharmacogn. Phytochem. 2018, SP1, 1576–1580.

Nithiyanantham S., Kalaiselvi P., Mahomoodally M.F., Zengin G., Abirami A., Srinivasan G. Nutritional and functional roles of millets—A review. J. Food Biochem. 2019;43:1–10. doi: 10.1111/jfbc.12859

Nutrihub & ICAR- Indian Institute of Millets Research (IIMR). Value Addition & Market Linkages in Millets – A success story from Nutrihub.

PIB Delhi. 2022. Ministry of Commerce & Industry. https://pib.gov.in/Press ReleaseI frame Page.aspx?PRID=1796514. Accessed on: 20th February, 2023.

PIB Delhi. Ministry of Finance. 2023. India's food grains production touched a record 315.7 million tonnes in 2021-22. https://pib.gov.in/PressReleasePage.aspx?PRID=1894899. Accessed on: 20th February, 2023.

Rao D.B., Malleshi N.G., Annor G.A., Patil J.V. Millets Value Chain for Nutritional Security: A Replicable Success Model from India. Indian Institute of Millets Research (IIMR); Hyderabad, India: 2017. Nutritional and health benefits of millets; p. 112.

Tiwari H, Naresh RK, Kumar L, Kataria SK, Tewari S, Saini A, et al. Millets for Food and Nutritional Security for Small and Marginal Farmers of North West India in the Context of Climate Change: A Review. International Journal of Plant & Soil Science. 2022;34(23):1694-1705.

# 3

# Climate Change and Millets: A Global Food Security for an Improving Livelihood

Kaushik Pramanik[1*], Debarati Sealand[2], Amit Layek[3]

[1] Department of Agricultural Entomology, Bidhan Chandra Krishi Viswavidyalaya, Mohanpur-741252, Nadia, West Bengal, India

[2] Department of Agronomy, Bidhan Chandra Krishi Viswavidyalaya, Mohanpur-741252, Nadia, West Bengal, India

[3] Department of Agricultural Entomology, Bidhan Chandra Krishi Viswavidyalaya, Mohanpur-741252, Nadia, West Bengal, India

**ABSTRACT**

An expanding population results in a constantly growing demand for food. Due to this worldwide concern, there is dispute over reserves like water and land. Millets are resilient to climate change because of their intrinsic malleability to high temperatures and drought. It is also patient of acid and saline soils and is perfectly fitted to negligible lands with minimum production. Compared to other cereals, millets have fewer pest and disease issues and are suitable for various cropping patterns. In terms of vitamins, dietary fibre, numerous vital minerals, high quantities of calories, proteins, and antioxidants, millets offer a high nutritional value. The majority of millets can be cooked, ground, fermented, decorated, germinated and extruded to create items like cookies, pasta, flour, snacks, and non-dairy probiotic drinks. So, there is a great possibility for tackling these positive qualities through various techniques like- enhanced crop management, genetic development, grain processing etc. Thus, the purpose of this chapter is to demonstrate the ability of millets as a future alternative food security crop to feed the world's expanding population. This ought to contribute to a clearer understanding of the significance of this crop for global food and nutritional security.

**Keywords:** climate change; nutrition; crop management; agricultural productivity; food security.

## Introduction

One of the most significant challengesconfronting the world is feeding everyone on the planet. This problem is caused by a variety of factors, such as shortages in the productivity of food owing to supply-demand inequalities and conflicts subverting different regions of the world. According to estimates, two-three

* Corresponding author.

billion people may experience starvation and nutritional imbalance by 2050 as a result of dwindlingthe rates of food production and the supplementarysprain of feeding thepeople that will approach 9 billion (Wheeler and Braun, 2013; Godfray *et al.,* 2010). Along with the staples cereals for example wheat, rice, and maize, millets are the significant one. Peoples, particularly those who reside in hot, humid climates, rely primarily on millet as a food source.

They are primarily planted in marginal locations of agricultural areas where major grains fail to produce significant yields (Adekunle, 2012). Because they can thrive in challenging environmental conditions like heavy drought and little rainfall. In angrier areas, millet serves as their chief source of protein and energy for the people. According to reports, millet serves both nutritional and therapeutic purposes in most of the dry regions (Obilana and Manyasa, 2002; Yang *et al.,* 2012).

Crop species with high nutritional benefits and the ability to withstand a variety of negative consequences of climate change might significantly improve nutritional and food security, particularly in developing nations. Millets are becoming more widely known for their higher levels of resistance to the effects of changingclimate and their superior nutritional qualities. The term "millet" suggests to a wide variety of species from several genera, the most notable of which are the proso, finger, foxtail, and pearl millet. Crop productivity, yields, and the completegrowth of our food structures are all clearly affected by changing environment and rising global temperatures.

## Constraints associated with millet cultivation

The majority ofmilletis produced in desert parts of Africa and Asia with poor and irregular rainfall (Murthy *et al.,* 2007). Any growth stage can experience drought, although post-flowering or season-ending dryness is more significant and better known than stress in the pre-flowering stages (Rai *et al.,* 1999). It is crucial to utilize integrated nutrient management techniques since they can considerably increase crop output and are cheap even for the poorest farmers. Another significant barrier to millet productivity is high-temperature stress. Due to several factors, increased air and soil temperatures cause a decrease in yields. Even though milletshave higher levels of thermotolerance than most other grains used for human consumption, heat stress can cause crop stands to fail in arid areas (de Wet *et al.,* 1992). The majority of millets are cultivated on poor soils with low natural fertility. As small or marginal farmers make up the majority of millet growers, nutrient or additional agricultural input application is also minimum, which leads to subpar productivity.

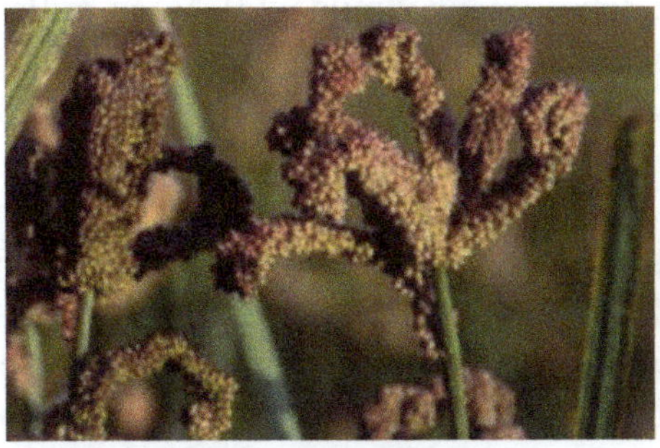

Finger millet

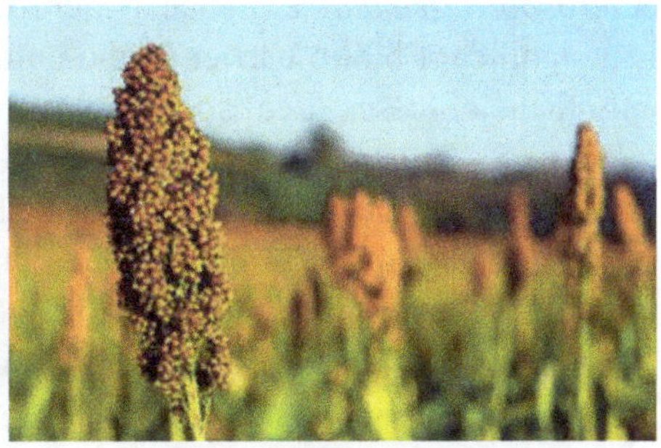

Sorghum

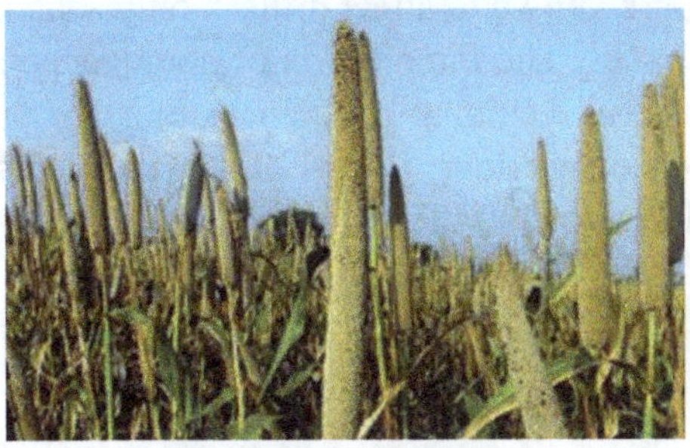

Pearl millet

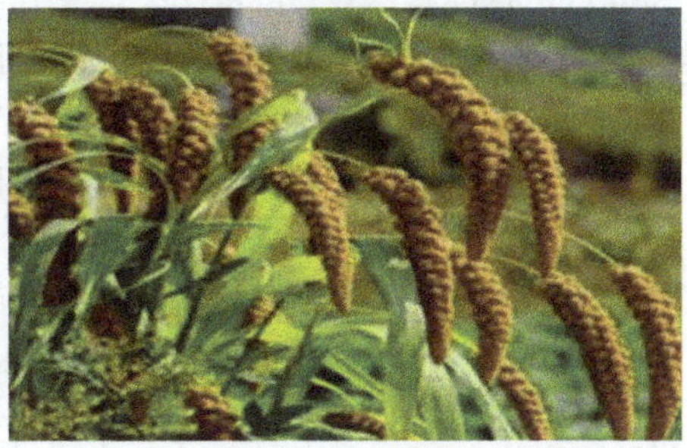

Foxtail millet

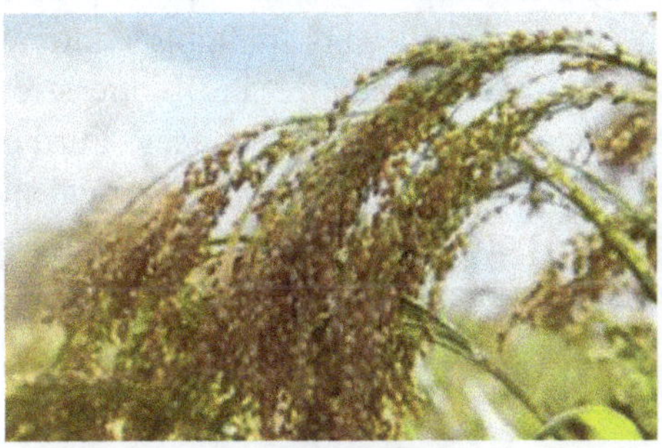

Little millet

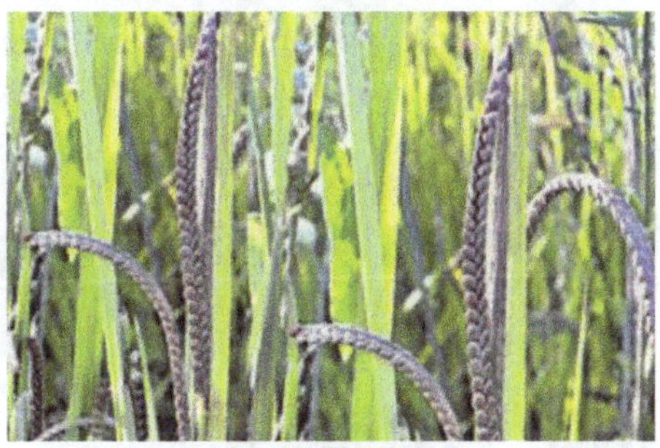

Kodo millet

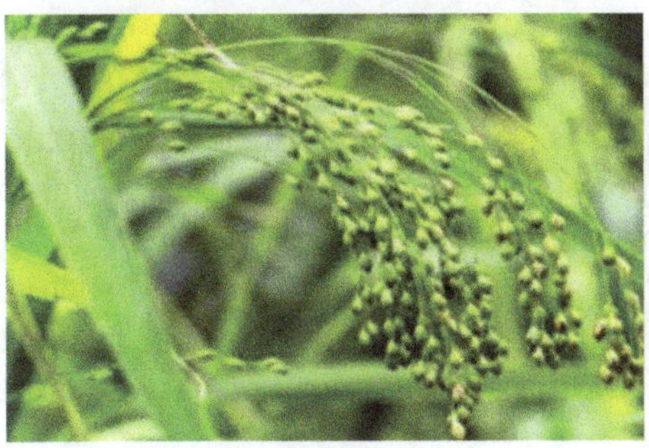

Proso millet

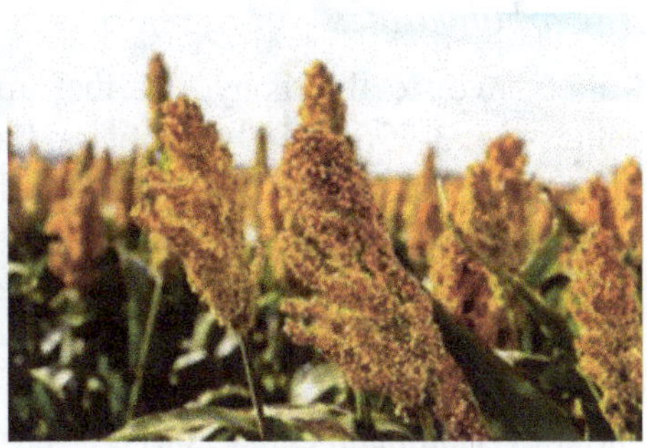

Barnyard millet

**Figure 1 :** Different types of millets commonly cultivated in various parts of the wotld

*Sclerospora graminicola* (Sacc.) Schroet-caused downy mildew (DM) in millets is a significant biotic barrier to the cultivation of millets, leading to serious crop and financial losses. Leaf spot or blast, which is brought on by *Pyricularia grisea* (Cooke) Sacc. is another newly discovered disease that significantly reduces the productivity of grain and forage in millets. Ergot, rust, and smut are additional ailments that damage millet. Besides this, witchweed, a parasitic and devastating weed, poses a significant menace to the cultivation of millets (Wilson *et al.,* 2004). The infestation of striga can result in up to 100 per cent grain production losses during drought circumstances. In India, insect-pests are not a serious problem for the cultivation of millets, but in sub-Saharan Africa, they are significant. Even though there are more than 100 pests that are known to affect millets, only a small number of them result in large financial losses. The importation of homogeneous HYVs has increased pest issues everywhere. Regional differences exist in the losses brought on by insect pests and their dispersion. As part of integrated pest management, biological, agronomic, andchemical strategies have been suggested for the management of major pests.

## Breeding in millets for improved food/nutritional security

Most of the time, rain-fed and low-input conditions are used to grow millets throughout Asia and Africa. Due to a changing environment, the limitations present in a given area are endlessly changing both temporally and spatially. Cultivars (varieties/hybrids) must therefore be capable to endureabiotic and biotic stress conditions in order to produce successfully under such circumstances. Further, the biological barriers to productivity development, particularly in Africa and North-western India, continue to be landraces' poor yield potential and those of the most improved varieties. Clearly, this necessitates the careful design of crop enhancement projects.

## Millets: A nutritious food crop

### *A) Carbohydrates*

Millets have a total carbohydrate, that is equivalent to or more than other grains. This value is 55. 3-75. 4 g/100 g for bajra. Bajra has a total soluble sugar concentration that ranges from 1. 4 to 2. 80%. In pearl millets, raffinose and sucrose account for roughly 29% and 63%, respectively, of the total sugars (McDonough *et al.,* 2000). Millets contain a variety of sugars, including stachyose, raffinose, and sucrose. Other sugars were found, including xylose, arabinose, galactose, and glucose. There was a reported range of 27–32% for the total amylose of various millet varieties (Hadimani *et al.,* 2001).

### *B) Protein and amino acids*

The protein percentageof millets ranges from 6 to 25%. Equated to other millets, kodo, proso, foxtail, and bajra has a higher range of lysine which is an important amino acid (McDonough *et al.,* 2000). Excludingtryptophan, leucine, lysine, isoleucine, and tyrosine, most cereals utilizedglobally have equal amino acid compositions. The tyrosine level of bajra is equivalent to that of barley (Ejeta*et al.,* 1987), but it is lower than that of rice and maize. Tryptophan and isoleucine, two crucial amino acids, are also present in millets (McDonough *et al.,* 2000; FAO, 1995).

### *C) Minerals*

The three main minerals found in millet are magnesium (Mg), potassium (K) and phosphorus (P). Abdalla *et al.* (1998) discovered that pearl millet grains had a high "P" concentration. In pearl millet genotypes, the proportion of phytic acid to total "P" ranged from 70 to 89%, with amean amount of 77%, whereas wheat grains contain 33–90% of their total phosphorus in the form of phytin 'P′ (Hamdy, 1971). Millets also have a greateroverall magnesium concentration than maize. Despite having a similar calcium content to other grains in millets, the bioavailability of "Ca" was low (Abdel Rahman *et al.,* 2005).

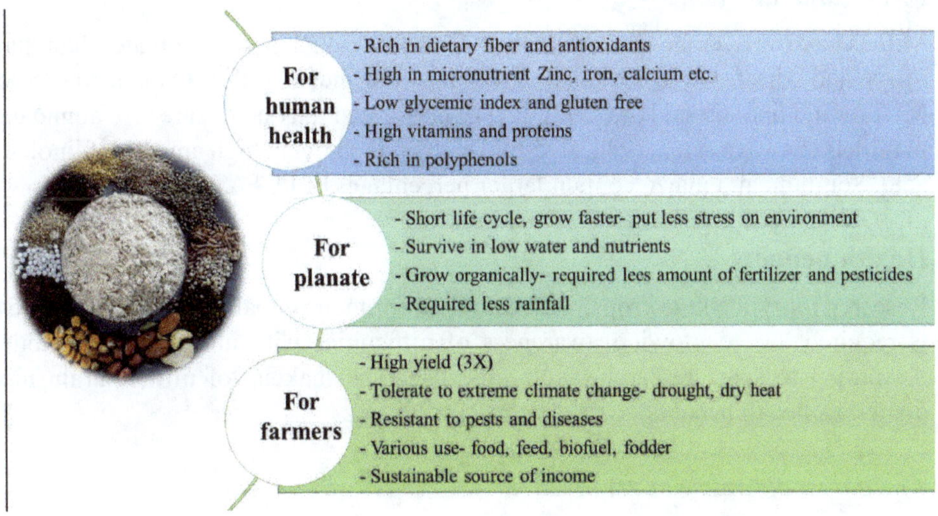


**Figure 2 :** Important properties of millet

### *D) Vitamins*

Although milletsare deficient in vitamin C, it is high in vitamin B (Nambiar *et al.,* 2011). The following vitamins are present in millets in varying concentrations: niacin, riboflavin, pantothenic acid, folic acid, thiamine, and pyridoxine. Niacin, riboflavin, and thiamine content decrease by around 50% after decortication (Nambiar *et al.,* 2011). Millet cultivars have very low levels of carotene, while improved varieties have slightly higher levels [0. 133 g/kg] or levels that are comparable to landraces and hybrids (Buerkert *et al.,* 2001).

### *E) Anti-nutritional factors (ANFs)*

Compared to other grains, milletshave a lower ANF content. According to Elyas *et al.,* (2002), in millets, the catechin equivalents of the tannins range from 0. 12% - 0. 24%. Different phenolic components, such as phenolic acids and flavonoids (flavones), are also available in millets in significant amounts. According to Dykes and Rooney (2007), the total phenolic acid concentration of millet grains is approximately 147. 8 mg/100 g. Flavones found in grains are also known as C-glycosylflavones, and their glycosylvitexin equivalent quantity ranges from 87 - 259 mg/100 g of C-glycosylflavone (Reichert *et al.,* 1980). Phytic acid contributes 65 to 85% of the total protein in millets (Raboy, 1990; 1997). The availability of different nutrients is impacted by phytic acid's propensity to combine with proteins and multivalent cations. Phytase, an enzyme that degrades phytic acid, is created during germination, making the bound minerals accessible (Geetha *et al.,* 1997).

### *F) Fat and fatty acids*

Millets have an average fat content of 4. 7- 4. 9%, which is much greater than that of rye and wheat, but lesser than oat (Alais and Linden, 1991). Oleic acid (25%; MUFA) and linoleic acid (45%; PUFA) (Unsaturated fatty acids) are also abundant in millets (Sawaya *et al.,* 1984). Despite having a relatively high amount of linoleic acid, Sorghum and maize contain larger percentages of PUFA (Rooney, 1978).

## **Health benefits**

Research into substitute crops, such as millet, for their probable health advantages is required due to growing awareness of difficulties with nutrition and health. According to some research results, the chemical makeup of millets grain has numerous health benefits:

### *A) Against coronary heart disease*

Total blood cholesterol (TBC) and low-density lipoprotein cholesterol (LDL-C) are both decreased when fibre-rich foods are consumed, and this is linked to a lower incidence of coronary heart disease-related death issues (Jukanti *et al.,* 2012). In addition, the oxidation of LDL-C is a major factor in atherosclerosis. The oxidation of LDL-C may have been inhibited by millet phenolics' chelation of scavenging of peroxyl radicals and cupric ions. Millet grains have a high caffeic acid content, and several phenolic components may work together to prevent LDL-C oxidation (Chandrasekara and Shahidi, 2011b).

### *B) Against Cancer*

The anti-carcinogenic benefits of millet's phenolic extracts included: (i) the highest singlet oxygen scavenging activity (25%) among various millets at 1 mg/ml; and (ii) an 80% reduction in UVA-tempted liposome peroxidation at 1 mg/ml (iii) millet extract reduced DNA scission brought on by hydroxyl and peroxyl radicals by around 60%. Additionally, millet extracts suppressed HT-29 human colon cancer cells over time and at different doses. Solvable extracts of millets include flavonoids such as luteolin, quercetin, vitexin, apigenin, and isovitexinthat may be employed as possible chemopreventive agents to stop the development of cancer (Chandrasekara and Shahidi, 2011a).

### *C) Against celiac disease*

An immune response to gluten results in the intestinal illness known as celiac disease, which is characterized by chronic small intestine inflammation. Since there are no treatments or medications for this disease, the only way to lead a regular, healthy life is to avoid gluten. People who are intolerant to wheat, barley, or rye are demanding more meals and drinks without gluten.

## Value addition in millets

A variety of procedures for the processing of millets can decrease anti-nutritional elements, enhance longibity, and improve digestibility. Such as dehulling reduces the amount of fibre, ash, fat, protein, and micronutrients while increasing the product's quality and sensory attributes. The milling characteristics of millets are enhanced by moist heating (heating, drying, and decortication), which also extends the longibityof flour (4–5 months) and lowers the microbial concentration on the grains. The amount of proteinsare decreased, but the quality is increased by malting. Additionally, it boosts vitamin content, lowers levels of polyphenols and phytic acid, and raises the accessibility of minerals. The process of blanching, which involves soaking grains in water that is 5:1(water to seeds) for thirty seconds, afterwards an hour of drying at 50 °C, is particularly successful in extending the longevity of flour and delaying the formation of fat acidity. By lowering polyphenols and phytic acid, the acid treatment enhances the product's superiority. The digestibility of proteins in-vitro is also improved by acid treatment. During storage, dry heat treatment lowers activity oflipase and minimizes lipid breakdown. The grain can be decorated by parboiling. Most often, parboiled, decorticated grains are utilized for a variety of snacks, particularly for diabetics.

The flour of milletsinured to produce numerous of synthetic foods (Yadav *et al.,* 2012). Traditionally, bajra flour is used to create dishes like porridge and flat, unfermented bread (chapatti). Processing millet flour results in dishes that are easier to digest and have a lower antinutrient content (Singh, 2003). Additionally, millet are used in India to make a variety of snacks with a long shelf life, including sev, laddoo, namkeen, and matari. Along with these classic dishes, millets make a wonderful raw material for the bread sector. The texture, grittiness, and top grain of millet cookies made with certain supplements are comparable to those made with wheat flour. Millet flour is used to make a variety of cakes and biscuits with good organoleptic properties (Singh, 2003). Ready-to-eat (RTE) foods can also be made with millet's flour. RTE products are made by extrusion, which involves heating at a high temperature for a brief period of time. These products are more digestible and likely contain inactivated antinutritional elements.

Although flaking is a modern market for millets, preliminary research has shown promise (Yadav *et al.,* 2012). Similar to millets, popping milletsare uncommon but have superior nutritional value. Popped millet is a supplementary or weaning foods for kids since it is a powerful source of calories, fibre, and carbs. Bajra is used for producing various sorts of healthy foods as it is rich in fibre, gluten-free status, and reasonably decent nutritional makeup. Additionally, lassi, buttermilk, "Cumbu Cool" (Tamil Nadu), rab/rabari (Rajasthan), and other beverages are made with pearl millet flour.

## Future prospects

Farmers in dry and semi-arid areas have few viable and affordable options for switching from millets to other lucrative crops. Smallholder farmers in these areas need appropriate, reasonably enhanced technology to maintain and boost millet's yield and productivity. Farmers want high-yielding cultivars, particularly hybrids, that provide high-quality grain and fodder that is both favoured by growers and consumers. The improvement of cultivars with higherproductivity, tolerance to significant abiotic challenges, and resilience to significant biotic stresses requires continuing crop improvement efforts that combine modern molecular tools and techniques with conventional breeding. Another important issue is the high soil salinity in pearl millet growing areas. By employing better crop management practices, the yield of OPVs and hybrids can be boosted even more and significantly.

Most of the Asian and African regions where pearl milletaregrown are very concerned about malnutrition. As a result, breeding efforts should focus on creating varieties and hybrids with higher amounts of nutrients. Development of varieties with reducedphenols, somewhat lower content of fat, and improved flour shelf life and maintaining quality is widely recommended as another area of attention (Nagaraj *et al.,* 2012). Incorporating these features into breeding, however, might cause the genetic advancement of other crucial traits to stall. The employment of diverse handlingskills, which need to be evaluated for their suitability at domestic, societal, and manufacturing scales, could better manage these characteristics. High starch varieties and hybrids could be a great addition to rice, maize, and other ethanol-producing crops. In addition to creating superior varieties, agronomic management technology needs to be improved. The explanation above makes it clear that there is significant room for investment in various technologies that will improve the lives of dryland farmers who grow and eat millet crops.

## Conclusion

Millets have largely persisted as a food grain crop with only a few unique foods and industrial uses, in contrast to other cereals like wheat, barley, rice, and maize that have been widely employed for food and manufacturing reasons. Due to difficult environmental circumstances, a scarcity of seed from upgradedvarieties, and the incapability of impoverished small farmers to espouse new crop production techniques, productivity has remained lower. As a result, a rise in millet's output will directly contribute to a decrease in poverty and an increase in food security. The lives of dryland farmers in Asia and sub-Saharan Africa will be significantly impacted by the progress and acceptance of HYVs and affordable crop production skills. The crop that can contribute to better health and nutrition is millet, which is also nutrient-dense. Millets are a cost-effective source of essential nutrients for human growth and development, including proteins, minerals, vitamins, carbs, and minerals. There is some evidence in the literature for the health-endorsing properties of millets; however, there is little data on the specific contributions of plant parts to illness prevention. All things considered, millets have the ability to help farmers in the semi-arid and arid tropics and other regions of the world with similar agroecologies achieve sustainable food and nutritional security.

## References

Abdalla, A. A., El Tinay, A. H., Mohamed, B. E. & Abdalla, A. H. (1998). Proximate composition, starch, phytate and mineral contents of 10 pearl millet genotypes. Food chemistry, 63(2), 243-246.

Abdel Rahman, S. M., Babiker, E. E. & El Tinay, A. H. (2005). Effect of fermentation on antinutritional factors and HCl extractability ofminerals of pearl millet cultivars. Journal of Food Technology, 3(4), 516–522.

Adekunle, A. A. (2012). Agricultural innovation in sub-saharan Africa: experiences from multiple stake holder approaches. Forum for Agricultural Research in Africa, Ghana.

Alais, C. & Linden, G. (1991). Food biochemistry. New York: Ellis Harwood Ltd.

Buerkert, A., Moser, M., Kumar, A. K., Fürst, P. & Becker, K. (2001). Variation in grain quality of pearl millet from sahelian West Africa. Field Crops Research, 69, 1–11.

Chandrasekara, A. & Shahidi, F. (2011a). Antiproliferative potential and DNA scission inhibitory activity of phenolics from whole millets. Journal of Functional Foods, 3, 159–170.

Chandrasekara, A. & Shahidi, F. (2011b). Bioactivities and antiradical properties of millet grains and hulls. Journal of Agricultural and Food Chemistry, 59, 9563–9571.

De Wet, J. M. J. D., Bidinger, F. R. & Peacock, J. M. (1992). Pearl millet (Pennisetum glaucum)-a cereal of the Sahel. In G. P. Chapman (Ed.), Desertified grasslands, their biology, and management. London: Academic Press. pp. 259–267.

Dykes, L. & Rooney, L. W. (2007). Phenolic compounds in cereal grains and their health benefits. Cereal Foods World, 52(3), 105–111.

Ejeta, G., Hassen, M. M. & Mertz, E. T. (1987). In vitro digestibility and amino acid composition of pearl millet (*Pennisetum typhoides*) and other cereals. Proceedings of the national academy of sciences, 84(17), 6016-6019.

Elyas, S. H. A., El Tinay, A. H., Yousif, N. E. & Elsheikh, E. A. E. (2002). Effect of natural fermentation on nutritive value and in vitro protein digestibility of pearl millet. Food Chemistry, 78, 75–79.

FAO. (1995). Chemical composition and nutritive value. In Sorghum and millets in human nutrition. Rome: FAO Food and Nutrition Series (No. 27). pp. 49–86.

Geetha, R., Virupaksha, T. K. &Shadaksharaswamy, M. (1997). Relationship between tannin levels and in vitro protein digestibility in finger millet (*Eleusine coracana*). Journal of Agricultural and Food Chemistry, 25, 1101–1108.

Godfray, H. C. J., Beddington, J. R., Crute, I. R., Haddad, L., Lawrence, D., Muir, J. F., . . . & Toulmin, C. (2010). Food security: the challenge of feeding 9 billion people. science, 327(5967), 812-818.

Hadimani, N. A., Muralikrishna, G., Tharanathan, R. N. &Malleshi, N. G. (2001). Nature of carbohydrates and proteins in three pearl millet varieties varying in processing characteristics and kernel texture. Journal of Cereal Science, 33(1), 17-25.

Hamdy, M. M. (1971). Interactions between phosphates and plant proteins. In Symposium: Phosphates in Food Processing, University of Guelph, Ontario, Canada. p. 83.

Jukanti, A. K., Gaur, P. M., Gowda, C. L. L. &Chibbar, R. N. (2012). Nutritional quality and health benefits of chickpea (*Cicer arietinum* L.): a review. British Journal of Nutrition, 108, S11–S26.

McDonough, C. M., Rooney, L. W. & Serna-Saldivar, S. O. (2000). The millets. In K. Kulp, & J. G. Ponte (Eds.), Handbook of cereal science and technology. New York, :Marcel Dekker Inc. pp. 177–202.

Nagaraj, N., Basavaraj, G., Rao, P. P. &Bantilan, C. (2012). Future outlook and options for target crops: the sorghum and pearl millet economy of India. policy brief No. 15. Patancheru: ICRISAT

Nambiar, V. S., Dhaduk, J. J., Sareen, N., Shahu, T. & Desai, R. (2011). Potential functional implications of pearl millet (*Pennisetum glaucum*) in health and disease. Journal of Applied Pharmaceutical Sciences, 1(10), 62–67.

Obilana, A. B. &Manyasa, E. (2002). Millets. In: P. S. Belton and J. R. N Taylor (Eds.). pp. 177–217.

Raboy, V. (1990). The biochemistry and genetics of phytic acid synthesis. In D. J. Morre, W. Boss, & F. A. Loewus (Eds.), Inositol metabolism in plants. New York: Alan R Liss. pp. 52–73.

Raboy, V. (1997). Accumulation and storage of phosphate and minerals. In B. A. Larkins, & I. K. Vasil (Eds.), Cellular and molecular biology of plant seed development. Dordrecht: Kluwer Academic Publishers. pp. 441–477.

Rai, K. N., Murty, D. S., Andrews, D. J. &Bramel-Cox, P. J. (1999). Genetic enhancement of pearl millet and sorghum for the semi-arid tropics of Asia and Africa. Genome, 42(4), 617-628.

Reichert, R. D., Youngs, C. G. & Christensen, D. A. (1980). Polyphenols in Pennisetum millet. In J. H. Hulse (Ed.), Polyphenols in cereals and legumes. Ottawa: International Development Research Centre. pp. 50–60.

Rooney, L. W. (1978). Sorghum and pearl millet lipids. Cereal Chemistry, 55(5), 584–590.

Sawaya, W. N., Khalil, J. K. & Safi, W. J. (1984). Nutritional quality of pearl millet flour and bread. Plant Foods for Human Nutrition, 34(2), 117–125.

Singh, G. (2003). Development and nutritional evaluation of value-added products from pearl millet (Pennisetum glaucum). Ph. D thesis. Hisar: CCS Haryana Agricultural University.

Wheeler, T. & Von Braun, J. (2013). Climate change impacts on global foodsecurity. Science, 341(6145), 508-513.

Wilson, J. P., Hess, D. E., Hanna, W. W., Kumar, K. A. & Gupta, S. C. (2004). *Pennisetum glaucum* subsp. *monodii* accessions with Striga resistance in West Africa. Crop Protection, 23(9), 865-870.

Yadav, O. P., Rai, K. N., Rajpurohit, B. S., Hash, C. T., Mahala, R. S., Gupta, S. K., . . . &Raghvani, K. L. (2012). Twenty-five years of pearl millet improvement in India. In: All India Coordinated Pearl Millet Improvement Project. Jodhpur. pp. 1–122.

Yang, X., Wan, Z., Perry, L., Lu, H., Wang, Q., Zhao, C., . . . & Ge, Q. (2012). Early millet use in northern China. Proceedings of the National Academy of Sciences, 109(10), 3726-3730.

# 4

# The Vital Role of Millets in Sustainable Agriculture: Ensuring Food Security and Enhancing Environmental Sustainability

Arjun Kumar Agarwal*

Department of Genetics & Plant Breeding, Ranchi Agriculture college, BAU, Ranchi-834006, (Jharkhand), India.

**ABSTRACT**

An increase in the globe's average temperature due to climate change is having an impact on agricultural productivity all around the world. Moreover, it directly affects biophysical aspects of life, such as the development of plants and animals, as well as many aspects of food supply and processing. For agricultural output to be maximized in order to satisfy the rising population's demands for food, it is critical to evaluate the consequences of worldwide climate change and use new tools and techniques to minimize their impact. Millets are the most helpful crop in this situation because they are nutrient-rich, climate change-tolerant, and have a huge potential to provide greater economic gains in marginal conditions than other cereals, even during the event of global warming with extreme temperature situations.

*Keywords*: Millets; Agriculture; Environment; Sustainability; Food security.

## Introduction

Millets have a long history of use in India. Numerous pieces of literature and documents have suggested that millets were a crucial component of ourceremonies, culinary traditions, dietary practices and society in general. According to experts, these were the first cereals to be farmed for household use and are among the earliest foods that mankind has discovered. Millet was reportedly one of the prized plants in the Hanging Gardens of Babylon. Millets, popularly called "Mota Anaj" in Hindi, are a group of highly variable small-seeded grasses, that have been cultivated and consumed widely around the world as cereal crops or grains for human food and fodder for thousands of years. There are around 6,000 different color-varieties of these grains in existence worldwide. They are one of the ancient foods dating back to the Indus Valley Civilization, around 3000 BC.

* Corresponding author.

They are grown in almost 131 countries today. Millets are the traditional food of 59 crore people in Asia and Africa. Millets have rekindled popularity in recent years because of their potential to support sustainable agriculture and food security. Millets are well-suited for usage in both rain-fed and desert areas because of their ability to grow in varied agro-climatic zones. Millets are suitable for cultivation in areas prone to water scarcity due to their low moisture demands and are renowned as drought-resistant crops. They also require little synthetic fertilizer and pesticide input and are highly resistant to insects, pests, and diseases. Additionally, due to their capacity to thrive in suboptimal soil conditions, they are a desirable alternative for small scale farmers who might not have access to quality inputs and fertile land.

Millets are not particularly well known, mostly because people are unaware of their many advantages for both consumers and producers. However, at a time when the globe is facing a pandemic, climate change, and a big issue with regard to food security, the nutri-cereals can play a key role if well-marketed, emphasizing their high nutritional content, minimal input and maintenance demands, and climate-resilient nature. There are still very few firms, farmers, and other stakeholders engaged in millets production, value addition, and commercialization in India because of a lack of understanding of the advantages of millets. To fully utilize their potential to boost farmers' incomes, create livelihoods, and guarantee nutritional and food security, challenges with the shortage of improved varieties, limited cultivation, short shelf lives, an insufficient amount of research, a lack of machinery, and market gaps must also be resolved. This year is the ideal time to publicize and raise knowledge of millets' advantages for consumers, cultivators, and climate.

## Millets for Sustainable Development

The International Year of Millet (IYM) was first proposed by India, and on March 3, 2021, the United Nations General Assembly (UNGA) approved a resolution designating 2023 as the IYM, which was supported by 72 countries, to make people aware of millets as a more cost-effective, environmentally friendly, and nutrient-dense substitute in response to the rising problem of food and nutritional security. India's efforts to promote the consumption and production of millet got a boost when the UNGA accepted the country's proposal and dedicated 2023 to spreading awareness about these grains. "The declaration has been crucial in helping India to lead the IYM celebrations, realise the PM's goal of making IYM 2023 a "people's movement," and establish India as the "global hub for millets."

The Indian government has emphasized millets because these crops are resilient to climate change, nutritionally superior, and water-efficient as well as due to their massive potential and integration with numerous United Nations Sustainable Development Goals (SDGs) or "The Agenda 2030" viz., zero hunger (SDG 2), good health and well-being (SDG 3), decent work and economic growth (SDG 8), responsible consumption and production (SDG 12), climate action (SDG 13) and life on land (SDG 15). These. Millets are significant due to their enormous potential to support livelihoods, boost farmer incomes, and guarantee global food and nutritional security.

## Millets area, production and productivity

Millets were one of the earliest food grains to be domesticated. They are often cultivated in arid and semi-arid regions and require a much less water than other major cereals.The three major millets producers in the world, making up more than 55% of total production, are India, Nigeria, and China. India is the world's leading producer of millets, producing more than 17 million metric tonnes annually, accounting for 20 per cent of global output and 80 per cent of Asia's production. The average productivity of millets in India (1239 kg/hectare) which is also greater than the average global productivity of 1229 kg/hectare. India is also among the top five exporter- India exported millets worth $64.28 million in 2021-22 and $59.75 million in 2020-21, according to the Agricultural and Processed Food Products Export Development Authority. The major millets cultivated in India are Pearl millet,Sorghum, and Finger millet, with a production share of 61%, 27%, and 10%, respectively. The largest millets-producing states in India include Rajasthan, Uttar Pradesh, Haryana, Gujarat, Madhya Pradesh, Maharashtra, Karnataka, Tamil Nadu, Andhra Pradesh, and Telangana (Table 1).

**Table 1:** Area under cultivation, production, and yield of millets

| Crop | Area (m ha) | Production (m tons) | Yield (kg per ha) |
|---|---|---|---|
| Sorghum(kharif) | 1.76 | 1.58 | 967 |
| Sorghum (Rabi) | 3.07 | 2.73 | 1002 |
| Sorghum (total) | 4.83 | 4.31 | 989 |
| Bajra | 7.55 | 9.22 | 1374 |
| Ragi | 1.01 | 1.67 | 1747 |
| Small millets | 0.459 | 0.33 | 809 |
| Total millets | 13.83 | 15.53 | 1248 |

*Source:* Final Estimates-2021-22, DES, Government of India

## Millets types and classification

In more than 20 States across the nation, differenttypes of millets are cultivated as kharif crops.The top producers are Rajasthan, Karnataka, Maharashtra, and Andhra Pradesh.In India, millets can be clubbed into major, minor, and pseudo categories.

1. **Major Millets:** Sorghum (Jowar), Pearl Millet (Bajra), Finger Millet (Ragi/ Mandua)
2. **Minor (Small) Millets:** Foxtail Millet (Kangani/Kakun), Proso Millet (Cheena), Kodo Millet, Barnyard Millet (Sawa/Sanwa/ Jhangora), Little Millet (Kutki), Browntop millet (ChotiKangani)
3. **Pseudo Millets:** Buck-wheat (Kuttu) and Amaranth (Chaulai)

**Millets' nutritional properties and health benefits**

The terms "coarse cereals" and "cereals of the poor" were once used to describe millets. Millets are regarded as "powerhouses of nutrition." In an effort to boost demand, the government designated 2018 as the "national year of millet." In the same year, these grains were officially rebranded as "nutri-cereals" due to their excellent nutritional potential and for the purposes of production, consumption, and trade. It is also included under the Prime Minister's overarching scheme for holistic nutrition (POSHAN) Abhiyan in the same year. In 2021, the Center launched the Pradhan Mantri Poshan Shakti Nirman (PM POSHAN), formerly known as the mid-day meal programme, in government and government-aided schools and recommended state governments incorporate millets into the mid-day meal diet to improve nutritional outcomes.

Millets are a great source of vital nutrients, including a variety of minerals and vitamins, proteins, and carbohydrates. They are also gluten-free, making them a good substitute for those who cannot consume gluten. Millets are said to be more nutrient-dense than wheat, rice, and maize since they provide several nutrients to the diet. Millets are high in dietary fibers, Fe, Ca, Mg, K, Zn, and vitamins such as B1, B2, and B3. The protein, fat, and carbohydrate composition of these grains ranges from 7 to 12%, 2-5%, 65-75%, and 15-20%, respectively. When comparing little millets to fine cereals, they are more nutrient-denser. They have greater levels of protein, fat, and fibre.

Millets are also "nutritional supplements" that have phytochemicals such as flavonoids, saponins, tannins such as phenols, tannins, flavonoids, alkaloids, terpenoids, and anti-nutrients that are essential for preserving good health and have a significant impact on the treatment of chronic illnesses. They include essential nutrients such as essential amino acids, carbohydrates, lipids, fibre, and folic acid, in addition to vitamins like thiamine, niacin, and riboflavin and micronutrients like iron, calcium, and potassium. The foods composed of millet nourish the body and protect it from a number of diseases, including diabetes, cardiac disease, cancer, allergies, digestive problems, and others. Despite the fact that millets are frequently farmed in dry and semiarid environments, their nutritional value and possible health advantages have received little attention.

Due to the presence of phytochemicals in millets, these grains are also considered to have antibacterial and DNA damage protective properties. Millets have a relatively high percentage of non-starch carbohydrates and soluble fiber, both of which aid in controlling weight. Millets are a great option for a diabetic diet because they slowly release glucose. Millets are a great source of slow-digesting carbohydrate and nutritional fibre that are helpful for the bowels and support the growth of billions of bacteria, including *Lactobacillus acidophilus*, *Actinobacteria*, and *Bifido* species. Millets include non-starch carbohydrates, which make up a significant portion of soluble fibre and function admirably as prebiotics by fermenting resistant starch to create short-chain triglycerides.

Due to their increased fibre content, millets have low glycemic index values. Even though food's glycemic characteristics vary depending on the kind of processing, food matrices, component composition, food shape (grain or flour forms), etc., most millet cuisines may be made to possess a low glycemic index (glucose level) and therefore can help in tackling lifestyle issues and medical conditions like overweight, hypertension, and diabetes. Anaemia caused by iron deficiency is one of the most serious health issues in pregnant women due to a lack of iron-rich foods.Similarly, lactating mothers also suffer from iron deficiency anaemia due to blood loss in the post-natal period. According to a study, including millet-based items in the diet throughout the prenatal and postnatal periods is essential for enhancing the nutritional quality of women during pregnancy and breastfeeding. The auxiliary food items made from millet are particularly nourishing for pregnant women and breastfeeding mothers. Foods made from millet improve the body mass index (BMI).

## Millets' advantages for preventing lifestyle disorders and providing nutrition

- *Benefits of Millets on Cardiovascular Disease and Type 2 Diabetes*

Millets are high in the amino acid leucine and contain slowly digestible carbohydrates and minerals, which dampen the otherwise abrupt rise in postprandial glucose levels and make them a nutritious food for diabetics. Type II diabetes, sometimes referred to as "non-insulin-dependent diabetes mellitus" (NIDDM), is brought on by an imbalance involving insulin sensitivity and insulin production. Heart problems are substantially more likely when NIDDM risk is higher. In terms of the likelihood of acquiring heart disease, low-density lipoprotein (LDL) and high-density lipoprotein (HDL) have variable effects. As a result, every 1 mg/dL elevation in LDL increases the risk of heart disease by 2%, whereas every 1 mg/dL elevation in HDL reduces the risk of heart disease by 2-3%. Triglyceride levels are another factor that raises the risk of developing heart conditions since there is a long-standing connection between having high triglyceride levels and an increased risk of heart conditions. Among all other methods for preventing heart disease, lowering LDL cholesterol has been shown to be the most effective. Thus, a diet that lowers LDL should be adopted in order to lower the risk of cardiac problems. Niacin-enriched millet lowers triglyceride and LDL levels and corrects irregularities in lipoproteins. Additionally, millets slow down the digestion of blood cholesterol. As a result, millet-rich diets are recommended as one method of lowering the risk of cardiac problems.

• *Millets' cancer-preventing properties*

Millets are rich in phenolic components, including phenolic acids, flavonoids, and tannins, which makes them potent nutrients capable of lowering the prevalence of colon and breast cancer in both humans and animals. According to in vivo research, a unique 35-kD protein called fibroin-modulator-binding protein (FMBP) isolated from foxtail millet blocks the proliferation of colon cancer cells by arresting cells at the G1 phase and causing the loss of mitochondrial transmembrane potential, which activates the caspase enzyme and causes colorectal cancer cells to go through apoptosis (programmed cell death).

• *Millets for Neurological Conditions*

Several studies have shown that excessive fat consumption in the human diet can not only increase the risk of heart diseases, but recent epidemiological research has revealed that dementia risk is also increased by a high-fat, high-calorie diet. Research indicates that polyphenols and their metabolites are crucial in controlling the amount of oxidative stress in the brain. Either by directly crossing the blood-brain barrier into the brain or by being transformed into tiny metabolic derivates with increased biological activity through the metabolism of intestinal microbiota, dietary polyphenols may have antioxidant and neuroprotective effects.

## How crucial are millets to eco-sustainable farming?

• *Millets as a climate-resilient crop*

Millets are pest-resistant, adaptable to a broad range of climates and moisture conditions, and require minimal input of synthetic fertilisers to flourish, making them environment-friendly in addition to their health advantages. They can even survive in locations that are prone to drought since they just need a little moisture for growth. In addition to being water-efficient, millets are $C_4$ carbon sequestering plants that help lower atmospheric $CO_2$ levels.

• *Viable choices for small and marginal farmers*

Millets are grown as crops with two uses: as food for people and as fodder for animals. The abundant crop and varietal diversification of millet-based farming systems fosters and enriches the agrobiodiversity of their ecosystems. Due to the low investment needed for the production of millets, they prove to be a sustainable and viable income source for small and marginal farmers.

- *High nutritional value and health benefits*

Millets are highly nutritious and provide food and livelihood security. Millets are known to be a storehouse of nutrition as they are good sources of calcium, zinc, magnesium, phosphorous, copper, vitamin, iron, folate, carbohydrates, micronutrients, antioxidants, and phytochemicals with nutraceutical properties. They are gluten-free and are also considered good for celiac patients. The promotion of millets is now being seen as an effective strategy for tackling malnutrition in the country. The nutrition and health benefits of millets hold special significance in today's times when people are gravitating towards healthier options.

- *Economic and food security*

Millet was once regarded as the "poor man's food grain" because it was less expensive than other grains. The millet output has grown as a result of India's National Food Security Program. Millets were produced in greater quantities throughout time, rising from 14.52 million metric tonnes in 2015–16 to 17.96 million metric tonnes in 2020–21 (Agriculture and Farmers Welfare Department). Due to the swiftly rising global demand for millets, its exports are growing dramatically. All stakeholders are benefiting from the increased commercial prospects brought about by the expanding demand for millets.

## Important millets and their significancein food security and environmental sustainability

### *Sorghum*

The grain sorghum (*Sorghum bicolor* L.), which originated in Africa, is a crop that contains a lot of carbs. It was cultivated between 3,000 and 5,000 years ago, following wheat, maize, rice, and barley as the world's greatest carbohydrate-rich crop. Nonetheless, many of the world's poor, who live in unstable agro-ecological zones and fight against hunger and malnutrition, depend on sorghum for their food supply. The most common millet crop farmed globally is sorghum (jowar). The main jowar producers are the United States, China, Australia, India, Argentina, Nigeria, and Sudan. Madhya Pradesh, Maharashtra, Karnataka, Rajasthan, Tamil Nadu, and Andhra Pradesh are the Indian states where jowar is mostly farmed.

Sorghum, commonly referred to as the "King of Millets," is an essential dual-purpose crop that is also the most drought resistant of the five major carbohydrate-rich crops in the world. Sorghum also has a worldwide reputation as a model crop due to its remarkable tolerance to minimal input levels. Although it is primarily grown as a significant feed crop for animal nutrition, sorghum also serves as a staple food for people. However, a lot of research has been done on sorghum for human food because of its excellent nutritional and physiological potential.

Sorghum is a grain that is rich in nutrients for human wellness and nutrition since it includes polysaccharides like carbohydrates, proteins, lipids, vitamins, fibres, and minerals. The main prolamins in sorghum protein are called kafirins. The majority of the minerals in sorghum are phosphorus, potassium, and zinc. Sorghum contains a significant quantity of phytochemicals that are good for your health, such as phytosterols, policosanols, and phenolic compounds. The two phenolic chemicals that are most prevalent in sorghum are flavonoids and phenolic acids. Since sorghum has a resistant starch, it appeals to diabetics and obese people. Those who are gluten intolerant may also use sorghum as a substitute for other foods.

In comparison to other major cereal crops like maize, sorghum often has cheaper production costs, including the cost of fertiliser, seeds, chemicals, land rent, etc., and yields higher net earnings. In terms of water usage effectiveness, and harvest index under water stress, sorghum likely performed better than maize. Sorghum can therefore play a key role in feeding the world's most helpless people given the increasing demand for a limited supply of freshwater, the increasing use of marginal agriculture, and changing climate patterns.

## Pearl Millet

Pearl millet (*Pennisetum glaucum* (L.) R. Br.) or bajra is the sixth most important cereal crop after rice, wheat, maize, barley, and sorghum. It is especially beneficial since it is nutritionally rich, climate resilient, and has a significant potential to provide more economic returns under difficult circumstances. It also serves as a source of fodder and cattle feed, producing more than half of the globe's millet. It is a staple food for 90 million people who live in poverty and is commonly grown on 30 million hectares of land in the dry and semi-arid tropical regions of Asia and Africa. On 7.55 million hectares, India produced 9.22 million metric tonnes of pearl millet. The leading producers are Tamil Nadu, Madhya Pradesh, and Haryana.

The two main productivity barriers caused by the various weather conditions are heat and drought. Because of its innate ability to thrive in such environments and tolerate abiotic pressures like drought, salt, and heat, pearl millet is mostly grown on marginal soils with irregular and untimely rainfall patterns and other environmental challenges (Serba and Yadav, 2016). It may increase the incomes and food supply of rural people in arid regions, and it is climate change resilient, which is essential to minimising the negative impacts of climate change. Because of its deep root system, pearl millet can flourish in a range of ecological conditions with little water supply. Because of its distinctive qualities, which include the $C_4$ plant's high photosynthetic activity, greater capacity for producing dry matter, and ability to survive in challenging agro-climatic conditions with limited input and greater economic returns, it outperforms all other cereals, including wheat, maize, rice, sorghum, and barley. It also has a number of benefits, including early maturity, resistance to drought, a low input demand, and a general lack of biotic and abiotic constraints.

It is nutritionally superior to other popular cereals and a great source of calories, carbohydrates, crude fibre, soluble and non-soluble fibre, proteins (8–19%), antioxidants, and fat (3–8%), with improved intestinal absorption. Moreover, it has a high mineral content (2.3 mg/100 g), which includes potassium, phosphorus, magnesium, iron, zinc, copper, and manganese, as well as vitamins like thiamine, riboflavin, and niacin. It is a very nutritious food that is non-acid-forming, non-glutenous, high in fibre, and includes a variety of nutraceuticals. It serves as a probiotic food for the bacteria in our bodies and eases constipation. Its grain contains niacin, which enables it to lower cholesterol as well. The antioxidant activity is enhanced by phytates, polyphenols, etc. Pearl millet, the crop of the future with the promise of both nutrient richness and climate adaptation, requires attention to developing nutrient-rich variants and varieties that are drought tolerant using various crop improvement techniques.

## Finger millet

Finger millet (*Elusine corocana*), also referred to as "ragi" or "Mandua" in Hindi, is a food crop that is widely cultivated in India and other nations in Africa and Asia. It is essential for safeguarding food security, advancing sustainable agriculture, and maintaining the environment's health. The popular name "finger millet" alludes to the branching of the panicle that resembles "fingers," and the genus name "Eleusine" is taken from the Greek goddess of grains. It could thus be one of Africa's oldest naturally domesticated tropical cereals. It is a crop that yields a lot, performs well in a variety of difficult environmental conditions, and is organic by nature.

Finger millet is a crucial crop for growers in arid and semi-arid areas because of its great drought tolerance and ability to thrive in tough conditions. It is also an ecologically beneficial choice because it uses less fertiliser and pesticide. It can be cultivated on low-fertility soils and doesn't require synthetic fertilisers, making it a blessing for the large desert and semi-arid regions. Finger millet seeds have earned the nickname "famine crop" because of their ability to withstand storage pests for up to 10 years, enabling year-round food security or even after a crop failure.

Karnataka, Uttarakhand, Maharashtra, Tamil Nadu, Odisha, Andhra Pradesh, and Gujarat are the major finger millet-producing states.

Finger millet is an important millet crop that is grown for feed and fodder. Its grains are a gluten-free cereal and a great source of protein, fibre, calcium, iron, and other minerals. Due to its high fibre content, finger millet is said to be an excellent laxative and prevent constipation.It is a healthy diet for people with diabetes, liver problems, high blood pressure, weak hearts, and asthma. It is mostly made up of unsaturated fat and has a low-fat level. It can combat the high prevalence of anaemia since it contains the most calcium and iron. In addition to being exceptionally high in micronutrients, particularly calcium, its seed coat also contains a significant quantity of phytochemicals, including dietary fibre and polyphenols. The high polyphenol content of the seed coat, which signals anti-oxidant activity, and the high fibre content, which encourages slow digestion and blood sugar stability, are the key reasons why the seed coat also exhibits anti-cancer and anti-diabetic properties. For the meals of pregnant and breast-feeding women, children, and the livelihood of marginal and small farmers, finger millet is essential. The levels of amino acids in finger millet are higher than those suggested by the FAO and WHO. Due to the presence of important amino acids like methionine, tryptophan, and lysine, finger millet grains are preferable to rice and wheat. Overall, finger millet is a versatile crop with several critical applications in sustainable agriculture, food security, and environmental health. Finger millet will probably take on a bigger role in feeding people all over the world as the need for food rises.

## Little Millet

Little millet (*Panicum sumatrense*), also called "Kutki" in Hindi, is an annual herbaceous plant that can reach heights of 30 cm to 1 m. Its leaves can grow straight or folded. The main states that cultivate little millet are Madhya Pradesh, Gujarat, Orissa, Maharashtra, Karnataka, and Gujarat. Little millet was originally planted in south-east Asia, but it is now grown all across India, especially in Madhya Pradesh, Orissa, Jharkhand, and Uttar Pradesh. It is a short-lived crop that grows quickly and can resist both drought and standing water. Its cultivation is limited to tribal regions and marginal grounds.

It is a great millet that is appropriate for individuals of all ages. It treats all stomach-related issues and aids in preventing constipation. It increases men's semen counts. Women who have issues with irregular menstrual cycles also benefit from it. Its high fibre content aids in lowering body fat accumulation. The 100 grammes of small millet contain 8.7 grammes of protein, 75.7 grammes of carbohydrates, 5.3 grammes of fat, 1.7 grammes of minerals, and 9.3 milligrammes of iron. It is especially beneficial for diabetics, who frequently experience blood glucose spikes after eating other grains, particularly rice and wheat (post-prandial). It digests a lot more slowly than wheat and rice do. Compared to rice, they have less carbohydrates. It contains a lot of fibre, which helps to control digestive health and boost metabolism. The increased intake of little millet also results in a decrease in the Body Mass Index (BMI), one of the main indicators of obesity.

It is a good source of antioxidants such as polyphenols, phenolic compounds, tannins, and flavonoids, which are vital for maintaining health and warding off illnesses associated with sedentary lifestyles like diabetes, heart disease, and obesity. Low-density lipoprotein (LDL) cholesterol, which can clog arteries and raise the risk of heart arrest and other heart issues, is significantly reduced by these antioxidants. It also provides a significant amount of bioactive nutraceutical components such as phenols, carotenoids, and tocopherols that play an important role in health, aging, and metabolic disease. It has a high content of resistant starch and insoluble dietary fibre, both of which support normal digestive health. Also, it aids in the treatment of typical gastrointestinal issues such as flatulence, bloating, constipation, and irregular bowel movements. It also contributes to the general wellbeing of the body's internal organs.

## Foxtail Millet

In various regions of India, foxtail millet (*Setaria italica* (L.) P. Beauvois) is also referred to as Italian millet, Kangu, Kangani, Koni, and Kaon. One of the earliest crops ever produced, it is said to be native to China. It is grown for hay, grazing, food, and grain. Foxtail millet is the second most produced millet in the world and continues to play a significant role in global agriculture, giving six million metric tonnes of food to millions of people, mostly on marginal or poor soils in temperate, subtropical, and tropical Asia and southern Europe. It will increase in height from sea level to 2,000 metres. Its grain is fed to chickens and caged birds as well as used for human consumption.

The production of foxtail millet is also regarded as being ecologically benign since it uses less water and fertiliser than other crops, making it a perfect crop for sustainable farming and the battle against a changing climate. It cannot stand standing water. Due to its early maturity, foxtail millet may sometimes avoid droughts despite its moderate drought tolerance. It is suitable for growing as a short-term catch crop due to its rapid growth. It can thrive in a variety of soils, climates, and elevations. It is a resilient crop that can thrive in several types of soil and endure harsh weather conditions like drought and high heat.

In order to increase nutrition and food security, particularly in rural and water-stressed regions, foxtail millet is being pushed by public and private groups as a superior nutritious substitute to other major grains like rice and wheat. A good source of carbs, dietary fibre, proteins, vitamins, and minerals, including iron and calcium, is foxtail millet. It is also devoid of gluten and easy to digest, making it a wonderful choice for those who are allergic to gluten. Beta-carotene, a precursor to vitamin A, and iron are all abundant in foxtail millet. It is a great meal for diabetics since it has a low glycemic index and is used to make burfi, a sweet product. Foxtail cultivars with yellow seeds are used medicinally as stomachics, astringents, digestive aids, and emollients. Moreover, it is used to treat dyspepsia, poor digestion, and abdominal food stagnation. Green seeds are diuretics that boost masculinity, whereas white seeds are chilling and used to treat cholera and fever. 12.3% crude protein and 3.3% minerals are present in this millet. In India, foxtail millet is frequently prepared as porridge, used to make rotis, and used in a variety of recipes. Moreover, it is used to make rawa, bread, and puffy treats.

### Proso Millet

Proso millet (*Panicum miliaceum* L.), is a prominent minor millet cultivated in India. Its origins date at least to 2000 B.C. It is planted around the world and is called by a variety of names, including broom corn millet, hog millet, Hershey millet, common millet, etc. India, Japan, China, Egypt, Arabia, and Western Europe are among the countries that cultivate it widely. Proso millet is a crop with minimal needs and no known diseases that damage it. Because of its shallow root system and resistance to atrazine residues, proso millet is a helpful intercrop between two crops that demand high amounts of water and herbicides.

While it has a protein level that is comparable to that of wheat, without gluten, it cannot be used on its own to make fermentation bread. The protein content is 11.6% of the dry matter and is substantially richer in the important amino acid leucine, isoleucine, and methionine. It is abundant in nutrients and minerals like magnesium and copper. Moreover, proso millet enhanced plasma levels and glycemic reactions. When ingested as food, proso millet offers several advantages. It is abundant in vitamins, proteins, dietary fibre, polyphenols, and minerals. Because it is gluten-free, it is perfect for those who cannot tolerate gluten. High levels of lecithin in proso millet help the neurological health system. Niacin, B-complex vitamins, folic acid, P, Ca, Zn, and Fe are among the vitamins, minerals, and important amino acids like methionine and cysteine are abundant in it. It lowers the risk of type 2 diabetes and has a low glycemic index. Unfortunately, it is mostly regarded as bird feed in many countries while being primarily used as food for humans in many other countries.

In addition to being excellent for human and animal health, proso millet is also excellent for the environment. Proso millet is a warm-weather crop. It is widely grown in warm climates across the world. It may be cultivated in locations with little rainfall because of its high level of drought resistance. It can tolerate stagnant water to some extent as well. It is a rare crop that goes through its whole life cycle quickly. Proso millet is a unique crop with a short growth season that is tolerant of dryness, making it a viable rotating crop for semi aarid regions. Proso millet may be produced in both rich and low soils, with soils of various textures ranging from sandy loam to clay loam; coarse sands are not suitable for proso millet farming. It is crucial for environmental sustainability, food security, and sustainable agriculture.

## Kodo Millet

The kodo millet, *Paspalum scrobiculatum* (L.), is extensively spread in wet environments across the world's tropical and subtropical regions. Among all the edible grains, it is the coarsest. Kodo millet is also called ditch millet, cow grass, and rice grass. It is believed that native paspalum, also known as Indian Crown Grass, was introduced in India over 3000 years ago. The grain has a protein content of 8.3%, a fat content of 1.4%, a carbohydrate content of 65.6%, and an ash content of 2.9%. The entire grain has a significant amount of fiber. It serves as the foundation for meeting dietary nutritional needs. It has a lot of fibre (14.3%), little fat (4.2%), and a lot of protein (11%).

Kodo millet is great for boosting the neurological system since it is very simple to digest and has a high lecithin content. Niacin, pyridoxine, and folic acid are particularly abundant in kodo millet, along with minerals including calcium, iron, potassium, magnesium, and zinc. Moreover, it has a lot of fibre and little fat. It has a high lecithin content and works wonders to fortify the nerve system. Kodo millets are suitable for gluten-intolerant people since they are free of gluten. Postmenopausal women with heart disease symptoms such as high blood pressure and cholesterol may benefit greatly from daily consumption of kodo millet.

Kodo millet has the lowest phosphorus level of any other millet and has the highest antioxidant properties of all other grains. Patients with diabetes are advised to use the grain as an alternative to rice. Most of the time, kodo millet is raised in warm, dry climates. Because of its strong drought tolerance, it may be cultivated in regions with irregular and sparse rainfall. It does well in regions with only 40 to 50 centimetres of yearly rainfall. Kodo millet is a significant crop that supports both human well-being and ecological sustainability. It is an essential food source for populations all around the world because of its adaptability, minimal input requirements, and high nutritional value.

## Barnyard Millet

Throughout Asia, notably in India, China, Japan, and Korea, barnyard millet (*Echinochloa* sp.) is a common millet crop that has been produced for centuries.

It is the fourth-most widely grown small millet, ensuring food security for a large number of underprivileged people worldwide. India is one of the major producers of barnyard millet in the world. The majority of barnyard millet is grown for human use; however, it is also fed to animals. *Echinochloa frumentacea* (Indian barnyard millet) and *Echinochloa esculenta* (Japanese barnyard millet) are two of the most popular varieties among the numerous cultivated and wild species of barnyard millet. It is also known as Japanese barnyard millet, ooda, sawan, and sanwa.

It is a short-lived crop that can tolerate diverse biotic and abiotic pressures and flourish in unfavorable environmental circumstances with almost negligible maintenance. In addition to these agricultural benefits, the grains are prized for their excellent nutritional content and reduced cost in comparison to main cereals like rice, wheat, and maize. It is a rich source of easily digested protein and dietary fibre with a decent quantity of both soluble and insoluble fractions and, most importantly, micronutrients including iron (Fe) and zinc (Zn), which are linked to a number of health advantages. Barnyard millet is a natural gift for today's sluggish human population because it contains low and slowly digesting carbohydrates. Linoleic acid is the predominant fatty acid in barnyard millet, followed by palmitic and oleic acids. Moreover, it exhibits a strong oxidative degradation of amylase, which promotes the creation of more resistant starches. As a result, it may be recommended to people with diabetes and coronary heart disease. The best results from barnyard millet come from lowering cholesterol and blood sugar levels. Each of these qualities makes it an excellent supplemental crop for marginal farmers as well as an alternative crop when the monsoon season fails in places where rice and other major crops are grown. Despite the tremendous nutritive and agronomic benefits of barnyard millet, this crop is nevertheless undervalued and neglected due to a lack of knowledge.

## Browntop Millet

Browntop millet (*Urochloa ramosa; or Brachiaria ramosa*) is a small-seeded annual grass used as a grain crop, particularly on poor soils in dry subtropical and tropical regions of the world. Browntop millet contains more nutrients than other millet varieties. Browntop millet has a good nutritional value. Browntop millet is gluten-free, loaded with vital minerals, and delicious in addition to being healthy. It contains 71.32 grammes of carbohydrates, 8.06–16.08% dietary fiber, 1.89 grammes of fat, 10–11% protein, and is a good source of zinc and iron. Moreover, it includes phytochemicals such as resins, quinones, tannins, and flavonoids. It could be utilised to create a number of value-added products and meals that are ready to eat. In comparison to other minor millets, such as proso and foxtail millet, brown top millets are a fantastic source of dietary fibre. It can be utilised in the treatment and prevention of a number of non-communicable disorders.

Brown top millet, a small millet that can be grown on degraded soils with very little water, is once again being grown by farmers. In addition, it is used as a cover crop in plantation crop groves to prevent soil erosion and increase straw output. It is raised as a catch crop with a rapid growth rate in between commodity crops. It is a crucial plant for the removal of contaminants from polluted soils due to its capacity to accumulate considerable levels of zinc and lead in root and stem tissues. As a result, browntop millet has enormous potential for reducing hunger, improving nutrition, and fulfilling sustainability goals.

## Summary

Millets are an important crop with a rich history, known for their tolerance to harsh conditions, low input requirements, and high nutritional value. They are crucial for ensuring food security and environmental sustainability. Millets represent one of the earliest foods that humans have ever known and may have been the first cereal grain to be domesticated for household use. Millets are small-seeded grasses that are drought resistant and grow well in arid regions under suboptimal conditions of soil fertility and water. Millets are distinctive in part because of their brief growth season. The main types of millet cultivated in India include sorghum, bajra, finger millet, and minor millets including foxtail millet, little millet, kodo millet, proso millet, browntop millet, and barnyard millet. They were repeatedly alluded to as "coarse cereals," but the Indian government has recently designated them as "nutri-cereals" in recognition of the nutritional content of the grains. The majority of the world's millet is produced in India. With a market share of almost 15% of international millets output, India is the world's top producer. Millets are primarily grown in 21 states across India, covering 12.53 million hectares and yielding 15.53 million tonnes at a rate of 1237 kg/ha. These are really nourishing meals that don't create acids and aren't glutinous. This makes them calming and easy to absorb. They have significant concentrations of dietary fibre, vitamin B complexes, important amino acids and essential fats, and vitamin E.

They include particularly high levels of minerals, including iron, magnesium, phosphorus, and potassium, and they release glucose at a smaller proportion over a longer duration, resulting in satiety and a decreased risk of developing diabetes. These grains have a large amount of carbs, 6 to 11 per cent protein, and 1.5 to 5 per cent fat. They aid in providing health advantages such as lowering blood sugar levels (diabetes), controlling hypertension, and preventing thyroid, cardiac, and celiac disorders.

Millets are important crops for farmers in semi-arid areas because they are both climatically appropriate and high in nutrients.Millets are understood to have considerable potential for food and nutritional security in the face of rising agricultural expenses, global warming, and a growing global population. Millets can grow in a variety of agro-climatic zones, making them suitable for use in both rain-fed and desert situations. Millets are known for withstanding drought and having minimal moisture requirements, making them appropriate for cultivation in places that experience water shortages. They are also very resistant to insects, pests, and illnesses and require little in the way of synthetic fertilisers and pesticides. Also, small-scale farmers who do not have access to good-quality inputs and rich land may find them to be an appealing choice because of their ability to grow in less-than-ideal soil types.

Overall, millets are a versatile crop that has many important uses in sustainable agriculture and human nutrition and health. As global food demands continue to increase, millets will likely play an increasingly important role in providing nutritious food to communities around the world.

## Conclusion

Millets are not widely consumed despite having significant advantages for both consumers and producers, mostly because they are not well known. However, nutri-cereals can play a significant role if well-marketed, focusing on their high nutritional value, low input and maintenance requirements, and climate-resilient nature at a time when the world is fighting a pandemic and climate change, as well as facing a significant challenge of food security. To fully realise their potential for raising farmers' incomes, generating livelihoods, and ensuring food and nutritional security, it is also necessary to solve issues with the lack of good quality seeds, limited cultivation, short grain shelf lives, inadequate research, lack of process technology, and market gaps.

## References

Bandyopadhyay, T., Muthamilarasan, M., & Prasad, M. (2017). Millets for next generation climate-smart agriculture. *Frontiers in plant science*, *8*, 1266.

Banerjee, P., Maitra, S., & Banerjee, P. (2020). The role of small millets as functional food to combat malnutrition in developing countries. *Indian Journal of Natural Sciences*, *10*(60), 20412-20417.

Das, S., Khound, R., Santra, M., &Santra, D. K. (2019). Beyond bird feed: Proso millet for human health and environment. *Agriculture*, *9*(3), 64.

Dayakar Rao B., Bhaskarachary K., Arlene Christina G.D., Sudha Devi G., Vilas, A. Tonapi. (2017). Nutritional and Health benefits of Millets. ICAR Indian Institute of Millets Research (IIMR) Rajendranagar, Hyderabad, PP 112

Maitra, S. (2020). Intercropping of small millets for agricultural sustainability in drylands: A review. *Crop Research*, *55*(3and4), 162-171.

Prabhakar, Prabhu C ganiger., Boraiah B., Sujata Bhat., Nandini C., Kiran., Tippeswamy V., Manjunath H. A. (2017). Improved production technology for Kodo millet. ICAR-AICRP on small Millets

Prabhakar, Prabhu C ganiger., Boraiah B., Sujata Bhat., Nandini C., Kiran., Tippeswamy V., Manjunath H. A. (2017). Improved production technology for Little millet. ICAR-AICRP on small Millets

Prabhakar, Prabhu C ganiger., Boraiah B., Sujata Bhat., Nandini C., Kiran., Tippeswamy V., Manjunath H. A. (2017). Improved production technologies for finger millet. ICAR-AICRP on small Millets

Prabhakar, Prabhu C ganiger., Boraiah B., Sujata Bhat., Nandini C., Kiran., Tippeswamy V., Manjunath H. A. (2017). Improved production technology for foxtail millet. ICAR-AICRP on small Millets

Prabhakar, Prabhu C ganiger., Boraiah B., Sujata Bhat., Nandini C., Kiran., Tippeswamy V., Manjunath H. A. (2017). Improved production technology for proso millet. ICAR-AICRP on small Millets

Rai, K. N., Gowda, C. L. L., Reddy, B. V. S., & Sehgal, S. (2008). Adaptation and potential uses of sorghum and pearl millet in alternative and health foods. *Comprehensive Reviews in Food Science and Food Safety*, *7*(4), 320-396.

Renganathan VG, Vanniarajan C, Karthikeyan A and Ramalingam J (2020) Barnyard Millet for Food and Nutritional Security: Current Status and Future Research Direction. Front. Genet. 11:500. doi: 10.3389/fgene.2020.00500

Sachdev, N., Goomer, S., & Singh, L. R. (2021). Foxtail millet: a potential crop to meet future demand scenario for alternative sustainable protein. *Journal of the Science of Food and Agriculture*, *101*(3), 831-842.

Satyavathi, C. T., Ambawat, S., Khandelwal, V., & Srivastava, R. K. (2021). Pearl millet: a climate-resilient nutricereal for mitigating hidden hunger and provide nutritional security. *Frontiers in Plant Science*, *12*, 659938.

Singh, S., Suri, S., & Singh, R. (2022). Potential and unrealized future possibilities of browntop millet in the food sector. *Frontiers in Sustainable Food Systems*, *6*, 974126

Srinivasan, N., Palanisamy, K., Mahomoodally, M. F., Zengİn, G., Arumugam, A., & Gopalakrishnan, S. (2019). Nutritional and functional roles of millets-a review. *Journal of Food Biochemistry*, *43*(7).

The Associated Chambers of Commerce and Industry of India. (2022). Millets: The Super Future Food for India. Associated Chambers of Commerce and Industry of India.

Vinoth, A., &Ravindhran, R. (2017). Biofortification in millets: a sustainable approach for nutritional security. *Frontiers in Plant Science*, *8*, 29.

# 5

# Role of Minor Millets in the Context of Climate Change and Genomic Resources

Ajay[1*], Nikumani Choudhury[1*]

[1] Department of Soil Science, Assam Agricultural University, 785013, India

**ABSTRACT**

Small millets are a very good potential agricultural crop for ensuring the security of the world's food supply. A substantial part can be played by millets in enhancing nutritional security and preventing diseases causedby poor nutrition because they are essential providers of nutrients. Their adaptability to climate changes and growing relevance in agriculture necessitate healthy food and feed. Small millets are a great option to supplement main staple foods for crop and food diversification due to their diversified adaptation to marginal areas, lower water demand, decreased susceptibility to stressors, and nutritional excellence in comparison to major grain staples. Millets have many morpho-physiological, genetic, and biochemical properties that make them more resistant to environmental stresses than other cereal crops. The nutritional content and capability to withstand abiotic stresses of the genetic diversity in the core and mini-core germplasm of small millets were characterized and can be incorporated into breeding strategies. The extensive morphological, taxonomic, and genetic variety of tiny millets seen in the wild species includes ploidy levels, life cycles, habitats, and reproductive strategies.

*Keywords*: Small millets; climate change: Genomic resources; food security

## Introduction

Millets area type of cereal grain of the Poaceae family. It's popular in underdeveloped nations across Africa and Asia. While it may appear to be a seed, millet has a nutritional profile comparable to sorghum and other grains. Millets have grown in favor in the West due to their gluten-free status and high protein, fiber, and antioxidant content. For the health and well-being of humans, millets serve as vital "nutritional reservoirs. " Due to their environmental endurance and adaptation, major millets (sorghum and pearl millet) in semi-arid tropical regions are important food and fodder crops. Despite being the world's oldest foods, they were abandoned in favor of the consumption of cereals mostly because of growing

* Corresponding author.

urbanization and changes in consumer taste. Millets' high protein content is one reason vegetarian diets tend to be low in calories.

They are commercial-scale good superfoods for the present and future generations, especially in rainfed areas, because of their great grain output potential with a short growing season, longer shelf life, and combined nutritional security. Climate change and increasing average world temperatures are predicted todirectly influence agricultural yields, crop productivity, and the long-term viability of the food system. Even though some assumptions indicate climate change may benefit select localities through higher production and harvests, this will not be enough to feed the world's growing population. Additionally, the majority of scientists think that present rates of global warming and greenhouse gas emissions will considerably diminish total agricultural output. As a result, limiting greenhouse gas emissions to manage global temperatures is critical to attaining food security. Yet, the agricultural sector is a major source of greenhouse gases such as methane in the environment. Increased emissions are predicted. The cultivation of millets, the greatest alternative among orphan crops, can address this problem as they can be grown on shallow, low fertile with pH ranges of 4. 0 to 8. 0 for different types of soil. Wheat and rice may both be easily swapped out for millet.

Millets have several morphological, physiological, molecular, and biological traits that make them more tolerant of environmental difficulties than other cereals. The molecular mechanics behind the plant response to abiotic stress encompass a wide range of activities, including senses, signaling, the transcription process, translation, or post-translational protein modification, controlled by both inherited and epigilotticfactors. Increased heat and drought caused by climate change are two of the main abiotic factors that negatively affect crop productivity and increase yearly losses on their own. "Climate change models anticipate that the stress caused by drought will continue to be a severe abiotic limitation on food production. Due to their poor economic competitiveness compared with other crops, the production of minor millets has progressively decreased in India over the last few decades.

Earlier, with the horticulture crops, and more recently, with the principal grains. Several factors contribute to this lower competitiveness, including a scarcity of higher-yielding varieties, superior seeds, improved farming techniques, appropriate food dispensation technology for ménages and communities, and a weak value chain. These constraints must be overcome towardgiving farmers in regions where major cereals may progressively decline due to climate alteration and minor millet may suggest a better option. The nutritious value of little millets is likewise high. According to aggregate statistics from FAOSTAT (2015), the total annual output of all millets (including major or small millets) is ejective to be 27. 83 Mt from the total harvested areas of about 31. 31 Mha. India is the world's top producer of millet, accounting for between 30 to 40% of total worldwide production. India produces about 11. 42 Mt of millet overall, with a harvest region of about 8. 8 millionha. The most widely used minor millet of India is finger also known as ragi, which is grown on almost 1. 6 million hectares and produces 2. 4 million tonnes annually at a productivity of an average of 1534 kg/ha (Figure 1) .

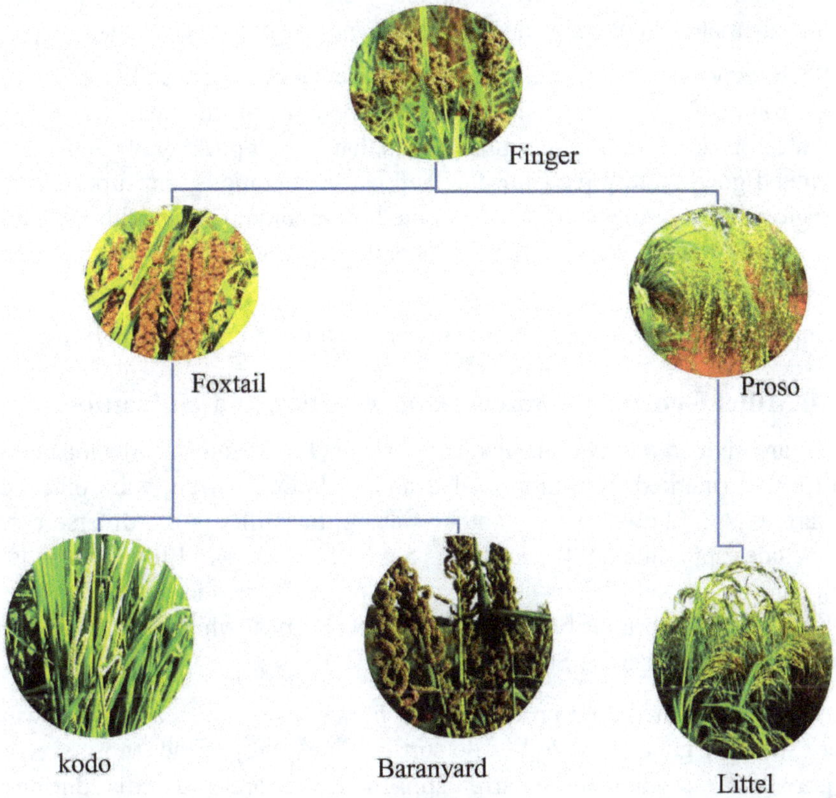


**Figure 1 :** The Importance of Small Millets in Climate Change and People's Livelihoods

The short biological cycle of small millets, a quality crucial for their climate change strategy, is minimizing risks in rainfed agriculture. In times of drought, their root systems are effective at drawing water from the ground. In comparison to the high-water requirements of rice and wheat, they may be successfully grown with less water and less rainfall, therefore India must revive these neglected crops due to depleting water supplies. They are a desirable crop alternative in mountain, hill, and tribal agriculture due to their capacity to provide a small yield in difficult farming circumstances, with poor soil and little to no input. small millets have a variety of advantages over cereal grains from a livelihood aspect. These include:

- Ecological advantages include compatibility with organic farming methods and eco-friendliness.
- Agronomic advantages, such as a high level of adaptation to short rainfall conditions, the capacity to survive relatively extended dry spells, the ability to recuperate quickly after late rain, the root system efficiency extracting soil moistness, a moderate sustained yield in marginal regions with poor management, and the absence of significant pest and disease issues.
- Socio-economic benefits include highly developed food cultures, grains that are comparably less expensive and therefore more affordable to the poor, grains thatcan be kept for a longer time, seeds that have a prolonged shelf life, high-valued good quality feed for dry land cattle operations, an important role in regional diet systems, especially in the hill, mountain areas with irregular and low rainfall, and opportunities for income generation for socially marginalized groups.
- Superior food quality, nutritional benefits, and nutraceutical qualities.

## Small Millet Genetic Resources: Conservation and Utilization

Millets are divided into two groups: large millet (Jowar and Bajra) anone end, and small millet (marked by minor seeded and including barren, sub-domesticated, and farmed spp.) however, on another side. Little millet is the diverse category that includes spp., like teff [*E. teff*], It is a well-liked crop in Ethiopia also is not a small consumer good. This is used to make "*injera*" a dish in the nation. The crop in "Kreb" consists primarily of barren and local types, which is how pastoralists have traditionally used the Sahel.

To maintain sustained seed production for human use as well as fodder, which is a very strategic good in these hostile surroundings, they gather those seeds from the grassland and manage the barren spp. In various areas of India, during years of drought, a barren barnyard (*E. Colona*), which is frequently foundedin paddy fields, is gathered for food. Finger millet is found in both cultivated and wild types. *Eleusine coracana* and *E. Africana* the spp., are most frequently employed in varietal development programs, though.

Tetraploid in nature (2n=4x=36), the cultivated *E. coracana* resembles mutually*E. indica* (n=18) or *E. Africa's* (n=36) morphologically. Cytologicdata suggest the cultivated *E. coracana* received one of its genomes from *E. indica*. As *E. coracana* or*E. africana* are both tetraploids and exhibit tight genetic relationships, it is possible that E. coracana descended as *E. africana* by natural selection. With little millets, artificial hybridization is exceedingly challenging due to the tiny size of the spikelets.

## Genetic Diversity

Little millets support a diverse range of morphological, taxonomical, and here ditary variations, as well as habitat, lifecycle, ploidy levels, or propagative behaviour. Genetic germplasm offoxtail or finger millet demonstrates a broad spectrum of the size of panicle, seed colour, and another plantstructural or morphological characteristics. Little millets were examined for morphometric diversity using standards from IBPGR. To date, 7, 127 finger millet accessions, 2, 821 foxtail millet accessions 1, 537 kodo millet accessions 1, 657 little millets, 939 proso millet accessions, and 988 barnyard millet accessions were characterized in the NARS system. A core (10% of an entirety reflecting the whole variation) and micro collection (1% of an existing array representing the diversity) are important collections of genes that may be used to characterize population dynamics, and genetic diversity, and find new alleles or genes. Most of these crops have "core" and "small core" collections, but a finger, foxtail, and Proso millet in particular were established.

Through a multi location assessment experiment of the core collections, a variety of distinct genotypes of foxtail and finger millet were carefully known for agronomical features, and nutritional content is high. Minor millets brought over from Africa, particularly finger millet, have a variety of desirable traits, including blast disease resistance, strong growing, early vigour, big size of panicle, higher grain number, higher density of grain, larger size seed, the weight of seed greater, or nutrition in grain also high. In finger millet, genotypes with advantageous physiological characteristics, like a low area of the leaf, and carbon dioxide fixation rates are higher, resistant to blast disease, and tolerant to drought found. The application value of morphological qualities such as lengthy types of glumeshas high photosynthetic rates of paniclecoupled with the greater weight of the seed is favourable for yield increase doneby breeding methods.

The substantial genetic heterogeneity of blast disease resistance against different isolates of M. grisea discovered at the field level and the limited assessment trials for germplasm demonstrate finger millet that there is plenty of potential for resistant breeding against the fungus. Through long-term field assessments at NARS centres, numerous potential consents of diverse minor millets are actuality discovered as sources of resistance to several additional stressors biotic, like helmintho-sporium blight, smut, and attack of shoot-fly. Less and more of the finger and foxtail millet germplasm accessions was found to have the desired traits of tolerance to drought, and tolerance to higher temperatures. Apart from the finger, and foxtail millet, minor millet germplasm has not yet undergone extensive genetic characterization. Little millets germplasm exhibits a great deal of variability, which makes it a significant source of genes and alleles for breeding efforts aimed at genetic improvement in these crops.

## Collection of Germplasm

The first small millets germplasm collection took place at the beginning of the 70s when the Foundation "Rockefeller" from the US make attempts to gathergermplasm ofminor millet for allowing breeders access to it. CGIAR and NARS currently maintain sizable collections of minor millets germplasm ex-situ underneath the sponsorship of the ICAR to promote long-term preservation. Over the 10, 000 +effectual accession of various minor millets is held by ICRISAT located in India; a greater number of these accessions belong tofoxtail, 1542, andfinger millet, 5957. NBPGR in Delhi or the AICRP improvement project on minormillets in Bengaluru house of the country's more than 15, 500 active accessions of minor millet germplasm.

Eight *Eleusine* species, including *coracana, indica, africana, mutiflora, tristachya, jaegeri, kigeziensis, floccifolia*, are represented by finger millet accessions. Bulkof the collections are from *E. coracana*, however, *E. africana* and *E. indica*, which belong to the secondary gene pool, may be viable sources to access genes for increased biomass output and tolerance to biotic and abiotic challenges. A significant fraction of the finger millet accessions preserved in gene banks across the world are landraces of *E. coracana*. There are eleven species of foxtail millet (genus Setaria) represented in the global germplasm collection in India, including *Setaria italica (subsp. italica and viridis), S. parviflora, S. sphacelate, S. verticillate, S. sphacelate (subsp. anceps), S. neglecta, S. lachnea, S. incrassate, S. Australians* About 10% of the germplasm for foxtail millet is made up of wild species, and there are barely any improved varieties or landraces of *S. italica.*

## Improvement of Minor Millets

Collection of germplasm shows considerable differences for several characteristics, such as duration in maturity, It is useful for breeding varieties there are appropriate intothree various majority group, earlier, middle, or late, based on late majority, ground, precipitation, temperature, moisture, day duration, and cropping needs that are peculiar to a place. For places with double or intense cropping, short-duration varieties would be appropriate, whereas regions with single cropping seasons would benefit from medium- to long-duration types. Minor millets have great nutritional potential, but because of anti-nutrition qualities such as phenol, tannin, phytate, or enzymatic resistor, as well as a higher concentration of amylases or proteases resistors hinder millet grains' ability to be digested, their usage is constrained.

Minor millets typically have greater levels of grain nutrients than the main cereals, although germplasm varies widely in terms of both grain nutrients and antinutrients. Breeding nutrients can be supported by utilizing the genetic heterogeneity already present in germplasm and hybridization-derived variants. dense cultivars against a background of greater yields. Little millets are less susceptible to severe biotic and abiotic pressures and are well suited to a variety of environmental conditions. Unfortunately, a few ailments and insect pests are significantly reducing yields, thus it is crucial to breed for cultivars that are disease- and pest-resistant. When blast infects millet, productivity may losetill 88% has been recorded. Due to the monsoon's failure, minors are mostly planted, severely impacted by drought, and planted such as rainfed crop. All minor millets experience lodging issues in addition to drought, mostly because of their soft stalks, crop management practices, and environmental conditions. Developed varieties were increasingly resistant to lodging is crucial in reducing productivity, and qualitative loss since lodggingis dependent on the genotype of the crop, also the impact of climatic issues. Shattering is another crucial characteristic of minor millets. Resistance to Shattering in minor millet is essential in reducing yield losses due to induced shattering, since shattering causes significant yield losses in tiny millets.

The development of varieties harvested by harvesters, improvement in the nutrition of fodder or grain to make a higher marketed price, varieties that are suitable for making good products like paddy grain, four, fakes, cod or hot exudeentrees, and the mixture of ready to cook, resistant to shade genotype of an orchard, agroforestry, quicker grown habit of genotype used in intercropping.

## Conventional Breeding methods

Minor millets are bred using a variety of breeding techniques, including mutation breeding, mass selection, pure, and pedigree selection suitable for self-pollinated varieties. According to reports on tiny millets cultivars issued over time, the bulk was released following the pedigree method, then selectedin topical germplasms and varieties. An essential breeding technique for tiny millets, notably for foxtail, proso, and, finger millets, involves hybridization to produce variety followed by selection in segregating populations. 45% of the finger millet varieties made available in India used the hybridization and selective breeding strategy, compared to 22% for foxtail or 29% for proso. Yet, because of their floral morphology and anthesis behavior, minor millets are not readily receptive to hybridization.

The contact method, in order to improve the possibility of natural cross-pollination with managed pollination whether using manual emasculation or heated water emasculation, the inflorescence of chosen cultivars is covered in a parchment bag prior to blossomingare available hybridization techniques for small millets. It was discovered that heated water therapy at 52°C for 5 minutes was successful in causing sterility in Finger millet (3–4 DAE), but only 48°C for 4 to 5 minutes in the barnyard. Emasculation and crossing techniques have been observed in minor millets. Developing effective emasculation and crossing techniques requires an understanding of floral biology and the pollination system. Yet, even for skilled hands, the variety of genetic research is constrained and minor millets improve as a result of the generally low success rate of creating the cross. Because of challenges in hybridization, the use of hybrids is restricted in minor millets. Hence, creating male sterile lines could serve as a practical way to apply heterogenesis, efficiently applied to crop improvement and the creation of cross seeds in commerce.

Just one male sterile line, which has a GMS system created from the source parental line IE 3318 by chemical mutation (EMS) has been documented so far in the finger millet species. Cross breeding is exceedingly tough to produce variety, and the crucial role is played by mutation. In India, 13 minor millet varieties, including 8, 3, and, 2, finger, kodo, or minor millets have been made available via mutation breeding. It is necessary to investigate how to make minor millet males sterile using chemical hybridizing agents (CHAs) . The efficacy and efficiency of a mutagen's ability to cause mutations that result in unwanted alterations or harm, such as sterility, death, injury, etc., determine the mutagen's value. By employing gamma radiation to irradiate a local cultivar of Proso millet. were able to identify two early maturing mutants from doses of 40 to 50, and 2mutants high-yieldby the treatments of 20 and 60 krad. For the best recovery of viable mutants in kodo, the dosage of 0. 4% EMS was suggested.

Employed 0. 2% of EMS for 8 hours in tef and found suitable mutant lines that demonstrated Al tolerance as well as significant variation in the mutant population. The characterization of minor millet germplasm and its application in the development and release of numerous cultivars, particularly resistant to abiotic and biotic stress, have both been successful using traditional breeding methods. Enhancing genetic gains in minor millet's improvement may be possible via the use of various omics techniques and genomics-assisted improvement.

## Modification of minor millets' inherited traits

The transformation of minor millets has mostly been accomplished via the agrobacterium-mediated method. Unfortunately, research on genetic transformation in millets is behind that of other important cereals like rice. There have been recent reports of transgenic millet that are expressing functionally active transgenes, and the improvement of transformation techniques has been published. Earlyresearch evaluated the performance of five transcription factors for the synthesis of the GUS reporter gene utilizing the biolistic method. Subsequent investigations in finger millet concentrated on the creation of transgenics for enhanceddrought, zinc content, salineresistance, herbicidaltolerance, or resistance to leaf blast. Subsequent work concentrated on characterizing phosphate transport and creating transgenic foxtail millet that is resistant to salt and drought. A few minor millets have used the transgene-based strategy due to the availability of efficient genetic transformation techniques. This has not yet been standardized in numerous millets; thus, it will not be possible to directly manipulate genes to help us overcome, knock out/down, or employ the CRISPR/Cas9 system. For genetic analysis and crop development research, key cereals like rice have routinely employed genome editing techniques like CRISPR/Cas9.

## Minor millets' genomic resources

### *Genetic mapping and Molecular Marker Resources*

To create genetic maps, gene identification, and plant breeding applications in addition to comprehending genetic diversity, many agronomically relevant genes and QTLs have been identified and tagged by molecular markers in field crops. SNPs and array-based molecular markers are acknowledged as next-generation high-throughput markers, whereas restriction fragment length polymorphism and SSRs are the most widely used and trustworthy molecular markers for the development of genetic maps. It is now possible to use the elevated genotyping by sequencing (GBS) approach thanks to the cost decrease that led to a rise in the use of direct sequencing technologies, regardless of the genetic information that is already available for the crop. It has aided in the simultaneous identification of markers like SNPs and large-scale genotyping of plant accessions. In genetic connection investigations involving minor millets, a range of molecular markers have been used, demonstrating their use in describing germplasm and identifying species. One of the main issues is the large-scale creation of molecular markers to cover the genetic mappings in finger millet and foxtail millet.

More than 150 highly informative SSR markers were found. These markers were important for the characterization of the germplasm, linkage mapping, and comparative genetic applications in other crops that were linked. Understanding genetic linkages, marker-assisted selection (MAS), and genetic analysis in foxtail millet and other small millets required the cross-species use of molecular markers like expressed sequence tag (EST) -SSR. For foxtail millet and finger millet, there are available genetic maps based on molecular markers. As minor millets germplasm contains a wide range of genetic variability for drought stress resistance, comprehensive phenotyping and genotyping of genetic variability overtaken under field-level drought conditions will be excellent for association and MAS investigations. to create genetic markers for MAS and to improve resistance to fungal blast disease in finger millet.

The current foxtail millet linkage map was created using SSR and RFLP marker data with reasonably uniformly distributed markers over all nine chromosomes. Similarly, to that, RFLP, AFLP, EST, and SSR marker data were used to create the genetic map for finger millet. Using finger millet and foxtail millet genetic maps to designate significant QTLs or genes has several drawbacks. There aren't enough uniformly distributed informative markers yet. For instance, the foxtail millet genetic map's average interval map distance (cM) between markers was 16. 4 cm. The foxtail millet's genome sequence proved useful for creating SNP markers, building genetic maps, and mapping a sethoxydim herbicide resistance feature that is adjacent to two markers separated by 1.1 cM on a map (2.4 Mb). More detailed mapping between two SNP markers revealed that a 100 kb area contains the sethoxydim-resistant phenotype.

## DNA synapsis and comparative genomics

Knowing the genetic relationships of closely related species allows us to make a priori predictions about the genetic makeup and functional similarities that can be applied across the species barrier. Comparative genomics is based on the concept that similar characteristics of closely related species are frequently contained within conserved DNA sequences. The two main elements of comparative genomics are synteny maps and genomic collinearity. The anchoring tools for creating a synteny map are a shared collection of orthologous probes or DNA markers. A synteny map can be used to translate genomic data from a thoroughly explored plant genome to even less known but related plant species.

Several crop taxa, including cereals, millets, and grasses, have produced comparative maps. The major cereal crops, including rice, corn, wheat, barley, sorghum, pearl millet, and minor millets including foxtail millet, finger millet, and tef, were compared using comparative genomic mapping to determine their genome connections. The availability of genome sequences for rice, Brachypodium, sorghum, maize, wheat, and foxtail millet may have made it easier to map traits using comparative genomics and find orthologous genes with important agronomic functions in less-researched crops. The use of comparative genomics is quickly becoming one of the key strategies in gene identification and for annotating gene activities in minor millets as a result of the growing number of plant genome sequences.

## Resources for nucleic acid sequences

Critical Reviews in Plant Sciences 65 abundance of nucleic acid sequence resources in a variety of significant crops has been produced by the rapid advancements in high-throughput next-generation sequencing (NGS) methods. The most appealing aspect of these technologies is their ability to quickly create millions of sequences, making them useful for a variety of agricultural plants regardless of the availability of genetic data, molecular markers, or genetic maps. There are currently over 16, 800 SSR primers for foxtail and finger millet available. Even though a significant number of SNPs were found in the foxtail millet genome, the mapped SNP marker resource for such crops has not yet been updated in the NCBI database. Around 0. 48 million updated nucleotide-sequence-based genomic resources exist for minor millets across all categories in the NCBI database.

The finger millet and foxtail millet genomes make up the majority of the accessible genetic resources. The NCBI database's primary genomic resources for tiny millets come from ProbeDB, GSS, nucleotide, and EST databases. The three most common categories of minor millet ESTs found in NCBI resources are tissue specificity, salt, and drought. The bulk of foxtail millet ESTs from spike tissues that are currently accessible at NCBI is somewhat connected to features linked to drought and salinity stress. In finger millet, the majority of the NCBI-accessible ESTs came from developing seed tissues, followed by ESTs associated with dehydration and water deficits and those originating from root tissues. The NCBI database contained 195 ESTs of proso millet in addition to foxtail and finger millet. They were all produced from leaf tissues that had undergone drought stress. The aforementioned genomic resource situation highlights the need for genomic resource enrichment, especially the accessibility of the attribute and stem-cell genomic information in small millets that support genetics.

## Study on bioenergy uses of foxtail genomes

The genomes of foxtail millet as well as its wild cousin, green foxtail, are both very short («515 Mb) and diploid. It has a huge variety of separate species and self-pollinating germplasm, as well as its unique physical characteristics. It was selected as either a model plant for relative genomic research of $C_4$ plants and biofuel feedstocks due to these advantageous characteristics and the genetic transformation techniques recently established. Molecular markers included in the foxtail millet genetic map are now accessible for comparative genomics research. Yet, the knowledge of the genome sequence continues to be crucial for foxtail millet genetic study. The Joint Genome Institute of the Department of Energy (DOE), USA, and Beijing Genomics Institute, China, accordingly, released 2 autonomous reference genome sequence drafts of the foxtail millet cultivar Yugu1 and Zhang gu, demonstrating >80% genome coverage. Nine chromosomes, or main scaffolds, were used to build the final genome sequence, which was about 405 Mb in size. Using RILs from the *S. italica S. viridis* population, a 992-locus SNP-based genetic map was created, and this genetic map served as the anchor for such genome sequence assembly of Yugu1. With a mere 1. 2% gap, 6, 791 contigs were created from this draft sequence.

Using the Illumina GA II platform, the sequence assembly was annotated by comparing it to 1. 3 million EST reads and 580 million RNA-seq hits across various tissue. SNP concentrations, a wide distribution of transposable elements, and significant chromosomal rearrangements and segregation distortions were the main findings of genome sequence annotations and analyses of the Yugu1 and Zhang gu cultivars. Nevertheless, the Zhang gu cultivar's draft genome sequence, which was published by the BGI, projected over 38, 801 odd genes, of which 81. 7% were discovered to be expressed genes. Subsequent investigation indicated that the Brachypodium, sorghum, rice, or maize genomes share considerable genome synteny with the foxtail millet genome. Using genome sequence data, the phylogenetic connections and genome evolution for foxtail millet in comparison to other grasses were projected. Foxtail millet was expected to separate from sorghum and maize. A tight evolutionary link between foxtail millet and other significant grasses, including Brachypomedium, rice, sorghum, & maize, was corroborated by the high genomic colinearity between these grasses. Research on biofuels will have a solid foundation thanks to the relevance of studies on genomic colinearity between the switch grass and foxtail millet genomes. The foxtail millet genome sequence would be a readily available resource that may be used for study on the $C_4$ photosynthetic system, the composition of grass cell walls used for bioenergy, the genetics of grass genome evolution, and other topics. 1, 517 distinct gene families were found in the foxtail millet genome and were projected to play a role in the plant's ability to adapt to semi-arid settings. The transcriptome data and the phylogenetic studies of 5 carbonic anhydrases (CA) genes there in the foxtail millet genome suggested that one of these CA genes may be crucial for the C4 photosynthesis pathway. The discovery of SNP markers to map quantitative features, such as herbicide resistance in the Zhang gu cultivar, was also done using the genome sequence information. However, the main difficulty that lies ahead is the use of the foxtail millet genome sequence in functional genomic studies and energy research. Foxtail millet lacks some essential resources compared to other well-known models plant systems like Arabidopsis and rice, despite its complete genome sequence thus emerging as a model plant for bioenergy grasses.

## Methods to improvegenomic or genetic resources of minor millets

The size, complexity, and cost of sequencing the genomes have traditionally restricted the growth of genetic studies in many under-researched crops, such as minor millet. As a result, there are fewer molecular markers available, which makes it more difficult to undertake genetic research on small millets. However, the accessibility of foxtail millet's entire genome sequences, improvements in reasonable NGS technology, or strength inthe analysis of bioinformatics have made it possible to create maps on genetic find higher-through output marker's on a broad level, enriching expressions of genetic factors.

To enable genetic improvement in small millets, this has concurrently promoted additional development of genetic resources, like population mapping and mutagenized populations. In reverse genetics or functional genomics, the creation of EMS and T-DNA places mutant resources in foxtail millet urgent necessity. The following discussion focuses on the cutting-edge genomic technologies that could be useful in enhancing tiny millet genomic resources. High-throughput markingtechniques, allow for fast genotyping of a variety of genetic selection or genetic sources in crop productionprojects, especially for lesser-studied crop plants. The constraints of polygenic QTL detection in crops may be addressed by the selection of a genomic strategy, that was also first modified from the breeding method for castles. In order to predict the projected breeding significance of genotypes within a population, the technique depends on observational studies of complicated traits with high-density marker scores.

## Prospects and challenges for the future

Due to their nutritional value, similarity in use and preparation to major cereal staples, and variety in how they can be adapted to challenging environments, small millets have had the potential to replace or augment these foods. Both in irrigated and rainfed environments, minor millets are used in a diversity of farming structures with great success. They have been designated as "famine reserves" because of their storage ability under typical store circumstances.

They can quickly produce both good feed and nutrient-rich grains. Their effective use in crop improvement initiatives is restricted by a dearth of germplasm and insufficient knowledge of genetic variation. To identify, genomes, and phenotypes that are characteristic and usable in small-scale milletgenetic improvement, it is crucial to prioritize germplasm collecting. minor millets variants have so far mainly been created using traditional breeding techniques. By using a male sterility system, taking use of heterosis, improving crops with the help of genomics, and improving agricultural management and mechanization, Minor millets' yield limitation can be overcome. Genomics-assisted breeding will make it easier to find new alleles and genes with improved agronomic performance and resilience to biotic and abiotic challenges to speed up the improvement of minor millet.

Cultured cells and bioengineering approaches used in associated crop plants have the potential to enhance minor millet improvement. Whether or there's prior sequence information, the quick advancement of sequencing technology can produce millions of before the site at even a low cost and in a short amount of time. An entire collection of small millets germplasm can be molecularly characterized using next-generation sequencing techniques. These methods could be used for plants whose genomes have not yet been decoded, such as minor millets, kodo millet, and job's tears. Comparative genomics also makes it possible to explore orthologous genes for significant features in much lower studies using the genetic sequences data for foxtail and paddy.

Minor millets' genomes can now be modified to increase production and stress resistance thanks to the development of genome editing technology. To move minor millet from the category of "minor and underutilized" crop, extensive and synchronized integrative cooperation across the domains of agriculture, pharmacology, nutrition, or technology addition to conventional breeding with genomics-assisted improvement. Also, to include food products made from small millets as a significant source of nutrients in diets, public-private partnerships, public education, and farmers' participation from all interested nations will be required. For minor millet more research and development are necessary to attain nutrition, and feedstuff, foodsanctuary in light of the changing climate change scenarios and the pervasive hidden hunger.

## Conclusion

Minor millets' nutritional profiles and climate-resilient characteristics have been extensively examined, suggesting that millets may be the preferred staple crop in countries where there is famine. Due to the lack of food in unusual circumstances, these places are severely afflicted by undernutrition, malnutrition, and untimely deaths. In the past, millet was the primary food source for many peoples in Asia, mainly India. Millets may be the most climate-resilient crop in the future. Millets are more resilient to many of the harmful consequences caused by global warming than other food crops are. They thrive in practically any kind of soil, including sandy and soils with different amounts of acidity. Fertilizers and irrigation are hardly ever needed. Under the impacts of global warming, millet could indeed promote equitable agriculture. They serve as the finest alternative to major cereal crops due to their tenacious nature and exceptional capacity to thrive in adverse conditions and places with limited water supply. There is a case for encouraging them to handle problems like hunger and food poverty, escalating drought and heat, and environmental deterioration in a sustainable manner. The creation of supporting agro-based policies, its improvement of climate warming adaptability through farming production, developments in small and marginal agricultural techniques, in addition to the general use of technological and scientific advances are all essential to the achievement of attempts to encourage regional livelihoods and provide nutrition and food security as well as the fight against poverty. Foxtail millet is the only small millet for which the total pool of genetic resources, including, genetic sequencing, marking, or expression sequencing, has been fully utilized. Despite this, the future seems promising thanks tothe latest entire maps of genes infoxtail cultivars, which would also act like a prototype plant canopy that could be crucial through empirical investigation outof a genomic and genetic standpoint. Several minor crops are already being impacted by the exponential growth inthe application of NGS technologies to the genetic material or expressionsequencing, and small millets' genetics and breeding will also greatly benefit from this development. This would allow for the large-scale production of SNP markers produced from NGS for more rapid and affordable genotyping of thousands of distinct genotypes.

Genomic improvement inminor millet is aided by a variety of genomic resources, as discussed earlier in the chapter in a brief description of minor millet. Moreover, comparative genomics and bioinformatic technologies will speed up the genetic advancement of millets, cereals, or bio-energy crops. Using the modules of foxtail, grass, and, paddy as well as synthetical relation, "comparative genomics" furthermore be useful for the genomic advancement of minor millet crops. Also, the creation of characteristics of inhabitants' mappings and the gathering of mutation makes it easier to identify novel genetic codes or recessives better at performing agronomically and resisting diversity in abiotic or biotic challenges. To sum up, the hitherto untapped genomic sources of minor millet and the scientific advantages offered by inexpensive genetic technologies stimulate the study into and care for abandoned millet, which may boost nutrition stability for millions of households in Asia and Africa.

## References

FAOSTAT. The future of food and agriculture: Alternative pathways to 2050; 2015;228.

Hassan, Z. M., Sebola, N. A., &Mabelebele, M. (2021) . The nutritional use of millet grain for food and feed: a review. *Agriculture & food security*, *10*, 1-14.

Kumar L, Naresh RK, Tiwari H, Kataria SK et al. Millets for food and nutritional security in the context of climate resilient agriculture: A Review. Int J Plant Soil Sci. 2022;34 (23) :939-953.

Louhar, G. A. N. P. A. T., Bana, R. S., Kumar, V. I. P. I. N., & Kumar, H. (2020) . Nutrient management technologies of millets for higher productivity and nutritional security. *Indian J. Agric. Sci*, *90*, 2243-2250.

Padulosi, S., Mal, B., Ravi, S. B., Gowda, J., Gowda, K. T. K., Shanthakumar, G., & Dutta, M. (2009) . Food security and climate change: role of plant genetic resources of minor millets. *Indian Journal of Plant Genetic Resources*, *22* (1), 1-16.

Saha, D., Gowda, M. C., Arya, L., Verma, M., & Bansal, K. C. (2016) . Genetic and genomic resources of small millets. *Critical Reviews in Plant Sciences*, *35* (1), 56-79.

Tiwari, H., Naresh, R. K., Kumar, L., Kataria, S. K., Tewari, S., Saini, A., &Asati, R. (2022) . Millets for Food and Nutritional Security for Small and Marginal Farmers of North West India in the Context of Climate Change: A Review. *International Journal of Plant & Soil Science*, *34* (23), 1694-1705.

Vetriventhan, M., Azevedo, V. C., Upadhyaya, H. D., Nirmalakumari, A., Kane-Potaka, J., Anitha, S. & Tonapi, V. A. (2020) . Genetic and genomic resources, and breeding for accelerating improvement of small millets: current status and future interventions. *The Nucleus*, *63*, 217-239.

# 6

# Millets in Organic Agricultural System

Nikumani Choudhury*, Ajay*, Md Salman A. Choudhury

Department of Soil Science, Assam Agricultural University,785013, India

**ABSTRACT**

A revolution in organic agriculture is being fueled by the world's need for nutrient-dense food, farmers' security, sustainable agriculture, and environmental preservation. India has already surpassed China to become the highest populated country in the world, therefore, it is a bit skeptical whether Rice and Wheat will be able to fulfill the quest of huge people while sustaining the ecosystem health also. This is where the organic millet cultivation comes to the rescue. Millets operate well on relatively poor soil, can thrive in dry conditions, and require minimal inputs. They are frequently seen growing on skeletal soil that is no deeper than 15 cm and are suited to a wide range of ecological circumstances. "Millets as Organic Matter, are slow to break down in soil just as in our digestive systems. Their slow composting nature helps in maintaining soil structure and retaining water, thus preserving soil health for extended duration"- Lynette Abbott, an eminent professor in Australian Institute of Agriculture. The effects of different solid as well as liquid organic supplements on the growth and production of transplanted finger millet (*Eleusine coracana* L.) were studied in a field trial at the Agricultural College cum Research Institute of Killikulam during the rabi season of 2019. The results revealed that all treatments had a significant influence upon the growth attributes and yield of transplanted finger millet over control. At 30 and 45 DAT, a considerable increase in growth and production was observed with the treatment of 100% poultry manure along with 3% panchagavya.

*Keywords*: Organic Agriculture, Millets, Organic Millet, Sustainable Agriculture

## Introduction

Millets is a collective term used to refer to the small grained, warm weather and annual grasses. Milets are classified under *graminae* family. Technical meaning of Millets is any of various small-seeded annual cereal and pasture grasses, according to Merriam-Webster dictionary. Millets are primarily cultivated for their edible seeds, but, it has also got considerable fodder values. Their nutritional abundance and ability to grow under harsh ecological conditions make them unique among the cereals. Millets can grow to a height of 1 to 4 feet and complete their life cycle in just one year. Exception arises in case of pearl millet, which goes up to a height

* Corresponding author.

of 5 to 10 feet. Most inflorescences are raceme-shaped, meaning that flowers are carried on stalks that are of similar length along an extended axis. Millets are also referred to as "coarse-grains" because of the rough surface of the grains. The color and size of the seeds vary among different kinds of millets.

Evidences are spread across the World, which says that cultivation of millet began first in the Korean Penninsula in around 3500-2000 BC or during middle Jeulmun Pottery period. Some other evidences point towards Asiatic region regarding the first cultivation of millets. Various speces of Millets were initially domesticated in the regions of, South East Asia, both Western and Eastern part of Africa notably and spread gradually throughout the World. In India, domestication of millets dates back to 1200 BCE, as in some of the oldest Yajuveda texts, different types of millets are recognized, viz, *priyangava* that refers to foxtail millet, *aanava* that refers to Barnyard milet and *shyaamaka* as Black Finger millet.

## Value addition in Millets

Millet based foods are classified into two types: RTE (Ready to eat) foods and RTC (Ready to cook) foods. Snacks, popcorn, biscuit and bread are examples of ready-to-eat foods while, instant foods (vermicelli, noodles, pasta, porridge, khichdi), South- Indian cuisines (idly, dosa, upma), multi grained flour, beverages such as malt drink mix and baby foods are examples of ready-to-cook foods.

## Types of Millets

Millets are categorized as Major and Minor millet based on the area of production and size of the grains. Sorghum and Bajra comes under major millet, while, the rest of them comes under minor millets (Table 1, Figure 1).

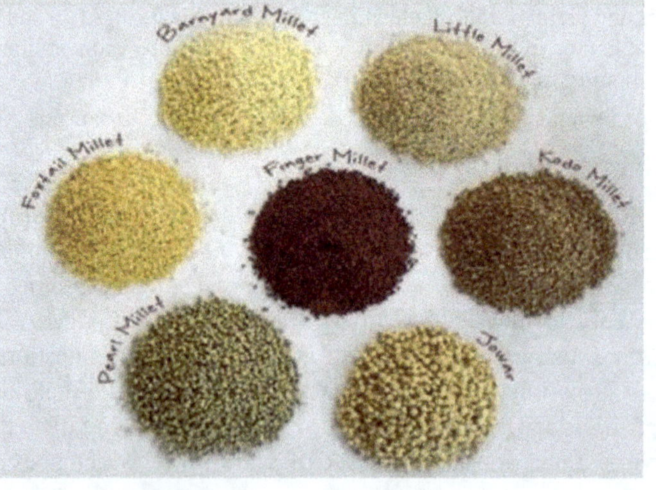


**Figure 1:** Different types of Millets and their characteristics

**Table 1:** Different types of Millets and their characteristics

| **Common name** | **Foxtail millet** | **Kodo millet** | **Barnyard millet** | **Proso millet** | **Little millet** | **Finger millet** | **Fonio** | **Tef** | **Pearl millet** |
|---|---|---|---|---|---|---|---|---|---|
| Other names | Italian millet | Koda millet | Billion dollar grass | Common millet | | Ragi, African millet | Acha | Teff, lovegrass | Bulrush millet |
| Scientific name | *Setaria italica* | *Paspalum scrobiculatum* | *Echinochloa esculneta* | *Panicum miliaceum* | *Panicum sumatrense* | *Eleusine coracana* | *Digitaria exilis* | *Eragrostis tef* | *Pennisetum glaucum* |
| Sub family | Panicoideae | Panicoideae | Panicoideae | Panicoideae | Panicoideae | Chloridoideae | Panicoideae | Chloridoideae | Panicoideae |
| Tribe | Paniceae | Paniceae | Paniceae | Paniceae | Paniceae | Eragrostideae | Paniceae | Eragrostideae | Paniceae |
| Ploidy level | Diploid | Hexaploid | Hexaploid | Tetraploid | Tetraploid | Tetraploid | Diploid or hexaploid | Tetraploid | Diploid |
| Chromosome number | 2n (= 2x) = 18 | 2n (= 6x) = 40 | 2n (= 6x) = 36 | 2n (= 4x) = 36 | 2n (= 4x) = 36 | 2n (= 4x) = 36 | 2n (= 2x) = 30 or 2n (= 6x) = 54 | 2n( = 4x )= 40 | 2n (= 2x )= 14 |
| Purpose | Food, biofuel | Food, feed | Food, feed | Food, feed | Food | Food, feed | Food, feed | Food, feed | Food, feed |

## Suitability of Millets to Organic Agricultural System

The repercussions of conventional farming systems are not out of sight to anyone. Excessive use of fertilizers, excessive tillage and the use of GMOs are jeopardizing the soil and environmental health to such an extent that it is not far when, one day, we will struggle to get contamination free food, water or in worse situations, food and water only. Natural resources are getting depleted or polluted, erosion loss of soil is increasing beyond the permissible limit (12t/ha), biodiversity is lost and the climate changed effects are getting more prominent. The World has witnessed the warmest February of the decade in the year 2023 itself as the mercury level rose to a greater value. 2023's february temperature went up to 29.4$^0$C, which is the highest since 1901. Agricultural scientists are fearing the failure of wheat, as wheat is a thermosensitive crop. Due to heat waves, in the year 2022, India's wheat production declined to such an amount that the country had to stop its exports. Otherwise, the exports would have been remunerative as Russia-Ukraine war was going on at that time, yet, India stopped it just to ensure food security to its countrymen first. If this kind of temperature increase prevails, which will prevail for sure, then it will be very difficult for the crops to survive in high temperature conditions. Indian Agricultural Research Institute has recently developed a heat tolerant wheat variety, but in the context of future, it doesn't seem enough.

With the increasing global population, the concern of food as well as nutritional security is also rising parallely. India now has more people than China, making it the world's most populous nation. So, it is a bit skeptical whether rice and wheat will be able to fulfill the hunger of crores of people. This is where the importance of millets lies in. Organic farming is founded on distinctive principles. It is a concept of collaborating with nature as well as a farming technique. "Green revolution" techniques are being criticized by many experts from environmental point of view. Therefore, a more sustainable production system, i.e. organic production system is gaining momentum these days. Organic Agriculture is a holistic production system that mainly encompasses four principles, viz, Health, Ecology, Fairness and Care. The main motto of Organic Farming is to ensure sustainability and escalating productivity alongside improving soil health.

Following green revolution, Millet cultivation and production has decreased to about 20 to 40 perecent because of the obvious reason i.e. introduction of HYVs of Rice and Wheat. The main reason of millet's unpopularity is the lack of technical understanding among crop growers and processors as adoption and diversification of new things are cultural challenges. Tribal regions of India were home to millets, but, people were not aware of its nutritional benefits (Shanthakumar *et al*., 2010). "Organic farming and millet cultivation were common practices in India for millennia. But we've forgotten about them in the past few decades, It's time to reintroduce them to society." says Byre Gowda, previous cabinet minister of Rural development, Law and parliamentary affairs. Millets are highly suitable to organic production system as it a low demanding crop. Millets, that are cultivated for both human consumption and fodder purpose, not only furnish food and livelihood stability to human beings but also assist in efficient farming specially for small and marginal farmers and residents of rain-fed/ remote tribal communities (Reynolds *et al.*, 2015). Organic cultivation and millet farming go hand in hand that influences agro-ecosystem health positively.

Millets can thrive in relatively poor soil, can grow in dry conditions, and require minimal inputs of minerals and soil tilth. As compared to the high water demanding crops, such as, sugarcane and banana, millets only require 25% of their water regime. Unlike Paddy, Millet not only lifts the burden of irrigation from states, but also helps in the saving of power, which can be used in some alternate production process. Millets possess the unique capability to withstand adverse soil and climatic conditions. Drought or inadequate soil moisture is the prime factor that limits the productivity of millets in arid as well as semi arid areas. Prolonged duration of abnormally low rainfall is termed as drought. From crop growth purpose, drought is classified into 4 types, viz, meteorological, hydrological, physiological and agricultural drought. When soil moisture is not enough to fulfill the requirement of a particular crop in a particular time, then it is termed as agricultural drought. Though abiotic stresses are largest contributor of substantial yield losses, millets relatively perform well in this kind of situations compared to other cereals, such as, wheat and rice. Rigorous study regarding the yield losses of millets due to drought is not made extensively, but, it is said by agronomists that the substantial loss of productivity depends on the drought severity. Nevertheless, millets are considered as drought tolerant, as, they produce few grains and little straw even in moisture stressed periods. Drought intolerant cereals, rice and wheat fail to do so, that is why, millets are advantageous over rice and wheat in dryland areas.

## Drought Adaptation Mechanism of Millets

Plants' mechanism to cope up drought constitutes 4 strategies, Avoidance of Drought, Escape of Drought, Tolerance to Drought and Recovery from Drought. First three of them are considered as major mechanism, while the last one has minor contribution to drought adaptation.

- **Drought avoidance**: Ability of the plants to maintain a favourable water regimee in the plant tissuse under moisture stress to prevent a water deficit is referred to as drought. It is linked to two different types of mechanisms: (i) Minimization of water loss through transpiration (for example, decreased stomatal conductance and leaf area reduction) and (ii) Maintenance of water uptake by plants during drought periods (e.g. high root/shoot ratio).

- **Drought Escape**: The scenario where plants acquire maturity stage before drought strikes is called drought escape. Early flowering, Faster growth, higher amount of nitrogen in leaves, and a greater capacity for photosynthetic energy are a few characteristics that help plants resist drought. In West Africa, where precipitation is scarce and irregular, it was discovered that pearl millet matches its phenology to the average distribution of rainfall. Development of primary panicle was occurred concurrently with an increasing rainy period in this case, reduction in the chances of a drought episode occurring before or at the commencement of flowering.
- **Drought tolerance**: Drought tolerance is associated with an increased amount of osmoprotectants and osmotic adjustment through reduction of osmotic potential by accumulating organic as well as inorganic substances.
- **Drought recovery**: The best example of Drought recovery is of *Eragrostis nindensi*, a herbaceous perennial plant that recover from the adverse effects of drought as it can stabilize the cell membrane at desiccated stage. These kinds of plants are termed as Desiccation-tolerant or resurrection plants.

## Morphological, Physiological, Biochemical and Genetic Mechanisms of Millets to tolerate Drought like situations

Morphological and Anatomical traits are mainly associated with root-shoot length and leaf area of millet plant. Three species of *Eragrostis* with varying degrees of drought resillience were evaluated by Balsamo *et al.* for their tensile strength of leaf. According to their research, a correlation exists between drought tolerance and tensile strength of leaf. Drought tolerant *E. curvula* possessed higher values than somewhat lesser drought tolerant *E. tef*, which again had greater values than drought susceptible *E. capensis*. In contrast to *E. capensis*, *E. curvula* and *E. tef* have widespread lignification in bundle sheath cells, according to structural examinations of the three species' leaves.

Osmotic adjustment is one of the numerous physiological features that is specifically controlled during moisture shortage, and it is a potential method for improving drought avoidance. Osmotic adjustment, which is described as the decrease in osmotic potential in cytoplasm as a result of accumulation of appropriate solutes such as Proline, Glycine-betaine, and organic acids, aids in the preservation of turgor in shoots and roots. Drought stress increases the levels of proline and glycine-betaine in the root and leaves of small millet. The authors speculated that disruption of protein synthesis, increased rate of protein breakdown, or partial hydrolysis may be accountable for the buildup of neutral amino acids in this millet under drought conditions. Another crucial factor is the plant's capacity to use water judiciously as millet grown areas are mostly water scarce.

Chemically reactive chemicals known as reactive oxygen species (ROS) are helpful for cell signalling at low quantities but harmful to cells when present in massive quantities. Abiotic stresses including salinity and drought are the crucial players to excessive generation of ROS. Plants produce antioxidants such as Glutathione, Ascorbic acid, and Carotenoids as well as ROS scavenging enzymes like Superoxide dismutase, Peroxidase, Catalase, and Ascorbate peroxidase to minimize the adverse effects of ROS. In order to help plants cope with unwanted ROS accumulation, SOD, POD, and CAT activity were increased in little millet during drought circumstances. Similar to this, when drought was introduced to tef plants, the activity of AP and monodehydro Ascorbate Reductase increased, compared to the control plants receiving considerable irrigation. However, when it comes to the agronomic traits of millet plants to deal with drought like situations, there is a dearth of research to draw any solid conclusion.

## Genes in Millets involved in tolerance to Drought

Millets' transcriptome sequencing following exposure to a dry environment offers information, in particular, on genes that are differentially regulated when exposed to abiotic stresses or a drought. In a transcriptome wide analysis of finger millet plants exposed to wate stress, 2824 genes with variable expression levels were discovered. When finger millet was exposed to drought, numerous genes were reported to be triggered by Parvathi *et al*., (2013) farnesylated protein ATFP6, Metallothionein, protein phosphatase 2A Farnesyl Pyrophosphate Synthase, and are among the up-regulated genes.

A genome scan and association mapping techniques were used to look at traits related to drought tolerance. When pearl millet was subjected to varieties of abiotic stimuli, such as salinity, drought, heat, a single enzyme called Carbonic Anhydrase was continuously up-regulated. The authors speculated that this specific gene helps the plant adjust to different abiotic stresses. mtlD, EcDehydrin 7, and Ecapx1 from finger millet, as well as Si ARDP from Wild Foxtail Millet, are other genes that have been linked to drought response in millets. Although it has not yet been documented for millets, the model plant *Arabidopsis thaliana* showed enhanced drought tolerance when two genes, SAL1 and ERA1, were suppressed via a process involving stomata closure, the era1 mutants become drought-tolerant (Table 2; Figure 2).

## Tolerance for salinity

Three types of Minor millets, foxtail millet, proso millet, and pearl millet, were grown and subjected to 3 degrees of salt stresses (1.5, 5.5, and 9.5ds/m) in the southern Khorasan region in eastern Iran. The Birjand pearl millet type, followed by foxtail millet, showed maximum production potential under both salt stressed and normal conditions. On the other hand, the Proso- millet cultivar from Ghaen showed greater salt tolerance (Gehrken, 1985).

## Tolerance to Heat

Because of its drought resistance and high temperature tolerance, pearl millet can well flourish in dry desert regions (Bidinger *et al.*, 2004). Pearl millet hybrids like HHB-67, HHB-68, and HHB-60 are suitable for dry areas.

**Table 2:** Differentially regulated Drough trelated Genes in Millets

| Source of the Gene | Gene Name |
|---|---|
| Foxtail millet | SiLEA |
| Foxtail millet | SiARDP |
| Finger millet | EcDehydrin7 |
| Finger millet | Ec-apx1 |
| Finger millet | RISBZ4 |
| Pearl millet | B carbonic anhydrase |

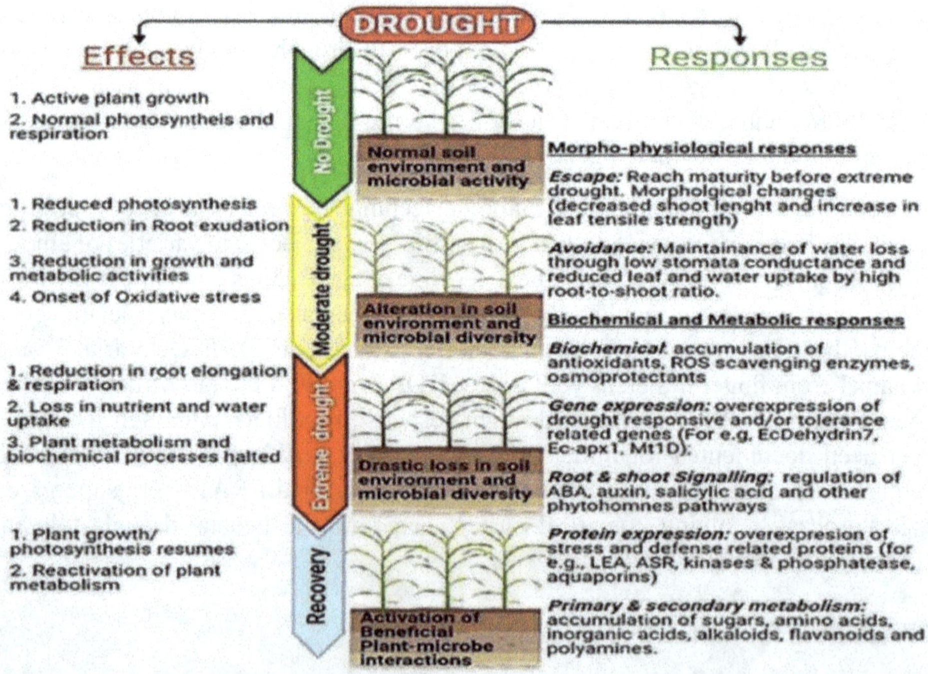


**Figure 2:** Drought responses and Adaptivity correlated to various morpho physiological, anatomical, and biochemical processes that offer tolerance to environmental stresses in millets

Millets are ecologically adaptable to a wide range of environments, frequently growing on skeletal soil that is only 15 cm deep. Rich soil is not necessary for their life and growth. They are therefore beneficial for large dryland areas. The majority of millets may be cultivated on low fertility soils, while others can be grown on acidic or saline soils. As is done in Rajasthan, millets like Bajra can also be cultivated in sandy soils. In actuality, finger millet thrives on salty soils. Whereas other crops, like rice, struggle to thrive on such soils, barnyard millet does well there. Many of them are also raised to recover soil. Poor farmers are the owners of poor lands, particularly in dryland India. On these lands, millets are the only crops that provide food security.

In reality, the fact that millets can thrive in Sahelian soils in West Africa, which produces 74% of total millets in Africa and about 28% of the world's millet basket, provides evidence of their ability to grow on deficient soils. Its ability to thrive in ecological zones with sandy, somewhat acidic soils, where average precipitation can be less than 500 mm, is a testament to their amazing resilience and ability to endure extremely difficult conditions. Because of this, millets may grow in regions that experience drought, such as Rajasthan and the Deccan plateau, and offer food and fodder for humans and animals respectively.

Due to low amounts of nitrogen and phosphate in soil, the root system of foxtail millet is altered. Foxtail millet increases biomass accumulation and root thickness despite having a smaller root system when nitrogen levels are low, likely for nutrient transfer. Foxtail millet's low phosphate content reveals its internal nitrogen status, which acts as a signal to control the production of nitrogen transporters and so characterises its innate relationship with nitrogen feeding.

In addition, brown-top millet, one kind of minor millet, has gained recent recognition for its enormous potential, wider versatility to grow in a variety of soils and climates, and ability to tolerate a mild level of environmental stresses. Brown-top millet is a facultative upland plant, favours sandy loam soils with a pH of 5-6.5 in full sun, but its unique quality is that it can also be cultivated in partial shade, ensuring wider yields and adoption possibility especially in agroforestry systems or fruit orchards.

Chemical fertilisers are not necessary for millets. This attribute makes millets the perfect crop to be included in Organic Farming systems. In reality, millets thrive in the absence of chemical fertilisers when grown on dry land. Because of this, the majority of millet farmers produce them in completely eco-friendly settings utilising farmyard manure. Farmers have recently begun utilising biofertilizers like vermicompost made in their own backyards and growth accelerators like panchagavya, aamritpani, etc. These methods make millet production environmentally benign while also keeping it under the farmers' control.

No pests are drawn to millet when it is grown using traditional techniques. They are considered Pest Free Crops. Majority of them are also unaffected by bugs that live in storage. As a result, they hardly ever need pesticides. Therefore, they greatly benefit the agricultural environment. Most millets, like foxtail, are pest-free and don't require a lot of insecticides. One of the main constraints that limit productivity in organic farming is the disease and pest infestation, as chemical pesticides are strictly prohibited and no organic pesticide can match the efficiency level of inorganic one. But with Millets, this problem is seemed to be negated by the crop itself. Even in storage situations, most millets, like foxtail, function as Antipest agents to keep sensitive pulses, like greengram, without the need for fumigants. "Millets are typically resistant to pests", according to Dayakar Rao, head scientist of Indian Institute of Millets Research Hyderabad. Yet, if planting is put off because of the monsoon's tardy arrival, shot fly attack has been documented. Farmers in Tamil Nadu's Jawadhu Hills, like Kuppusamy, claim that neem-based natural insecticides and byproducts of cows can be used to combat pests.

The efficacy of seed protein extracts to stop the growth of *Macrophomina, Rhizoctonia*, and *Fusarium* was tested in vitro on Bajra, Jowar, Barnyard millet, Foxtail millet, and Small millet,. All three of the tested phytopathogenic fungi are effectively stopped in their growth by protein extracts from pearl millet.

While millets can give many benefits (food, financial and nutritional security), including security of livelihood and ecosystem, rice and wheat can only successfully produce food security in India. Used as a double purpose crop (food and forage) they yield considerable economic values in mixed farming systems. The majority of millets have edible stems or stalks, which are preferred cattle fodder. Millets offer superior fodder than corn because they have more tillers or branches. Crops like pearl millet and sorghum are frequently produced solely for their value as animal feed. Millets also serve as a source of fodder and are rich in nutrients, which results in nutrition security. In addition to producing fibre and fuelwood, millet fields are home to a variety of crops, as it well supports intercropping. According to Kuppusamy, farmers in the Jawadhu Hills cultivate foxtail and kodo millets in a small area for their own use as well as a small amount of millet and vegetables for sale. The millets' companion crops, legumes, are similarly vigorous leaf shedders. This litter fall serves as organic manure and keeps the soil fertile. As a result, millet fields utilise soil fertility for their growth as well as returning it to the land.

Majority of millets farmed using conventional methods represent a farming system, not merely a crop. Most of millet cropfields are naturally bio diverse. Millets are a desirable crop for more intensive cropping systems due to their fast maturation and all season growth characteristics. This is how millet cultivation has historically been done throughout the nation. In the same area, six to twenty crops are planted simultaneously. renowned “Baranaja” cropping techniques in the Himalayas are evidence of this. Twelve different crop kinds are incorporated in this millet led system. In Rajasthan, “Saat Dhan” is home to a wide range of millets. A comprehensive agricultural method, the “Pannendu Pantalu” system of South grows millets alongside pulses and oilseeds.

There is always been conflicts among agronomists whether organically grown crops are nutritious enough or not as no kinds of mineral nutrients are applied in organic farms. Millets are called as Nutri cereals or Nutri grains since they’re very nutrient-dense, gluten free, non acid forming, and readily digestible. Compared to rice or wheat, millets are far superior nutritionally. The calcium content of finger millet is 30 times higher than that of rice. Little millet and Bajra are so rich in iron that Rice is well behind in the race. Millets are now referred to as Adbhut Anaj and nutri cereals, sometimes known as “miracle grains”.

Given that finger millet contains 16 times as much calcium as maize does, some people think it may someday replace rice as a main food source. This is significant for humans since it means that essential minerals are readily available. Also rich in micronutrients are millets. Two minerals that are crucial for human health are iron and zinc. Researchers should investigate raising the iron content of minor millets grains to address the widespread malnutrition in this population. Moreover, millets are easily digestible and gluten-free, reducing the risk of intolerance, stomach ulcers, or high cholesterol.

An alkaline-forming food is millet. To attain optimal health, an alkaline-based diet is frequently advised. The calming alkaline properties of millet aid in preserving the body’s optimal pH balance, which is essential to ward off infections (Table 3, Table 4).

**Table 3 :** Nutrient composition of millets (per 100 g)

| Food grain | Carbohydrates (g) | Fat (g) | Protein (g) | Energy (KCal) | Mineral Matter (g) | Crude Fibre (g) | P (mg) | Ca (mg) | Fe (mg) | Zn (mg) |
|---|---|---|---|---|---|---|---|---|---|---|
| Finger millet | 72.00 | 1.39 | 7.39 | 328.0 | 2.71 | 3.60 | 283.0 | 344.0 | 3.92 | 1.90 |
| Kodo millet | 65.90 | 1.41 | 8.30 | 310.2 | 2.60 | 9.04 | 188.6 | 27.6 | 0.53 | 2.71 |
| Proso millet | 70.41 | 1.10 | 12.58 | 341.3 | 1.90 | 2.23 | 206.4 | 15.4 | 0.80 | 2.52 |
| Foxtail millet | 60.90 | 4.37 | 12.30 | 330.0 | 3.30 | 8.01 | 290.0 | 31.6 | 2.89 | 1.62 |
| Little millet | 67.04 | 4.76 | 7.78 | 341.0 | 1.53 | 7.66 | 220.5 | 17.0 | 9.30 | 1.41 |
| Barnyard millet | 65.56 | 2.20 | 6.22 | 309.3 | 4.40 | 9.81 | 280.3 | 21.7 | 5.01 | 2.42 |
| Sorghum | 72.60 | 1.92 | 10.40 | 349.4 | 1.64 | 1.62 | 222.2 | 25.4 | 4.12 | 1.83 |
| Bajra | 67.54 | 5.02 | 11.61 | 360.0 | 2.32 | 1.23 | 296.5 | 43.3 | 8.01 | 3.00 |

**Table 4 :** Essential Amino acids in Millets (mg per g of N)

| Millet | Arginine | Histidine | Lysine | Tryp-tophan | Phenyl Alanine | Tyrosine | Methionine | Cystine | Threonine | Leu-cin | Isoleucine | Valine |
|---|---|---|---|---|---|---|---|---|---|---|---|---|
| Foxtail millet | 222 | 130 | 150 | 60 | 425 | - | 180 | 100 | 190 | 1045 | 480 | 4306 |
| Proso millet | 290 | 120 | 190 | 55 | 310 | - | 167 | - | 152 | 762 | 416 | 410 |
| Finger millet | 302 | 130 | 222 | 110 | 315 | 223 | 210 | 140 | 247 | 699 | 400 | 476 |
| Little millet | 249 | 120 | 113 | 60 | 330 | - | 189 | 90 | 190 | 760 | 375 | 350 |
| Barnyard millet | 270 | 130 | 150 | 50 | 438 | - | 180 | 110 | 198 | 655 | 360 | 412 |
| Sorghum | 240 | 160 | 150 | 70 | 300 | 180 | 98 | 90 | 210 | 880 | 270 | 340 |
| Bajra | 310 | 140 | 190 | 110 | 290 | 208 | 150 | 110 | 140 | 750 | 260 | 330 |

## Millets' Flavonoids Compound and Nutraceutical Development

The varied collection of secondary plant metabolites known as flavonoids and phenols serve an important role in coloration and defence against other herbivorous animals. It has antioxidant qualities and has the ability to scavenge free radicals produced during metabolic reactions. Ragi (finger millet), in particular, is a good source of phenols and flavonoids. The ability of polyphenols to bind free radicals, chelate metal catalysts, aid in the activation of antioxidant enzymes, eliminate tocopherol radicals, and guard against damage to biomolecules and membranes. The phenolic chemicals caffeic acid, protocatechuic acid, Gallic acid, Polymeric Tannins, Vanillic acid, Gentisic acid, Syringic Acid, Para-coumaric Acid, ferulic acid, 5n-alkylresorcinols, and tran-cinnamic acid are all present in millets in good amounts. Quercetin, catechin, luteolin, apigenin, orientin, isoorientin, daidzein, vitexin, myricetin, sponarin, isovitexin, violanthin, tricin, and lucenin are flavonoids that are frequently found in millets. Several different types of chemicals have potential as neutraceuticals. The chemical extracted from millets and its raw extracts have attracted lots of attention in the recent years for use in neutraceuticals as functional foods.

The secondary metabolites that are present in millet grains contain a variety of biological characteristics, including antibacterial and antifungal effects. The millet grain's seed coat is richer in phenolic and flavonoid chemicals, which have significant health benefits like preventing cancer, neurodegenerative illnesses, and cardiovascular issues. The human body benefits from a type of phytonutrient called lignans, which is present in millet. These lignans undergo a transformation into mammalian lignans under the control of interstitial beneficial flora, which protects against hormone related cancers like breast cancer and lowers the risk of heart related ailments. According to Chandrasekara and his coworkers, phenolics in millets may be useful in stopping the development and spread of cancer in lab animals. Ferulic acid has powerful anti-inflammatory, free radical scavenging, and antioxidant properties. Antioxidants dramatically reduce tissue deterioration and promote wound healing. According to Rajasekaran *et al.* (2004), finger millet has positive antioxidant effects upon dermal wound healing in diabetes induced rats with oxidative stress mediated inflammatory control.

For diabetic patients, finger millets' phenolic extract is advantageous since it is an efficient inhibitor of the enzymes -glucosidase and pancreatic amylase, which lower blood glucose levels. Aldose reductase inhibitors limit the buildup of sorbitol and lower the incidence of diabetes-related cataract disorders.

Due to its high amount of dietary fibre, finger millet possesses a lower glycemic index. Both forms of soluble and insoluble dietary fibres are present in finger millet. Because insoluble dietary fibres are not digested in the small intestine, they protect against diabetes, coronary heart disease, gastro-intestinal problems, and colon cancer. As a result of the high calcium of foods made from finger millet, millet-based diets are advantageous for children's bone mass growth alongside adults' prevention in osteoporosis and other bone diseases. Millets' greater iron content protects against anaemia as well.

Millets are a good storehouse of magnesium, which has a profound effect of lessening the symptoms of migraines and heart attacks. Millets are abundant in phytochemicals, particularly those that contain phytic acid, which is believed to reduce cholesterol. In hyperlipidemic rats, finger millet lowers plasma triglycerides, which may help avoid cardiovascular disease.

When someone with a genetic predisposition consumes gluten, they develop celiac disease, an immune-mediated enteropathy. Due to their lack of gluten, millets are a great alternative for those with celiac disease and gluten sensitivity who are aggravated by the presence of gluten in wheat or other cereal grains (Saleh *et al.*, 2013).

We now have a scourge of cardiovascular disease, diabetes, and hypertension because to recently acquired lifestyles. For the aforementioned illnesses, millets have come back as a feasible alternative to taking a lot of expensive anti-diabetic and anti-hypertension medications, which also have substantial long-term adverse effects. In our internal environment, minor millets serve as a prebiotic feeding microflora. Millets will hydrate the human intestine and prevent constipation. Minor millet has significant levels of tryptophan, which is a precursor to serotonin, a mood-stabilizing chemical. Millet's niacin (vitamin B3) can help reduce cholesterol.

Postmenopausal women can benefit most from minor millet if they consume it regularly. Millet's high insoluble fibre content has been linked to reports that women who consume it can prevent gallstones. It has also been shown by researchers that giving children whole grains, such as small millet, can lessen their symptoms of asthma and wheezing. Millets are a boon from net zero emission point of view also, since they have the capacity to sequester carbon due to the presence of Phytoliths. Noncrystalline minerals called phytoliths develop inside the cells and cell walls of various plant components. The phytolith content of plants varies greatly, ranging from 0.1% to 10%. When a plant dies, its phytoliths are discharged into the soil and other sediments, where they are stable over a wide pH range (pH 3-9) and in a variety of habitats and climatic situations. Phytoliths can obstruct the tiny quantity of organic carbon (0.2% to 5.8%) absorbed from ambient $CO_2$ during photosynthesis while a plant is growing. Hence, 1.5 billion tonnes of $CO_2$ that are annually captured and occluded inside phytoliths has been identified as a substantial long-term terrestrial carbon sink.

All kinds of plants throughout the plant kingdom contain phytoliths. The *Restionaceae, Arecaceae, Zingiberaceae, Bromeliaceae, Orchidaceae*, and *Cyperaceae* groups of monocotyledonous plants are particularly prone to phytolith deposition. Yet, *Poaceae*, the biologically advanced and most thriving family of grasses, deposits the heaviest and most recognisable phytoliths. The Carbon content in phytoliths of foxtail millet and common millet were analyzed by Xinxin and his co researchers in 2011 in the dry farming regions of China. The findings showed that (1) common millet and foxtail millet, measured on a dry mass basis, contained 0.136% 0.070% and 0.129% phytolith occluded C respectively; and (2) based on the average annual production of foxtail millet and common millet over the previous ten years, phytolith occluded C accumulation rate of common millet and foxtail millet was roughly 0.020 ± 0.010 and 0.023 ± 0.01 t $CO_2$ $ha^{-1}$, respectively.

Potential for carbon sequestration in millets such as Pearl millet, Jowar, Small millet, Finger millet, and Foxtail millet at three different growth stages was investigated by Vidhya *et al* in 2022 in typical millet growing regions in India. Crop samples were splitted into aboveground biomass (AGB) and belowground biomass (BGB) for measurement of carbon occluded within phytoliths at three growth ages: 30th day, 60th day, and 90th day after sowing (phytOC). According to this study, the 60th day was when phytolith accumulation peaked and carbon was most completely occluded. Finger millet displayed the highest phytOC output, flow, and production rate among the millet crops.

*How millets are helpful in maintaining soil health in organic production system*

- According to Lynette Abbott, an eminent professor of Western Australia's Institute of Agriculture "Millets, an organic material, take a long time to decompose in soil, just like they do in human bodies." Their methodical composting helps preserve soil structure and water storage, soil health for an extended length of time.
- Due to their highly branched character, millets, like the majority of grasses, have a fibrous root network that contributes to the preservation of soil integrity.
- Millets, however, are the best crop to grow during fallow times. This is due to millets' propensity to develop symbiotic relationships with mycorrhizal fungi, which invade the plant's root system and enhance its capacity to absorb nutrients and water. The two nutrients, phosphorus and nitrogen, which are essential for crop growth, but are only found in trace amounts in the soil during the fallow season, can also be readily absorbed by these fungi.

## Some Case Studies on Organically Produced Millets in various states of India

In order to maintain crop yields and soil natural properties, a long duration experiment was conducted at the Agricultural Research Station in Vizianagaram for 6 years, beginning in 2014 during the Kharif season. The main motto of the experiment was to study the effect of using organic sources of nutrients versus conventional methods on soil health, Yield and quality of finger millet. Green manure (sunhemp), neem cake, FYM, and biofertilizers (*Azospirillum spp* and P Solubilizing Bacteria) were used as organic inputs in the aforementioned research.

Six years experimental data shows higher yield both in terms of grain and straw in the inorganically grown millet plot over the organically grown one. But, in the case of soil health, an opposite scenario was encountered. After the sixth year of the experiment, the pH and Electrical Conductivity of the soil remained unchanged from their initial levels under both treatments. In the organic plot, the Organic C% has increased in comparison to the initial value. Application of FYM and continuous in-situ incorporation of green manures increased the Organic Carbon%. The organic carbon buildup could be attributed to application of manures and the subsequent addition of plant leaf residues along with debris. In both the organic and inorganic treatments, the soil available macronutrients N, $P_2O_5$, and $K_2O$ showed an increasing trend over their initial status. Mean pooled data of available N and P were encountered to be significantly higher in the organic plot when compared to the control plot. In terms of biochemicals, total phenol content and total antioxidant activity were found to be highest in inorganic plot grains, whereas protein content, TSS, and tannin content were highest in organic plot grains.

During 2007-2011, a trial was conducted with different doses of organic manure in combination with biofertilizer and Rock Phosphate, as well as intercropping of pulses for incorporation to sustain soil health and production of Little millet+pulse cropping system. The results showed that a combined application of 5t FYM/ha with the recommended dose of straight fertilisers resulted in significantly higher grain yield and B:C ratio (1.64). Amongst different organic culivated packages, enriched FYM with biofertilizer application as well as in-situ incorporation of sunhemp and balance of P & K via natural minerals, yielded higher amount of grains than other organic manures. However, it was quickly proceeded by the application of vermicompost enriched with biofertilizers.

To determine the best nutrient management techniques for the organic growing of finger millet (*Eleusine coracana*) in the southern region of Karnataka, a field experiment was carried out in 2014 kharif season at the Agricultural cum Horticultural Research Station of Bhavikere, University of Agricultural cum Horticultural Sciences, Shivamogga. Application of farmyard manure at 10 $tha^{-1}$ +

Biodigester Liquid Manure @75 kg $ha^{-1}$ produced significantly higher grain yield, straw yield, and harvest index of value 0.46 as well as higher growth and yield related traits like length of stalks, number of tillers per hill, leaves per plant, and finger length. This treatment also produced a higher gross return and benefit cost ratio of 2.63 than application of FYM at 5 $tha^{-1}$ + Biodigester Liquid Manure.

A Field Trial was carried out at Kanke to determine the effect of seed inoculation of biofertilizers *Azospirillium*, *Bacillus*, and *Pseudomonas*, as well as micronutrients $ZnSO_4$ and boron @ 3 g/kg seed at three different fertilizer levels of 50, 75, and 100% RDF. Application of 100% RDF, micronutrients, and seed inoculation of biofertilizers resulted in considerably higher yield in terms of grain, which was found to be 128 and 59% higher than the absolute control and application of the recommended dose of FYM only (7.5 t/ha), respectively. Yield in terms of Straw also followed a similar pattern.

Agricultural College and Research Institute, Killikulam undertook a field trial to investigate the effects of different solid as well as liquid organic nutrients on the growth and production of transplanted finger millet during the rabi season (2019–2020). The experiment was run in RBD three times with ten treatments each. Treatments included three distinct liquid organic nutrients (3% jeevamrutham, 3% panchagavya, and 3% beejamrutham, respectively) in addition to two different solid organic supplements (100% poultry manure and 100% FYM). Over RDF and control, each treatment had a discernible impact on the growth characteristics, yield characteristics, and yield of finger millet transplanted. At 30 and 45 DAT, the application of 100% poultry manure plus 3% panchagavya considerably increased growth and yield.

During Kharif 2019, research in Finger millet was done in red sandy loam soil at the UAS, Bengaluru with various liquid organic nutrient management practises. When compared to all other treatments in the experiment, application of Amritapani along with Sanjivak @ 125% N equivalent $ha^{-1}$ produced significantly taller plants, high tillers, more leaf area, and dry matter concentration at harvest. Higher net returns and B:C ratios (Rs. 95740 $ha^{-1}$ and 3.53, respectively) were encountered when Amritapani along with Sanjivak @ 125% N equivalent $ha^{-1}$ was used.

Despite the fact that finger millet is resistant to a variety of abiotic and biotic stresses, blast caused by *Magnaporthe grisea* is one of the most damaging diseases, resulting in significant yield loss. Amongst various bioagents tested for blast disease control in organic cultivation, seed inoculation with *Pseudomonas florescence* @ 10 gm/kg of seed followed by 2 times spraying of *Pseudomonas florescence* @ 10 gm/lit water was found to be effective. This recommendation was recognised at the national level in 2011 and was widely spread among finger millet growers, particularly organic farmers, throughout the country.

Another emerging disease in small millets is banded sheath blight caused by *Rhizoctonia solani*. Amongst various treatments tried in all six small millets, for 3 years in a row, from 2015 to 2017, Application of talc formulated *Pseudomonas*+ *Trichoderma*+ *Bacillus* together @1kg each in 25kg FYM or Vermicompost with 15 days incubation was found helpful by researchers for banded/sheath blight management in all six millets.

2 spraying of *P. fluorescens* @ 0.6% (first spraying at half flowering stage, and second spraying after 10 days of first spraying) are recommended for the control of neck as well as finger blast diseases in organically grown finger millet. For all 3 blast diseases in finger millet, seed treatment with *P. fluorescens* @ 6g/kg seed and 2 spraying of *P. fluorescens* @ 0.6% (first at half flowering stage and second spraying after 10 days of first one) are recommended.

*Pseudomonas fluorescens* as Seed coating along with Soil application of value added FYM or Vermicompost + single spray @ 6 g/litre at 50% flower initiation is recommended for barnyard millet brown leaf spot and smut diseases.

AICRP, Ranichaurias centre has maintained a bio control repository consisting of 42 *Pseudomonas* strains and 30 *Trichoderma* strains for management of small millets diseases in Uttarakhand.

- *Trichoderma aesperellum*: - Effective against barnyard millet banded sheath blight.
- *Pseudomonas fluorescens*: - Effective against finger millet foot rot and blast, as well as barnyard millet smut and brown spot.
- *P. fluorescens*: Inhibits *Pyricularia grisea*,

When compared to late sowing, early sowing when the monsoon onsets, results in a lower infestation of shoot fly in Kodomillet. Intercropping Red gram or Arahar and kodo millet in a 2:1 ratio significantly decreases shootfly attack in field when compared to solo cropping of kodo millet. The organic pest management experiment during 2008–2010 revealed that application of Karanj cake in soil alongside spraying of Karanj oil 4% or NSKE 5% were considerably effective in controlling kodo millet shootfly.

Spraying of 1500 ppm Azadirachtin at 15 DAS decreased shoot fly infestation and was comparable to 5% NSKE spraying at 15 DAS, according to the experimental data of management of Shoot fly in eco-friendly manner in Kodo millet & Little millet in Dindori, Madhya Pradesh (2015-2017). The control plot had a higher percentage of dead hearts.

Because millet is grown primarily during the warm and humid season, unwanted vegetation proliferate and deprive this plant species of vital minerals and moisture, reducing yield significantly. Because of their marginal nature, most millet lands have poor soil fertility; weed removal of nutrients exacerbates the situation. Weed growth is encouraged during the early crop growth stages by bigger row spacing and slower initial growth of millet plants. As a result, early weed control in the critical period of crop-weed competition is regarded necessary to optimise yield.

Green manures are grown chiefly for their contributions to soil health and nutrition; however, they may also have a significant impact in weed management in organic agriculture.

i. Green manures, like smoother crops, outcompete weeds for water, nutrients, and sunlight.
ii. Green manures induce diversification in the cropping system, and thus limits opportunities for any unwanted vegetation to adapt to that niche cropping cycle.
iii. They possess an allelopathic effect, which means it releases chemicals that inhibit weed germination, growth, and development. Sunhemp, Alfalfa, Lucern, Cowpea, and Velvet bean were discovered to have an allelopathic effect upon weed vegetation.
iv. Agronomic practices such as tillage, mowing, and incorporation inhibit the termination of green manure crops.

Allelopathic crops can be included in cover cropping, intercropping, green manuring, mulching, smother cropping, or can be used in rotational manner to control weeds.

i. Sorgoleone, an allelopathic chemical released by jowar root hairs, is responsible for weed suppression in field.
ii. "Sorgaab," a water extract of mature jowar plants that is obtained after 24 hours water soaking, is effective as a natural herbicide.

Triketone, Cinmethylin, Bialaphos, Glufosinate, and Dicamba are some of the nature based products that is commercially used as herbicides.

## Conclusion and Future Prospects

The use of chemical fertilisers in modern agricultural methods has increased food grain production's self-sufficiency but also introduced a number of new problems. Most of the crops' output had been dropping. Countries are promoting organic inputs as source of nutrients for crops and as a soil ameliorant as a result of rising prices for chemical fertilisers and worries about the sustainability of intensive agricultural systems. By renewing and bolstering natural processes and farm ecosystem services, organic farming uses less external inputs and seeks to maximise crop output rather than optimise it (Shukla *et al.*, 2011).

No crop could possibly be more suited to being integrated into the organic production system in the current environment than millet. Millets can ensure food security, nutritional stability, and sustainability, serving a dual purpose. Millets are important for the livelihood of people in developing countries, particularly because of their substantial contribution to these nations' food security. Millets possess multidimensional aspects: they use 70% lesser water than rice, takes only half time of wheat to reach maturity, and require 40 percent less energy to process. Millets offer an alternative to current climate-smart crops because of their superior ability to adapt to harsh environments compared to the world's leading crops today.. The United Nations has designated 2023 as International Year of Millets in consideration of all these advantages. 2018 has already been proclaimed the National Year of Millets in India. Millets are being referred to as "siridhanya" or rich grains in Karnataka. The name "Siri" means "rich" in Kannada. They began establishing local grain distribution of millets through PDS. Karnataka is currently one of the nation's top producers and consumers of millets. With a great demand for millets, it also dominates the market.

India is world's top producer of millets. Tribal regions of Central India and the Himalayas, which are home to millet crops and millets cultivated in these areas are by default organic, grown with organic manures only. Millets were once poor farmers' insurance against the vagaries of the Indian monsoon. The resource inputs, whatever minimum is needed for millets are abundant in our country. However, more efforts from Government and research from Agricultural Universities are needed to make millet popular in the housholds as well in the crop fields. Breeders, agronomists, policy makers, and donors must work together in a real way to increase millets' productivity, both on an individual and institutional level.

As millets are receiving more attention, it is crucial to revive the nation's production of nutritional cereals. The only way to achieve the program's goal of doubling millet farmers' earnings is by using a targeted and comprehensive approach to planning, strategy, and execution. First off, given the inelastic nature of land supply, millets farmers can significantly increase productivity of millets by reducing yield gaps, including fallow and wastelands under millets cultivation, improve TFP through technological advancement and development of HYVs and hybrids, develop bio-fortified millets varieties, and establish seeds villages and seed hubs. By lowering the cost of production, millets farmers' revenue can also be successfully raised in dryland environments.

The most crucial factor in absorbing the extra output produced in the techniques outlined above is the demand creation for millets. Through creating demand through value addition and the growth of the millets subsector, farmers will receive fair prices and see their income from millets quadruple. With the development of steady price policies, increase of millets' procurement through MSP, incentivization of organic millet growers, development of marketing infrastructure using cutting-edge supply chain models, online marketing channels for organic millets, easy certification of organically grown millets and giving of insurance to all nutri-cereal crop firms, they can be brought into the mainstream of organic agriculture and diet.

## References

Basavaraj Naik, T., Kumar Naik, A. H., & Suresh Naik, K. P. (2017). Nutrient management practices for organic cultivation of finger millet (*Eleusine coracana* L.) under southern transitional zone of Karnataka, India. *International Journal of Current Microbiological Applied Sciences*. **6**(11). 3371-3376.

Bidinger, F. R., & Hash, C. T. (2004). Pearl millet. *Physiology and biotechnology integration for plant breeding*. 225-270.

Choudhary, S. K., Kumar, R., & Gupta, S. K. (2019). Integrated farming system (IFS) is possible way out for double farmer's income. *Journal of Pharmacognosy and Phytochemistry*. **5**. 282-289.

Gehrken, U. (1985). Physiology of diapause in the adult bark beetle, Ips acuminatusGyll., studied in relation to cold hardiness. *Journal of insect physiology*. **31**(12). 909-916.

Hemalatha, M., & Paramasivan, M. (2020). Influence of organic supplements on growth and yield of finger millet (Eleusine coracana L.). *Journal of Pharmacognosy and Phytochemistry*, *9*(3), 1564-1567.

Kuo, H. C., &Nakhata, C. (2019). The impact of electronic word-of-mouth on customer satisfaction. *Journal of Marketing Theory and Practice*. **27**(3). 331-348.

Lokesh, K., Dudhagara, C. R., Mahera, A. B., & Kumar, S. (2022). Millets: The future smart food..

Palai, J. B. Role of Minor Millets in Malnutrition Elevation in India.

Parvathi, M. S., Nataraja, K. N., Yashoda, B. K., Ramegowda, H. V., Mamrutha, H. M., & Rama, N. (2013). Expression analysis of stress responsive pathway genes linked to drought hardiness in an adapted crop, finger millet (Eleusine coracana). Journal of plant biochemistry and biotechnology, **22**, 193-201.

Rao, B. R., Nagasampige, M. H., & Ravikiran, M. (2011). Evaluation of nutraceutical properties of selected small millets. *Journal of Pharmacy and Bioallied Sciences*. **3**(2). 277.

Reynolds, T. W., Waddington, S. R., Anderson, C. L., Chew, A., True, Z., & Cullen, A. (2015). Environmental impacts and constraints associated with the production of major food crops in Sub-Saharan Africa and South Asia. Food Security. 7(4). 795-822.

Saleh, A. S., Zhang, Q., Chen, J., & Shen, Q. (2013). Millet grains: nutritional quality, processing, and potential health benefits. *Comprehensive reviews in food science and food safety*. 12(3). 281-295.

Shanthakumar, G., Yenagi, N. B., Shekhar, G. C., & Halikatti, S. I. (2010). Food security and income enhancement of rural poor through improved production technology and value addition of nutritious small millets: A case study from Northern Karnataka. *Minor Millets in South Asia: Learnings from IFAD-NUS Project in India and Nepal*. 69.

Shukla, A., Patel, B. R., Patel, A. N., & Patel, A. R. (2011). Organic farming for sustainable agriculture. *Kisan World*. **38**(3). 39-42.

Singh, A., Kumar, M., & Shamim, M. (2020). Importance of minor millets (Nutri Cereals) for nutrition purpose in present scenario. *International Journal of Chemical Studies*. **8**(1). 3109-3113..

Singh, R. P., Qidwai, S., Singh, O., Reddy, B. R., Saharan, S., Kataria, S. K., ... & Kumar, L. (2022). Millets for food and nutritional security in the context of climate resilient agriculture: A Review. *International Journal of Plant & Soil Science*. 939-953.

Subramanian, A., Nirmalakumari, A., & Veerabadhiran, P. (2010). Trait based selection of superior Kodo millet (*Paspalum scrobiculatum* L.) genotypes. *Electronic Journal of Plant Breeding*. 1(4). 852-855.

Tadele, Z. (2016). *Drought adaptation in millets* (pp. 639-662). InTech.

Tang, N., Jiang, S., Yang, Y., Liu, S., Ponnusamy, M., Xin, H., & Yu, T. (2018). Noncoding RNA s as therapeutic targets in atherosclerosis with diabetes mellitus. *Cardiovascular Therapeutics*. **36**(4). e12436.

Verma, V. C., Acharya, S., & Verma, B. C. (2020). Millets for Sustainable Agriculture and Nutritional Security.

# 7

# Breeding for Genetic Improvement of Millets

Madhuri Pradhan[1*], Manasi Dash[2]

[1] Department of Agriculture and allied sciences, C.V. Raman Global University, Mahura, Bhubaneswar, India

[2] Department of Plant Breeding and Genetics, College of Agriculture, Odisha University of Agriculture and Technology, Bhubaneswar, India

**ABSTRACT**

Millets belong to the diverse groups of small-seeded grasses that are cultivated all over the world. In the semi-arid tropics, millets play an essential role as staple foods, particularly in Asia and Arica. Previously, they were regarded as unimportant secondary crops. Recently millets are gaining popularity due to their superior nutritional value and their capacity to withstand climatic stresses such as heat and moisture stress. Millets have not received a significant amount of breeding attention yet. Due to the difficulty of hybridization in small-sized flowers, hybrids development has not been completely exploited. By utilizing existing sources of genetic material, breeding tactics may be designed to boost the nutritional content of millets without sacrificing yield or desirable traits. In the era of high-quality food materials, breeding techniques should prioritize combining enhanced quality with high yield and climatic resistance.

*Keywords*: Climatic resistance, High yield, Millets, Nutritional content

## Introduction

It is anticipated that the global population will reach 9.8 billion by the year 2050, which will need a 60–70% boost in food production from the present stage. This will present a tremendous problem in terms of being able to provide for a growing population. Then again, rice, wheat and maizeare the three grains that contribute more than sixty percent of the human diet's energy intake from plant sources. This percentage is much higher in a number of Asian countries. Despite the fact that these primary cereal grains are an essential component of several diets, they have a lesser concentration of mineral elements. Almost 2 billion people around the world are affected by the "hidden hunger" that is caused by a lack of micronutrients. This is mostly as a result of our significant reliance on a relatively small number of primary foodstuffs.

* Corresponding author.

Hence, there is a necessity for a significant change of the existing agricultural and food systems in the direction of greater diversity (crops and diets). This can be accomplished by encouraging the production and utilisation of traditionally significant underutilised climate-resistant and nutrient-rich crops for the purposes of sustainable agriculture andnutritiousfoods. A category of cereal crops belonging to the grass family Poaceae, small millets are also referred to as minor millets. They have very small seeds. Included in this category are finger millet, foxtail millet, proso millet, barnyard millet and kodo millet. Small millets are well-known for the climate-resilient properties that they possess, such as their greater adaptability to a wide range of ecological circumstances, lower water requirements, reduced risk of harmful pests and illnesses, and least susceptibility to pressures due to environmental factors. Rainfall enables semiarid regions' rainfed areas to produce significant amounts of small millets. As a result of the transition away from traditional crops and towards cash crops, they are only planted on a tiny area, which only accounts for a fraction of the total millet output around the world.

Several of these millets produce stable yields in unfavourable conditions, and they provide a substantial contribution to the overall food demand. Small millets grains are quite adaptable have the ability to be readily included in diets that are primarily based on rice or maize, or they can be used as a substitute for rice in dishes that already exist. They are also used as important food components in a number of traditional dishes and beverages, and they are ingredients in a range of products that are cereals that contain both multiple grains and do not contain gluten. Millets are also ingested as fermented beverages, which increases the obtainability of nutrients such as protein and mineral bioavailability, as well as the digestion of the food and reduces the amount of antinutritional elements.Consumers are looking for more nutrient-dense foods that are not only tasty but also healthful as a response to the rising prevalence of sedentary lifestyles and the health problems that are connected with them.The fact that millets provide a significant amount of energy, a high amount of fibre, protein having a balanced amino acid profile, numerous vital minerals, vitamins, and antioxidants, and possess a low glycaemic index makes them an excellent candidate for the role of healthy food choice (GI).These characteristics are what give rise to the terms "Smart-Food Crops" and "nutri-cereals" when referring to these plants.The nutrient profile of millets is highly dependent on the specific variety and type.

The expanding population of the world, which is largely dependent on a diet that is primarily composed of cereals but is lacking in micronutrients, poses a significant challenge in the form of nutritional insecurity. In the semi-arid tropics and drought-prone regions of Asia and Africa, millets are the principal suppliers of energy and represent an extremely promising agricultural entity. Because of their resistance to climatic shifts and their ability to thrive in dry conditions, they quickly rose to prominence in the agricultural industry. Millets have a superior nutritional profile than other cereal grains due to the high levels of protein, essential amino acids, vitamins, and minerals that are present in their grains. The presence of antinutrients in millets, such as phytic acid, polyphenolic compounds, and various tannins, continues to be a barrier to the process of biofortification. By a process known as marker-assisted selection (MAS), which uses DNA markers, there is a significant opportunity to reduce the content of antinutrients, to boost the productivity and accuracy of traditional plant breeding. Research on millet at the molecular level is quite limited, and only a very small number of molecular markers have been reported. It is necessary to conduct additional genome-wide analyses of small millets in order to create genetic maps and MAS. Traditional breeding techniques, biotechnological tools, and advancedtechnologies can all be used in conjunction to increase yield, improve quality, and lower the antinutrient levels.

## Nutritional value of millets

Millets are typically referred to as "small seeded grasses," but they are more frequently known as "Nutri Cereals" these days due to the amazing nutritional benefits they contain. There are a few different classes of minor millets that fall under this category.In terms of their protein and fat content, millets are comparable to rice and wheat, but they outperform these grains in terms of their availability of other nutrients. Proteins, dietary fibre, vitamins, calcium, iron, zinc, phosphorus, potassium, and other necessary amino acids are all present in large amounts in millets (Kumar *et al.,* 2018). Wheat and rice both include a fair amount of carbs. As stated bythe Indian Council of Medical Research (ICMR), small millet has 1,229% more iron, 840% more fat, and 350% more fibre than foxtail millet when compared to rice. Moreover, foxtail millet contains more fibre than small millet.

Nevertheless, the abundance of phytates, polyphenols, and tannins reduces the bioavailability of minerals by chelating multivalent cations including iron, zinc, calcium, magnesium, and potassium. This limits the amount of minerals that can be absorbed by the body. Millets have come to be recognised in recent years for the health-promoting nutritional values that they contain; as a result, they are regarded as a treasure trove of nutrients. In addition, the necessary amino acids, sulphur-comprising amino acids, such as cysteine and methionine, can be found in millet proteins in quite high quantities. However, the amount of tryptophan and lysine that cereal proteins contain can vary depending on the variety. On general, cereal proteins contain a low amount of these two amino acids. Millets contain a higher proportion of the important amino acids. Moreover, millets include a high quantity of dietary fibres in addition to a low glycemic index (GI) polysaccharide content (Figure 1).

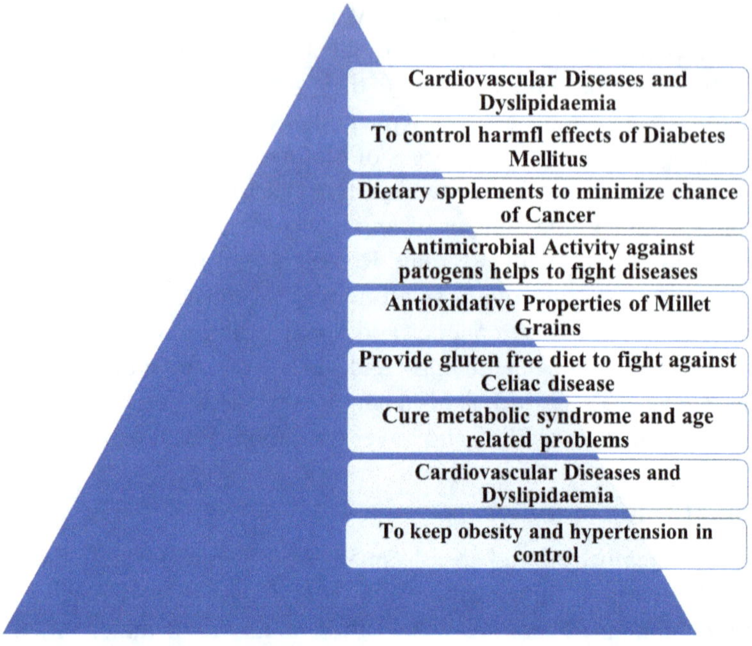


**Figure 1:** Different types of health benefits of millets

## Production constraints and breeding objectives

In general, yield and the characteristics that contribute to yield are the importantcharacters in the improvement of small millets. As a result, selection for yield in and of itself has been the primary base for increasing productivity; nevertheless, interactions between genotype and environment have a significant impact on these traits.As a result, determining the consistency of yield across a variety of conditions and researching the physiological variables (such as harvest index, water use efficiency, and so on) that are connected with yield and adaptation are both critical steps in the process of targeting yield enhancement.

Germplasm collections display important variation for a variety of traits, one of which is the duration of maturity. This variation can be used to breed cultivars with specific maturation timesdepending on the location-specific requirements of soil, rainfall, temperature, humidity, day-length, and cropping patterns.There is a considerable amount of variety in germplasm, which includes both grain nutrients and antinutrients. Using the existing variety that is found in germplasm as well as the differences that are a result of hybridization can help assist the breeding of nutrient-dense cultivars in the context of higher yielding backgrounds.

Millets of smaller size have greater resistance to main biotic and abiotic stresses, and they cangreatly adapt to a wide range of environmental conditions. The majority of millets are planted as rainfed crops, which means they are significantly impacted due to lack of rainfall.lodging cause serious problem in small millets andthis is mostly due to the soft stem, as well as factors related to crop management and the environment.There is no clear estimate available for the yield loss that can be attributed to lodging in small millets; nevertheless, big grains such as rice and wheat have reported losses of up to fifty percent.It is caused by the bending of plants when they reach maturity as a result of increased panicle weight, soft stem, and inadequate anchorage roots.

It is vital to produce cultivars with superior lodging resistance in order to reduce losses in both yield and quality. Shattering is highly observedin small millets. Small millets experience significant yield losses as a result of grain shattering, hence developing small millets that are tolerant to or resistant to shattering will be essential to preventing yield losses caused by shattering. Creating cultivars that can be harvested by machines, improving the nutritional worthof grain and fodder to command a premium price, creating varieties that can be used to produce high-value foods like rice, flour, vermicelli, flakes, hot and cold extruded snacks, noodles, and ready-to-cook mixtures, developing genotypes that can withstand shade in orchards and agroforestry, developing quick-growing varieties for intercropping, and other such special traits (Table 1).

**Table 1:** Breeding objectives of millets

| S. No. | Breeding objectives |
|---|---|
| 1 | High yield |
| 2 | Lodging resistance |
| 3 | Shattering resistane |
| 4 | Drought tolerance |
| 5 | Salinity tolerance |
| 6 | Nutrient responsiveness |
| 7 | Bold grain |
| 8 | Early maturity |
| 9 | Blast, head smut, grain smut, leaf spot and sheath blight resistance |
| 10 | Shoot fly resistance |
| 11 | Grain quality |

## Challenges and framework for millet improvement

Millets were domesticated early and are climate robust, but the green revolution and other programmes to boost agricultural yields primarily concentrated on rice and wheat. As a result, the traditional millet harvests vanished from the ordinary families' food baskets. Millets have fallen into the category of neglected and underutilised crops as a result of ignorance and carelessness, which has been further exacerbated by the inadequately established agribusiness and food processing models. For instance, the price of millets is more than twice as high in India, the world's top producer of millet, as compared to other major grains like rice, wheat, or maize. The growth of millets is hampered by absence of appropriate routes between the producer, distributor, and dealer as well as by consumer awareness. To establish millets as the predominantcrop in the agriculturesector, joint effortsplay an essential role. Both internationally and locally, there has to be an encouragement for the expansion of wholesome and nutrient-dense food crops. The Food and Agricultural Organization (FAO) of the United Nations has designated 2023 as the "International Year of Millets" in light of theirsocioeconomic and nutritional potential (Figure 2).

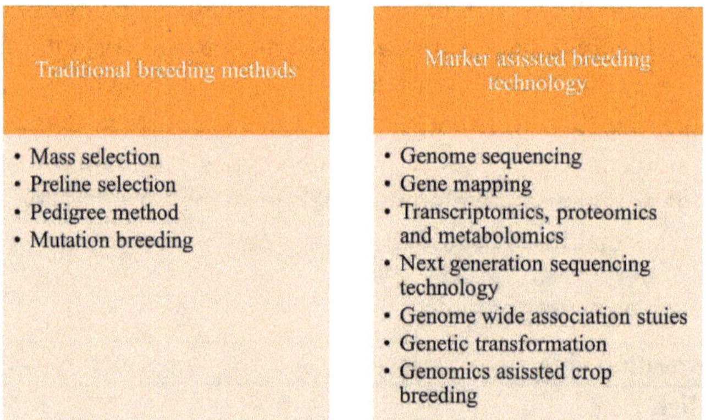


**Figure 2:** Different breeding methods for improvement of millets

## Conventional approaches for millet improvement

The breeding techniques used for self-pollinating crops, such as pure line selection, pedigree selection, mass selection, and mutation breeding, are used for small millets. According to reports on small millets cultivars issued over time, the bulk of them were released after selection from local landraces and cultivars, then pedigree selection. A key breeding strategy for small millets is hybridization to increase variety followed by selection in a population that is segregating. 45% of the cultivars of millet that were made available in India used the hybridization and selection breeding approach for finger millet, 22% for foxtail millet, and 29% for proso millet. Millets, on the other hand, are difficult to hybridise because of their floral shape and anthesis behaviour. Small millets can be hybridised using both the contact method, in which selected plants' panicles are wrapped in parchment bags before flowering to increase the likelihood of accidental cross-pollination, and controlled hybridization, which can be accomplished by either hand emasculation or hot water emasculation. In finger millet inflorescences (3–4 days after emergence), induction of male sterility by hot water treatment at 52 °C for 5 min was successful, however in barnyard millet 48 °C for 4-5 min was successful. Little millets have been known to use emasculation and crossover methods. In order to create effective emasculation and crossing protocols, it is helpful to understand flower biology and the pollination system. Even with skilled hands, the success rate of generating the cross is typically relatively low, which restricts the number of genetic studies and small millets' ability to increase productivity.

Due of challenges in hybridization, there is a limited amount of hybrid vigour that can be utilised in small millets. So, using heterosis, which is effectively used in key crops for the generation of commercial hybrid seeds, would be a viable choice. So far, only one male sterile line (INFM 95001) of finger millet, with a genetic ale sterility system created from the source parental line IE 3318. A variety of male sterile lines for foxtail millet are developed in China. Till now, only partially genetic male sterile lines are applied to hybrid seed production successfully. Other small millets have no reports of male-sterile lines. In self-pollinated crops, where hybridization is exceedingly difficult to produce variety, mutation breeding generally played a crucial role. In India, 13 small millet cultivars, including finger millet (8), kodo millet (3), and little millet (2), have been made available through mutation breeding. It is necessary to investigate how to make little millets male sterile using chemical hybridising agents (CHAs). High frequency and spectrum of beneficial mutations can be obtained by mutagenic effectiveness and efficiency of a mutagen.

The absence of sufficient variability in the existing germplasm collection has led to the employment of induced mutation techniques in teff to produce variability for critical traits like lodging resistance. Small millets germplasm has been successfully characterised by conventional breeding methods, which have also been used to create and release a number of cultivars with various properties, such as resistance to and tolerance for biotic and abiotic challenges. Enhancing genetic gains in millets improvement may be possible using genomics-assisted improvement using several omics techniques.

## Genomics assisted millet improvement

Genetic resources can be utilised in millet improvement programmes by using advanced genomic technology.There are many examples, including genome sequencing, the development of novel molecular markers, functional genomic studies, genome-wide association mapping, genomic-assisted breeding, and biotechnological developments (Goron *et al.,* 2015).Germplasm resources are quite important source of valuable genes and are used effectively in traditional breeding methods to enhance a number of crop plants.The first step in finding genotypes that contrast for desired characteristics is to characterise the germplasm for those traits.

Most agronomically significant characteristics are controlled by a number of genes or quantitative trait loci (QTL). For effective crop breeding, it is crucial to quickly find each QTL locus using molecular markers. High-throughput sequencing-based genotyping technologies can quickly accomplish this on a whole-genome scale. The discovery of QTLs is currently done using a variety of techniques, such as genome-wide association studies (GWAS), QTL-seq, MutMap, SHOREmap, NGS, etc.

Through the use of genetic markers, such as single nucleotide polymorphisms (SNPs), simple sequence repeats (SSRs), cleaved amplified polymorphic sequences (dCAPS), restriction fragment length polymorphisms (RFLPs), and amplified fragment length polymorphisms(AFLPs), the genetic diversity within a population can be assessed. For crop genetic improvement, a reliable genetic transformation system must be established. For pearl-, foxtail-, and finger millet, a successful Agrobacterium mediated transformation system has previously been constructed. The millet transgenic research is expected to be accelerated to an extremely high altitude by currently used silencing techniques which negate the expression of candidate genes.Virus-induced gene silencing has been demonstrated to be effective in foxtail millet and other cereal crops.To hasten millet grain biofortification and quality enhancement, these strategies must be used effectively.

## Future prospects for millet improvement

Millets are very nutrient-dense that are fed to undernourished poor communities in Asia and Africa. Millets can be further improved by having good grain characteristics and considerable amounts of nutrients that contain necessary amino acids, minerals, and vitamins. Nutrient bioavailability can also be increased by reducing antinutrients or by using new promoters. Molecular markers make it easier to identify unique millet germplasm that contains the right nutrients. Controlling these variables will be aided by the discovery of gene-based trait-specific molecular markers that are specifically connected to nutritional traits. The introduction of next-generation sequencing technology favours the quick sequencing and characterisation of the millet genome's traits. Omics research on millets as cereal crops needs to advance more quickly in order to increase their use in the battle against micronutrient deficiency. To make millets more helpful for feeding a burgeoning population, recent advancements in RNA interference and genome editing technologies like clustered regularly interspaced short palindromic repeats (CRISPR) must be used.

## Conclusion

Millet grains must be revived since malnutrition and vitamin deficiencies are spreading alarmingly, especially in developing nations. Increased instability is brought on by fluctuation in environments, absence of public awareness, bad policies, and sluggish economic growth. Agriculture and food security are facing new challenges brought on by the climate and global warming. Small-scale farmers in underdeveloped countries suffer the most in this situation. The cultivation and consumption of millet must become more widely accepted at this time, when there will be an extra 2-2.5 billion people on the planet near 2050. Furthermore, the time has come to increase funding for millet research. Millets possess the capacity to guarantee food, nutrition, and health security by sustaining a constant supply even amid the unfavourable effects of climate change. Government coordination is also necessary, including subsidies for millet farmers, the creation of the public and private collaborations for promotion of millets, and increased public awareness.

## References

Amadou I, Gounga ME, Le GW. Millets: Nutritional composition.; some health benefits and processing-A review. Emir J Food Agric. 2013; 25:501-508.

Collard BCY, Mackill DJ. Marker-assisted selection: an approach for precision plant breeding in the twenty-first century. Philos Trans R Soc Lond B Biol Sci.2008; 363(1491): 557–572.

Goron TL, Raizada MN. Genetic diversity and genomic resources available for the small millet crops to accelerate a New Green Revolution. Front Plant Sci. 2015; 6:157.

Kumar A, Tomer V, Kaur A, Kumar V, Gupta K. Millets: a solution to agrarian and nutritional challenges. Agric Food Security. 2018; 7:31.

Mamo T, A Singh.Millet Breeding. In Crop Improvement, interactive e-learning courseware. Plant Breeding E-Learning in Africa. 2016.

Nagaraja A, Kumar J, Jain AK, Narasimhudu Y, Raghuchander T, Kumar Bijendar. Compendium of Small Millets Diseases. Bangalore: AICSMIP, UAS, GKVK. 2017;1–80.

Patil HE. Breeding for Quality Improvement in Small Millets: A Review. International Journal of Genetics. 2018; 10(9):507-510.

Saleh ASM, Zhang Q, Chen J, Shen Q. Millet grains: nutritional quality.; processing.; and potential health benefits. Compr Rev Food Sci Food Saf. 2013; 12:281-295.

Santra DK, Khound R, Das S. Proso Millet (*Panicum miliaceum* L.) breeding: progress, challenges and opportunities. In: Al-Khayri J, Jain SM, Johnson DV, editors. Advances in plant breeding strategies: cereals. Cham: Springer; 2019; 223–57.

Seethatram A, and Krishne Gowda K T. Production and utilization of small millets in India, (In) Food uses of small millets and avenues for further processing and value addition. Project coordination cell, All India Coordinated Small Millets Improvement Project, ICAR, G.K.V.K. Campus, Bangalore. 2008.

Sushma Tiwari, Sanjeev Kumar Yadav, Vinod Kumar Sahu and Tripathi, M.K. Current Status and Future Prospects of Marker Assisted Breeding for Genetic Improvement of Minor Millets. IntJCurrMicrobiolAppSci. 2018; 7(12): 2587-2590.

Vinoth A, Ravindhran R. Biofortification in millets: a sustainable approach for nutritional security. Front Plant Sci. 2017; 8:29.

# 8

# Millets: A Biotechnological Perspective

Jyoti Prakash Dash*

Maharaja Sriram Chandra Bhanjadeo University (Erstwhile North Orissa University), Orissa.

**ABSTRACT**

One of the earliest grains in the globe to be cultivated is milletsand are referred to as $C_4$ crops. But these are underexploited yet potent crops. Being rich in dietary fibre, resistant starch, antioxidants, Niacin, β-carotene and essential amino acids, gluten free proteins and several micronutrients, vitamins and minerals, they prove to be a potent crop for obtaining the nutritional requirements of humans. Apart from this, their ability to reduce glycaemic load and lower blood cholesterol level as well as other health benefits makes them a good fit for human consumption, while providing a helping hand to accomplish the Sustainable Development Goals. Millets have several advantages including rich nutrition, health benefits, good fodder value, low maintenance, and several other ecological benefits; despite various biotic as well as abiotic stresses halt their production. To help come out of this, biotechnology has emerged as an effective tool. As such, various biotechnological approaches including genetic engineering, genomics, proteomics, metabolomics, transcriptomics etc. can prove beneficial to achieve sustained production of millets. This work therefore discusses various properties of millets as well as the role of biotechnology in enhancing millet production.

*Keywords* : Millets, Nutrition, Health, Sustainable Development Goals, Bio-technology, Genomics, Proteomics, Metabolomics, Transcriptomics.

## Introduction

Global population growth is acceleratingand consequently a steep shortage in food supply and increased malnutrition has taken place. UN FAO is the world body responsible for food and agriculture (FAO, 2009) and states that, "In cases where everyone, at all instances, has monetary, social, and physical access to sufficient, secure, and nutritious food to satisfy their nutritional needs and dietary choices for a healthy and energetic existence, then there is food security". *Availability of food, it's access, utilisation*, and *stability in the availability of food, access and utilization* are the four pillars of security of food. But in contrast, Conflict, extreme

* Corresponding author.

weather, fluctuations in the economy, and rising disparity are among the leading causes of insecurity regarding food and nutritional deficiency.

Consequently, a number of crucial steps have been made in order to deal with this issue.As a result, To "Eradicate extreme poverty and hunger," the first Millennium Development Goal (MDG), was created(United Nations, 2015a) and the 2030 objective for the sustainable development goals was to "put an end to starvation, shortages of food, and all possible kinds of nutritional deficiencies". Furthermore,Ending starvation, achieving food security, improving nutrition, while encouraging agricultural sustainability are all among the objectives of the second Sustainable Development Goal (SDG), for "Zero Hunger." (United Nations, 2015b).Yet all these are running unsuccessfulwhich is noticeable from the FAO, 2019 report titled the State of Food Security and Nutrition in the World, which demonstrates that over 820 million individuals worldwide endured hunger in 2018, particularly in the African continent, the Americas, particularly Latin America, and Asian nations.

On Putting more light, there are approximately two thousand million or more individuals, encompassing eight per cent of the overall population of nations with developed economies, do not have a decent level of food security (e.g. North America and Europe). Added to this, one more issue of concern is the growing level of malnutrition. And to prevent this, one of the solution is to ensure accessibility of healthy diets to each and every individual of the growing population. However, the updated estimates reveal the fact that almost 3.1 billion individuals are still impotentof affording it. Moreover, the advent of COVID 19 pandemic and it's consequences has halted the path of sustainable development goals 2. And consequently, this will lead to an increased malnutrition in children (FAO, 2022). To further worsen the scenario of food security,those hardest hit by the world wide epidemic who have unrecoverable income losses and the haphazard economic rebound in 2021 across nations have all contributed. Food prices have increased in recent years in light of the widespread nature of the COVID-19 epidemic's supply chain bottlenecks, escalating expenses for transportation, and other complications. Also as hoped about the world to emerge out of the pandemic effects, it has rather fallen into the tighter grips of it. Furthermore, in various nations, the war in Ukraine is also impacting the state of food and nutrition and those which are already facing food and hunger crisis are no exception, rather are more susceptible to it' affect. This war between the two of the world's biggest producers of staple cereals and agriculture, has further disrupted the supply chain to increase the inflation of food price.

A jump of 8.0 percent in 2019 to 9.3 percent in 2020, in the prevalence of undernourishment has been seen, that, in accordance with "The State Of Food

Security And Nutrition In The World 2022",had also continued it's increase in 2021. According to projections in the same report, there will be amid 702 to 828 million hungry individuals will be there in 2021 worldwide. In addition, out of 768 million underfed person worldwide in 2021, 425 million reside in Asian regions specifically, 278 million individuals in the African continent, and lessin the nations of Latin America as well as the region of the Caribbean with almost 57 million. All these data indicates the failure of the present food systemhas failed to make available therations and nutritional protection to one and all. Food system, whichusually is a combination of agronomical manufacture, stowage, processing, delivery and eating has feedback loops or unintended consequences striking at various stages. As such, the drivers including demand, economics, legislation, climaticalteration as well as the consequences like wastage ofrations, loss of nutrients, safety in food, access, global change in climateportraysa collective role in deciding the achievement of healthy and sustainable diets. Nonetheless production of waste cannot be ignored as estimations reveal the fact that one third of food remains uneaten. In addition, nutrient losses occurring through-out the food system during production, processing or cooking, storage and transportation cannot be ignored and are a serious issue of concern. Therefore, we need more radical changes to achieve sustainable and nutritional diets. Further, in order to access and afford food, state and intercontinental governments, business and law-making play their significant part guaranteeing food as well as nutritional security at both individual and national level (Macdiarmid & Whybrow 2019).

The failure of the dietary system to operate properly leads to insecurity over food, which is a unique convergence of several factors. Amongst, climate change is one such impacting factor that can never be ignored. According to "The 2012 Intergovernmental Panel on Climate Change","climate change is one of the persistent encounters faced by us". The 13th SDG "Climate action" therefore has aimed to "Take immediate actions to combat climatic alterations and its repercussions" (United Nations, 2015b). Moreover, the intensification of extreme climatic conditions is a major disrupter of supply chains in general and in particular, it's impact is disastrous in the low-income countries. Climate change has caused a rapid upsurge in the worldwide temperature norm, which has had a detrimental effect on progressof livestock besides plants as well as various aspects of the processing of food and dissemination. Further, variations in climatic conditions consequently having several negative impacts that includes dry spells, storms, and flooding, and immensely scorching temperatures have caused a serious food catastrophe, establishing themselves as a major factor in the rise in world hunger (FAO, 2018). Literatures suggest that an elevation in atmospheric $CO_2$ levels and rising temperature provokes crop yield reductionas well as reduces a variety of staple crops' nutrient density (Myers *et al.,* 2014, Lizumi *et al.,* 2017, Challinor *et al.,* 2016) while the impact of which is reliant on both the variety in whole foodas well as the use of suchprimary crops to obtain nutrition. However it's impression is expected to bein smaller amounts in advancednations owing to high diet diversity as well as fortification of these crops with micronutrients while their processing is being carried out.

In contrast, the developing countries will be significantly impacted upon as these crops are the principle source of micronutrients. In order to maximise the yields that are acceptable culturally and viable economically, there is a requirement of complex decisions in the choice of the finest cultivars that would guarantee nutrient quality and climate change resistance (e.g. drought-resistant varieties). Owing to it's direct impact on crop yields, fish and livestock productivity, the food availability is severely affected by climate change. Particularly the countries that depend on rain for agriculture will be hit more severely on account of climate change. Such a country whose economy is majorly dependent on agriculture is highly frailto change in climate and it's associated consequences which subsequently results in reduced production of various staple crop like rice, maize and wheat. Climate change and it's associated impact would lead to downfall of production which will subsequently increase the food price. Millions of the impoverished people of regions like South Asia that already experience high levels of malnutrition and destitution will be immediately impacted by this.

In such a delicate world scenario where nutritional security is an issue of great concern, we need to look up for crops which apart from being nutritious are readily available and affordable. Amongst, various millet species which are under exploited yet potential can be the saviour. Apart from this, the role of biotechnology in general and food biotechnology in particular cannot be ignored. Biotechnology holds great and significant potential in solving various issues which are of significant concern to humankind. Be it the production of vaccine for the destructive COVID 19 or the production of insulin, monoclonal antibodies, genetically modified plants etc. This chapter therefore focuses on the various millet species and other vegetable and fruit species which are under exploited yet potential and how biotechnology can use them to address the issue of food security.

## Cultivation of millets

One of the most prominent reason for looking towards millets is that their contribution is much less towards global warming as compared to other cereals. Even though the content of micronutrients in these cereals is found to be higher, contrastingly their contribution towards global warming is also significant. As such, nearlyfour tons $CO_2$eq/ha, wheat is the chief contributor of global warming after maize and rice tributing 3.4 tons $CO_2$ eq/ha. Moreover, the carbon equivalent emission of rice, wheat and maize are 956 kg C/ha, 1000 kg C/ha and 935 kg C/ha respectively (Jain *et al.,* 2016) which cannot be ignored as such. In contrast, the comparatively lower carbon footprints establishes millets as a potent alternative against other cereals. As suchit could help in the dropping down the carbon trail on earth (Prasad and Staggenborg 2009).

FAO 2014 states that, "Japanese Barnyard, Pearl, Proso, Foxtail, Finger and Kodo remains the mostgrown millets throughout the world". Being grown in diverseportions of the earth, their cultivation requires dissimilar growing environment. One of the peculiar characteristics of millets is their ability to grow in water deficient regions. Moreover, the ability to tolerate biotic and stresses from both livingsources and non-living sources as well as the ability to generatea significantharvest in lands having low-quality with least input permitstheir growth in arid regions. Further more, the thermophilic as well as xerophilic nature of millets permits their growth in variousportions of the world in diversifyingsoil types. As such, in terms of their worldwide importance, pearl millet remains in the6$^{th}$ position (FAO, 2014) and has the ability to use the moisture content of the soil efficiently and hence can be grown in dry climate as well as poor sandy soil. Pearl millets are therefore grown in regions where the yearly rainfall is between the 200–500 mm range (Guigaz, 2002). Hence it becomes a vital crop that can guarantee food security in areas like India as well as Africa (Passot *et al.,* 2016).

In the instance of an Indian production, finger millet places itself in the 6$^{th}$ position in production in India (Devi *et al.,* 2014). It is susceptible to growth in soils having high alkalinity as well as higher environmental temperatures. As such, 11°C to 27°C of temperature range and pH range of 5 to 8.2 in the soil as well as medium rainfall are the ambient parameters required for their cultivation (Upadhyaya *et al.,* 2008). On the other hand, according to Roshevits 1980 and Baltensperger 1996,"Originating in Central and Eastern Asia, the proso millet eventually propagated to the nations of India, Russia, the region known as the Middle East, as well as the European continent", has a cultivation period of 60–75 days and has a mean yearly rainfall requirement below 600 mm (Zarnkow *et al.,* 2010). Similarly in India,in the European nations, East Asian countries like the People's Republic of China, Indonesia as well as the Korean peninsula, the foxtail millet is cultivated. It is nutritious and displays the necessary resilience to pests and diseases (Vetriventhan *et al.,* 2012).

"The only two barnyard millet types that are still grown commercially are Indian and Japanese varieties" (Yabuno 1987). Being cultivated in Africa, India and it's neighbouring countries, it reside in the second place in terms of production with an annual production of 87,000 tons (Padulosi *et al.,* 2009) and is a crop that can withstand dry conditions and has excellent nutritional values (Wallace *et al.,*

2015). Similar to this, the Indian-born Kodo millet thrives in warm and humid subtropical environments (Arendt and Bello 2011, Hulse *et al.,* 1980) and has the greatest drought resistance potential in comparison to all the other minor millets.

## Nutritional value of millets

Widespread occurrence of chronic diseases and numerous health disorders has taken the world into its grip. The sole cause of such a condition is none other than an imbalanced nutritional diet. The FAO reported nearly 800 million people to be undernourished, which accounted 10.9 percent of the world population in 2015 (FAO, 2015) and housing the biggest undernourished inhabitants of the globe, India is no exception. This is evident from the fact that 15.2 percent of India's population remains under the shadow of undernourishment (Kumar *et al.,* 2022). Moreover, corresponding to the Global Hunger Index report of 2017, India places itself within the top hundredpoor countries (Grebmer *et al.,* 2017). Similarly, obesity and deficiency of vital nutrients is also a major health concern. Reduction in coarse grain consumption along with an increased consumption of polished grains particularly rice has pushed 51 million people into the claws of diabetes and an increase in this number up to 79.4 million is expected by 2030 if such a trend continues.

Therefore, looking to resolve such a serious problem, several researchers had investigated upon various species of millets and had found positive results. Foxtail millet (with high fibre, vitamins and minerals content) has a superior value of nutritionthan wheat and rice. Furthermore, by virtue of it's stearic and linoleic acid content, it is helpful in providing a sound lipid profile (Gowda *et al.,* 2022). As such, in an experiment by Lee *et al.,* 2010, decreased triglycerides level was observed in hyper-lipidemic mouse fed with foxtail millet which exhibits the beneficial effect of ingesting foxtail millet. Similarly in another study, "Foxtail millet significantly lowered blood sugar levels in streptozotoc-induced diabetic rodents by seventy percent." (Sireesha *et al.,* 2011).

Conversely, Hegde *et al.,* 2002, informed a decrease in fasting blood glucose on consuming various extracts of kodo millet. Moreover, while formulating infant and geriatric products, Kodo millet proves to be beneficial owing to its easy digestibility. In addition, it contains a lot of the B-complex vitamin and other inorganic elements (Gowda *et al.,* 2002).

Generally, the ability to lower glycaemic load is found in all the millets but it is highest in the barnyard millet (Krishna Kumari and Thayumanavan 1998). Owing to their high carbohydrate content of 49-65 percent (Sood *et al.,* 2015) and high dietary fibre. The barnyard millets are effective at avoiding constipation, lowering blood cholesterol,and cutting glycaemic load. Apart from this, the barnyard millet has crude fibre content of 14.7g/100g, iron content of 18.6 mg/100g and mineral content of 4.0g/100g which is highest among all the millets and hence can help in preventing the various deficiency diseases.

In case of proso millet, the protein content is 10.6 g per 100g servings. Moreover, the protein present is free from prolamin and glutelin which together constitute the gluten and hence is beneficial for those who cannot tolerate or are sensitive to gluten as well as thosein the grip of celiac disease (Kumar *et al.,* 2022). Apart from having lower glycaemic index and a good dietary fibre content, (Park *et al.,* 2008) it is can also provide niacin, folic acid, Vitamin B2, B3 and B9 as well as several minerals including iron (Fe), zinc (Zn) and magnesium (Mg) in sufficiently good quantities (Gowda *et al.,* 2022).

"Contrarily, finger millet includes 2.5–3.5% minerals, between 65 and 75 percent carbs, fifteen to twenty percent fibre in the diet, and anywhere from 5 to 8 protein." (Chethan and Malleshi 2007). It also contains amino acid in proper amountas well as higher proportion of threonine and lysine comparison to others. Micronutrients (Ca, Fe, Zn etc.) as well as B-vitamins are also richly found (Antony *et al.,* 1996 and Senthilvel *et al.,* 2008).One of the healthiest cereals, finger millet has a decent supply of naturally occurring calcium that can help enhance bones and lower the possibility of future bone breakages. Being considered as a nutritious food, it can be a good replacement for rice and wheat (Ambati and Sucharitha 2019).

In case of pearl millet, the energy value it exhibits is comparable to the cereal crops. Pearl millet has high amylose starch (20–22%), as well as insoluble dietary fibre by virtue of which it shows a lower glycaemic response (Gowda *et al.,* 2022). Furthermore, the higher prolamin content proves to be beneficial for people with gluten sensitivity. However it has reduced content of sulphurous amino acids (Zhang *et al.,* 2014 and Nambiar *et al.,* 2011). Additionally, Omega-3 fatty acid is present in good quantitywhereas, Pearl millet has also adequate levels of alpha linolenic acid. Micronutrients such as Fe, Zn, copper (Cu), K, Mg, P, manganese (Mn), and B-vitamins are also abundant in pearl millet (Zhang *et al.,* 2011).

## Millets in health

In order to have an optimum heath, an alkaline based diet is usually recommended. Millet being an alkaline forming food, proves to be highly beneficial in protecting from illness owing to its ability to maintain a pH that is healthy for the body (Sarita and Singh 2016). Millets hold great potential in solving various health issues related to human and accordingly various studies on the health benefits of millets have revealed their significant impact on human health. The nutrients present in millets like starch (resistant), antioxidants like avenanthramides, flavonoids, etc. establishes millets as a health beneficial food (Miller, 2001 and Edge *et al.,*

2005). Consuming millets reduces the occurrence of various health issues and consequently strengthens the functioning of the muscles and neurological systems, raises one's level of energy, improves immune function in respiratory health, cuts the likelihood of cancer, defends against coronary artery disease, advances the process of digestion, lowers the risk of Parkinson's disease, removes the impurities from body, and increases immunity. (Scalbert *et al.,* 2005; Chandrasekara and Shahidi, 2012; Manach *et al.,* 2005).

## Cardio vascular diseases

Helping to lower blood pressure, millets with rich magnesium content also acts to decrease the menaceof cardiacarrestsparticularlyin instances like Arteriosclerotic vascular disease (ASVD). Additionally, element potassium in the millets has the ability to vasodilate, which helps to keep the level of blood pressure modest and reduce coronary risk. Plant lignans, which are converted from animal lignans, offer protection from certain sorts of cancer and heart problems.Moreover high fibre present in millets lowers the cholesterol in level. As such, in case of proso millet, the consumption of it's protein concentrate effected levels of the lipid as well as significantly elevated the HDL cholesterolin plasma (Park *et al.,* 2008). Moreover, Kumari and Thayumanavan 1998, while investigating theimpressionof starch from barnyard millet found a reduction in cholesterol, triglycerides and sugar in blood, in contrast to rice as well as other minor millets in mice. Feeding Proso under high fat conditions on the other hand exhibited enhanced adiponectin in plasma and cholesterol (HDL) in diabetic mice (type-2) (Park *et al.,* 2008). Furthermore, according to (Lee *et al.,* 2010), the millets particularly the finger variety as well as the proso millet variety, by virtue of their ability of reducing triglycerides in plasma may help in the preclusion of diseases of heart and blood vessels (Cardiovascular diseases) in hyperlipidemic rats. Pearl millet is regarded as an excellent diet for cardiovascular wellness because of the strong antioxidant properties of several phytonutrients and lignin in pearl millet, which helps to avoid illnesses related to the heart.

## Diabetes

Along with hyperglycaemia and significant variations in carbohydrate, lipid and protein metabolism, Diabetes mellitus remains the most common endocrine as well as chronic metabolic disorder resulting in a reduction in the secretion of insulinfor the individuals with instances of type-1 diabetes but when type 2 is present, there exists a resistance to the effectiveness of insulin as well asit's secretion. (Saleh *et al.,* 2013). Presence of fibre in higherquantitiesin pearl millet leads to the protractedliberationof glucose into the blood as a result of slow digestionsuccessfully maintaining sugar levels steady for a prolonged time in people with diabetes.

Dietsgrounded on finger millet have demonstrated lower glycaemic response due to their exceptional dietary fibre content along with their power to inhibit the enzyme amylase (Kumari and Sumathi, 2002). Additionally, it promotes the skin's natural ability to heal wounds, and in a few rat tests, it proved beneficial in efficacy of antioxidation and maintained healthy sugar levels. (Rajasekaran *et al.,* 2004). In addition, antidiabetic molecules known as polyphenols in finger millets also act as major antioxidants and are proved to be highly beneficial for diabetic patents in terms of aldose reductase (AR) - inhibiting activity. Similarly, in case of type 2 diabetics, Barnyard millet, particularly the dehulled variety with a glycaemic index of 50 was found to be beneficial (Ugare *et al.,* 2011). However, foxtail millets' Water-based extractions have great ability to prevent hyperglycaemia (Sireesha *et al.,* 2011). Therefore, all these studies indicate the potential use of millet grains in preventing and treating diabetes.

## Celiac disease

Millets are anexcellent supplier of fibre and subsequently may help in the prevention of various gastro-intestinal disorders that include constipation, excess gas, bloating and cramping. Moreover, the gluten induced immune mediated enteropathic celiac disease in susceptible individuals (Catassi and Fasano, 2008) can be overcome by the consumption of millets. The substitution of staple crops(e.g. wheat as well as barley) with thosethat are free from prolamin and glutelin (e.g. rice as well as sorghum) and especially millets may be helpful for those who are sensitive to gluten (Thompson, 2009). In such a scenario, millets can play the role of a potent alternative owing to their gluten less nature and can be a fortunate thingfor the personwho is in the anguish of celiac (Taylor *et al.,* 2006; Chandrasekara and Shahidi, 2011b and 2011c; Taylor and Emmambux, 2008).

## Cancer

There has been a lot of development in medical science in the last few decades. Despite such development, cancer still remains a headache for researchers and remains one of the most dangerous disease in the world. However, some antinutrients, including phenolic acids, phytates, and tannins, have shown promise in lowering the chance of cancer of the breast and colon. Additionally, millets' phenolic substance stopped cancer in vitro from developing and progressing (Chandrasekara and Sahidi 2011c). Sorghum's polyphenols and molecules of tannin have characteristics that are both anti-mutagenic as well as anti-carcinogenic (Grimmer *et al.,* 1992). Additionally, sorghum consumption was found to reduce the prevalence of cancer of the oesophageal cavity in manyvarious regions of the globe (Van Rensburg, 1981). The free radicals well known for their cancer inducing property, were neutralized by the antioxidants found in millets and also cleans up other toxins from the body. In addition, neutralizing enzymatic activity as well as the presence of Quercetin, curcumin, along with beneficial catechins help in avoidance of foreign agents and toxins by stimulating proper excretion (Reddy, 2017).

## Obesity

Linked to a number of persistent diseases like diabetic complications, elevated blood pressure, and cardiac issues, obesity remains one of the most common disorder for the world population in general and the Indian population in particular. Literatures indicate the reduction of obesity with the consumption of high dietary fibre (Alfieri *et al.,* 1995). Additionally, consumption of millets prominentin alimentary fibredrops the ventureof emerging chronic ailments because it enhances bowel activity and delays down the breakdown and absorption activities (Ali *et al.,* 1982). Additionally, the millets possess the highest level of dietary fibre than any grain. Chethan and Malleshi 2007 states that, "finger miller is a good source of fibre as it has 15.7% insoluble dietary fibre, 1.4% soluble dietary fibre in finger millet" . Hence millets can be looked upon as a good crop to eradicate obesity as literatures suggesting their efficient role against obesity can be found in abundance. Consequently, they can address the issue of hunger as well as nutrient management. Thus consumption of millets is a good way to reduce the incidence of obesity as well as it's associated diseases and disorders.

Though millets have proved to be the a potent crop for eradicating hunger, poverty, nutrient deficiency and various health disorders, there remains certain constraints in their cultivation. Among them are the onset of fungal diseases (Ceasar and Ignacimuthu 2008), weather fluctuations, little or inconsistent rains, and the predominance of soils that are deficient in nutrients (Sharma and Ortiz 2000). Apart, resistance to abiotic stress like drought and saline also hinders their nutritional quality and quantity. All these factors contribute to the decline in the production of the millets as well as substantial loss to the farmer. Further these common factors push the agriculturists backwards in general and in millet production particular. Therefore, efficient and effective technologies must interfere in millet production so as to ease the above mentioned constraints for the welfare and wellbeing of the mankind. As such, biotechnology can play a very significant and prominent role here. It is evident from the current status of biotechnology that it has been continuously helping humans in various fields like medicines, food technology, for producing vaccines, production of biosimilars etc. And agriculture is no exception. Similarly biotechnology can come into play in cases of millets and resolve the various hindering factors associated with their production.

## Millet biotechnology

### *Genetic manipulation of millets*

Millets are one of thechief supplier of calories as well as proteins especially throughout the African as well as Asian continent (O'Kennedy *et al.,* 2006). Moreover, estimations regarding yield of cereals, including millets point for a food demand increase from two and a half to four and a half tonnes per hectare for 2025 (Borlaug, 2002). In addition, fungal diseases have constrained millet production. Therefore, to confer a high degree of resistance and increase yield, gene editing as a specific application of science is required (Ceasar and Ignacimuthu 2008). Further, by virtue of genetic engineering, improved nutrition as well as enhanced toleration to stresses that are abiotic in nature can be accomplished. There are a variety of methods for transforming a plant. But according to literatures available, the biolistic method has been used in most than the versatile agrobacterium mediated gene transfer (Latha *et al,.* 2006).

Pearl millet has been the most extensively studied millet for transformation studies. The first attempt for transforming pearl millet was done using biolisticwhere target explants were immature embryos (Taylor *et al.,* 1991). In this study, the promoter gene was"maize alcohol dehydrogenase (adh1)"that carried a β-glucuronidase gene. Furthermore, GUS histochemical assay was used to confirm the transformation. This operation was done using the pMON 8678 plasmid. Later, Taylor et al 1993, utilized two different plasmids, one being the pBARGUS plasmid and the other being the pAHC25 plasmid. Similarly, Lambe *et al.* (1995) successfully utilized the biolistic setupusing a couple of plasmids that include p35SGUS and pROB5 for millet transformation. The former carried the code for GUS where as the code for deliberating defiance to hygromycin was carried by the later. Similarly, Girgi *et al.* (2002) used a couple of transformation methods which included the PDS with particle gun 1,000/He and PIGwhere GUS and bar genes (reporter and marker) under uq1 promoter were used. However the transformation frequency was low. In another approach, in order to transform pearl millet, a transformation system independent of genotype was easily developed and employed by Devi and Sticklen 2002 rice Act1 (rice actin) promoter containing uidA gene carried by the pAct1-F plasmid was used for this purpose. Additionally, Goldman *et al.,* 2003, attempted to increase the transformation frequency by using inflorescences, apical meristems and embryogenic tissue. O'Kennedy *et al.* (2004) utilized a pNOV3604ubi plasmid for phosphomannose isomerase alteration. Using such technology, millet of pearlwhich demonstrates endurance against downy mildew has effectively been acquiredby several researchers (Girgi *et al.,* 2006).

Due to seed yield loss in finger millet owing to pathogenic fungus, *Pyricularia grisea,* remains a major hindrance in it's cultivation (Ceasar and Ignacimuthu

2008). In response, Gupta *et al.* (2001) originally conducted a study comparing the efficacy of an aggregate that comprised five promoters, including that of the Flaveriatrinervia (Ft) gene and the gene for the small subunit of ribulose 1, 5-biphosphate carboxylase obtained from rice. The results indicated that Actl and uql provided the best transformation. The successful use of *agrobacterium* in the transformation of foxtail millet has additionally been shown by numerous researchers. (Liu *et al.,* 2005, Fang *et al.,* 2007) (Table 1).

**Table 1 :** Genetic manipulation of millets

| Promoter gene | selectable marker | Method of transformation | Name of the millet | Results | References |
|---|---|---|---|---|---|
| Adh1, uidA | CaMV35S, bar | Biolistic | Pearl millet | Expression of plasmid pAHC25 was twice higher than pBARGUS plasmid | Taylor *et al.* (1993) |
| CaMV35S, uidA | CaMV35S, hptII | Biolistic | Pearl millet | Stable expression of hph gene, | Lambe *et al.* (1995, 2000) |
| CaMV35S, uidA | CaMV35S, bar | Biolistic | Pearl millet | Succesful integration of bar and GUS gene | Girgi *et al.* (2002) |
| Act1, uidA | ---------------- | Biolistic | Pearl millet | Transient expression of β-Glucuronidase gene | Devi and Sticklen (2002) |
| uq1; CaMV35S, uidA; gfp | uq1, bar | Biolistic | Pearl millet | Stable integration of herbicide resistance gene | Goldman *et al.* (2003) |
| CaMV35S/ActI/ UqI/ RbcS/Ft | ------------- | Biolistic | Finger millet | Increased GUS activity | Gupta *et al.* (2001) |
| CaMV35S, uidA | CaMV35S, npt II | Agrobacterium mediated | Foxtail millet | 6.6 percent transformation frequency of GUS gene | Liu *et al.* (2005) |
| CaMV35S/ActI/ UqI/ RbcS/Ft uidA | ----------------- | Biolistic | Barnyard millet | Increased GUS activity | Gupta *et al.* (2001) |

*Adh1*- alcohol dehydrogenase gene promoter, *CaMV35S*- cauliflower mosaic virus 35S promoter, *Act1*- rice actin gene promoter, *bar* -phospinothricin acetyl transferase gene, *hpt* - hygromycin phosphotransferase gene, *nptII* neomycin phosphotransferase gene, *Uq*1 ubiquitin gene promoter from maize, *RbcS* rice ribulose 1,5 biphosphate carboxylase small subunit gene promoter.

## OMICS driven Biotechnology solving Abiotic Stress

Being sessile in nature, both biotic strainsas well as abiotic strains are heavily applied to the vegetation. As such the stressors that are abiotic in nature are dryness, saltiness, flooding with water, extreme temperatures etc and contribute in excess of 50 percent towards the decline in output of major crops (Bray *et al.*, 2000). Further, merelyten percent of all arable area is devoid of any abiotic stress but the rest of the cultivable lands faces a bunch of abiotic stress (Dita *et al.*, 2006). Adapting to such stressful condition for survival and reproduction is very complex and is regulated by the crop's physiological, cellular and molecular activities. Therefore scientists have been working very hard to comprehend and utilize the stress toleration mechanism since a long time. However, with the advent of OMICS technology as well as the characterizing of each of the genes functionally, it has been discovered that strong regulations govern how well plants can adjust to environmental pressure. (Muthamilarasan and Prasad, 2014; Kissoudis *et al.*, 2014; Lopez *et al.*, 2008). Significant research has been done to reveal the mechanism behind stress tolerance in model plants like Arabidopsis as well as other plants like woody species, cereals, garden speciesas well as millets (Bokhari *et al.*, 2007; Alvarez *et al.*, 2008; Caruso *et al.*, 2009; Degenkolbe *et al.*, 2009; Shulaev *et al.*, 2008; Watkinson *et al.*, 2008; Zellar *et al.*, 2009; Ginzberg *et al.*, 2009; Dwivedi *et al.*, 2012).

Due to their status as important regional crops, millets have got atinyconsiderationin spite of their relevance. Thus, their genetic and genomic evolution has received very little attention. Due to irregular, infrequent, and scarce rainfall that eventually becomes a significant constraint for crop yield, millets also frequently experience dry spells. This is due to the fact that millets are raised using a input which is low as well as an agriculture method that is fuelled by rain. In addition the abiotic stresses like drought, salinity act as a great hindrance to their cultivation and hence it becomes important to mend the millets to endureabiotic strains.

## Genomics for millets

Genomics involves the molecular assisted selection (MAS) for developing molecular markers as well as manipulating quantitative trait loci (QTL) consequently producing improved cultivars. One beneficial aspect of these genomic resources is that they eliminate the tedious and lengthy direct screening of germplasm produced in greenhouse and open environments. In addition, they support research on crop species' syntenies. According to Rajaram *et al.*, 2013 study, a synteny has been demonstrated between the foxtail millets chromosomes, pearl millets, and other grasses. However, the use of such technology in millets for identifying or finding markers of DNAas well ascreation of linkage maps still lags backsideand pearl millet, finger millet, foxtail millet etc. have all been researched for the creation of genomic components (Dwivedi *et al.,* 2012).

Genetic and physical maps as well as genome sequence acts as a treasure for accurately identifying and classifying the genes as well as QTLs responsible for different agronomic qualities. According to Lata 2015, "This in turn facilitates Marker Assisted Breeding as well as crop improvement". The first RFLP based map comprising a total of hundred and sixty genes for foxtail millet was created by Wang *et al.* in 1998. Following this, several researchers successfully created different SSR markers based on EST or genomic data to be used for phylogenesisas well as genotypicinvestigationsregarding foxtail millet, as well as for various genotype applications. (Heng *et al.,* 2011, Jia *et al.,* 2009, and Jia *et al.,* 2007). Similar ILP markers were created by Gupta *et al.* 2011 and Muthamilarasan *et al.* 2014a, and were found to be helpful in research on the genomic relationships between millets and non-millets, transferability between taxa, classification of the germplasm, as well assimilarity mapping. Moreover developing the genomic resource on a large scale for the foxtail millet was made possible when the genome sequence of the *Setaria*was made accessible (Bennetzen *et al.,* 2012; Zhang *et al.,* 2012. As such several researchers had identified several SSR marker (Xu *et al.,* 2013), eSSRs (Kumari *et al.,* 2013), (miRNA)-based molecular markers (Yadav *et al.,* 2014b), SNPs associated with toleration to dryness (Lata *et al.,* 2011a) etc. The approaches like AFLP, ISSR as well as SSRs have extensively been utilisedfor theassessement of the relatives that are genetically as well as phylogenetically linked, studying the geographical structure related to taming between foxtail as well as it's wild version (Li *et al.,* 2012;Le Thierry d'Ennequin *et al.,* 2000;Wang *et al.,* 2012). Additionally, web tools have been developed to support this technology, including the transcription factor database (FmTFDb) as well as the marker database (Bonthala *et al.,* 2014 and Suresh *et al.,* 2013).

## Transcriptomics

Transcriptome is the presence of total mRNA within a cell whereas Transcriptomics deals with their investigation (Lata *et al.,* 2015). Genomic profiling studies become exceptionally significant to spot potential genes that contribute to numerous biological procedures and stress regulatory networks as well.The transcriptomic method typically aids in analysing and estimating the magnitude of adjustments triggered by abiotic factors at the level of the whole being. Foxtail millet, despite having an elevated water use ability, is still a naturally drought-adapted cereal. (Lata *et al.,* 2013 and Zhang *et al.,* 2007). Moreover using transcriptomic approach, foxtail millet has been analysed and 2,824 genes which are responsive to drought condition with differential patterns of expression have been discovered (Qi *et al.,* 2013).

Further, this study revealed the presence of LEA proteins, HSPs, aquaporins etc in abundance and possiblythey areaccountable for foxtail millet's ability to endure dry conditions. Similarly, the F-box protein was found to portraya noteworthypartboth in drought and ABA response in a study by Yin *et al.*, 2014. Another observation intending to investigate the *Setaria* genome identified 586 'response to water' genes that may be significantly playing a partin reaction to strain and adaptation (Zhang *et al.*, 2012). Similarly, several genes that express themselves differently in response to drought have been discovered by early studies using cDNA microarray along with suppression subtractive hybridization (Zhang *et al.* 2007).

Conversely, pearl millet remains a drought and heat tolerant plant andis able to acclimate to a broad spectrum of soil situations and can endure extreme dampness and elevated temperature variations.With the intention of improving stress resistance in pearl and related crops, methods for doing so can be developed with the aid of the detection and classification of such genes from pearl millet, for instance. In reaction to extreme salinity, drought, and the frigid pressure in pearl, Mishra *et al.*, 2007, acknowledged 2,494 distinctively modulated genes. In the instance of finger millet, Rahman *et al.* 2014, revealedquite a fewbrininess responsive genes and similarly to understand how calcium is accumulated in this cereal, Singh *et al.* 2014, successfully carried out the detection and confirmation of the calcium mineral sensor family of genethroughoutthe transcriptome.

## Proteomics

Proteome is the total protein formedas well astailored by an organism and proteomics on the other hand refers to the analysis of proteins on a big scale that areformed by an organism under certain condition or at a certain stage. Proteomics studies are therefore carried out to reveal the underlying mechanisms of proteins in an organism. Moreover, the proteome is the link between the transcriptome and metabolome of an organism. Instead, proteomics gains relative importance as a result of the possibility that levels of messenger RNA and retention of proteins might not always be interconnected(Gygi *et al.*, 1999). In order to identify the proteins that are modified post translationally, proteomics that is based on mass spectrometry approaches are usually employed (Barkla *et al.*, 2013). Though there has been advancements in the field of proteomics, there application in crops against stress is still restricted (Reddy *et al.*, 2012, Canovas *et al.*, 2004). Further,twenty-nine uniquely expressed proteins allegedly involved in signal propagation, photosynthesis, metabolic activity, and reaction to stress were found, among others, in a proteomics study salt-treated of just seven days old resistant "Prasad" seedlings. (Veeranagamallaiah *et al.*, 2008). Additionally, it has been stated that 52 different varieties of millet called finger millet were successfully used for protein profiling, SSR analysis, and RAPD-PCR (Kumar *et al.*, 2012).

## Metabolomics

One of the newest omics approaches, metabolomics, identifies all of the low molecular weight substances in the environment. These enzymatic reaction substrates or by-products frequently have a direct impact on an organism's appearance (Lata, 2015). A direct report of an organism's functional physiology at a specific age or state can be obtained through metabolomics. Target investigation, the metabolic profile analysis, and fingerprinting are additional thought-provoking methodsthat may eventually be used for phenotype analysis transgenics, finding how genes operate, examining for considerable analogy, and keeping track of responses to stress. Metabolomics is therefore basically a link between genotype and phenotype (Lata, 2015). On the application of metabolomics in millets, there is a very small amount of research. As a consequence, model plants and typical grains have been the focus of nearly all of the metabolomics field research. There is research on three different types of proso millet that uses gas chromatography and, more specifically, the GC-TOFMS to measure the variety of the phenolic acids as well as main metabolic products (Kim *et al.,* 2013).

## The phenomics approach

Any organism's molecular and morphological features, with an inclination to alterwhen exposed to environmental changes or genetic alteration, are collectively referred to as 'Phenomes' and their measurement is known as Phenomics (Lata, 2015). There is an information separation among phenotype and genetic makeup (Furbank and Tester, 2011). As a novel constraint in the improvement of plants and stress biology, high-volume physiological processes and phenotype determination has also emerged (Yang *et al.,* 2013). Therefore the formulation of basic principles for phenomics characterization has become very important as well as necessary for analysing any non-living strain in crops. Therefore phenomicsapplication has also been done in case of millets. Development of a dry down approach in pearl millet for increasing water stress and the development of a drought resistance indicator are two examples (Vadez *et al.,* 2012) can be cited as a good example. Similarly, Lata *et al.,* 2011b, established LP as an important marker for oxidative stress.

## Conclusion

Millets being a vital source of various nutrients like protein, carbohydrate, fats as well as vitamins and minerals. Therefore, millets can be a very potent crop in eradicating the nutritional deficiencies the world is facing. Furthermore, it can help globe to accomplish objectives for sustainable development for eradicating hunger and undernourishment. On the contrary, climatic alterations have devastating influence on the agricultural system. Consequently there occurs disruptions in agriculture and supply of food. This in turn challenges the safety of food and nourishmentas well as questions the sustainability of livelihoods. Millets being cheap and having high nutritional value, several health benefits and lower contribution to global warming can help achieve the sustainable development goals. Despite such high qualities, millets still remain one of the most underexploited and under-researched crop. This may be due to the unawareness of people about the nutritional potency of millets. Another imperative reason is the occurrence of various biotic and abiotic stress. As such, attacks by fungus and pests as well as occurrence of drought and salinity are having an overwhelming impact. In such a scenario, researchers are looking for various ways to resolve this issue. Amongst, biotechnology introduces itself as a potent factor in addressing the issue of both types of stressors including living as well as non-living for the ease production of various crops in general and millets in particular. Genetic engineering as well as various other biotechnological interventions including OMICS has a significant impactin enhancing the millet production consequently helping greatly in achieving the objectives of sustainable growth. However, very little biotechnological research has been done in case of millets. Therefore more in depth studies need to be done in order to help biotechnology achieve nutrition, eradicate deficiency diseases, achieve a healthy life, reduce the impact of climaticalterations through millet crop development.

## References

Alfieri, M.A.H., Pomerleau, J., Grace, D. M., Anderson, L. (1995). Fiber intake of normal weight, moderately obese and severely obese subjects. Obesity Researc 3h, (6), 541-547.

Ali, R., Staub, J., Leveille, G. A., Boyle, P.C. (1982). Dietary fiber and obesity. In: Vahouny, G. V. and Kritchevsky, D. (ed) Dietary Fiber in Health and Disease Plenum Press, New York, 192-194.

Alvarez, S., Marsh, EL., Schroeder, SG., Schachtman, DP. (2008). Metabolomic and proteomic changes in the xylem sap of maize under drought. Plant Cell Environment, 31, 325-340.

Ambati, K. and K.V, Sucharitha. (2019). MILLETS-REVIEW ON NUTRITIONAL PROFILES AND HEALTH BENEFITS. International Journal Of Recent Scientific Research, 10, 33943-33948.

Antony, U., Sripriya, G., Chandra, TS. (1996). Effect of fermentation on the primary nutrients in finger millet (Eleusine coracana). Journal of Agriculture and Food Chemistry, 44(9).

Arendt, E., Dal Bello, F. (2011). Gluten-Free Cereal Products and Beverages; Academic Press: Cambridge, MA, USA.

Baltensperger, D.D. (1996). Foxtail and proso millet. In Progress in New Crops; Janick, J., Ed.; ASHS Press: Alexandria, 182-190, VA, USA.

Barkla, BJ., Castellanos-Cervantes, T., de Leo´, JLD., Matros, A., Mock, H-P., Perez-Alfocea, F., Salekdeh, GH., Witzel, K., Zörb, C. (2013). Elucidation of salt stress defense and tolerance mechanisms of crop plants using proteomics-Current achievements and perspectives. Proteomics, 13, 1885-1900.

Bennetzen, JL., Schmutz, J., Wang, H., Percifield, R., Hawkins, J., Pontaroli, AC., Estep, M., Feng, L., Vaughn, JN., Grimwood, J., Jenkins, J., Barry, K., Lindquist, E., Hellsten, U., Deshpande, S., Wang, X., Wu, X., Mitros, T., Triplett, J., Yang, X., Ye, CY., Mauro-Herrera, M., Wang, L., Li, P., Sharma, M., Sharma, R., Ronald, PC., Panaud, O., Kellogg, EA., Brutnell, TP., Doust, AN., Tuskan, GA., Rokhsar, D., Devos, KM. (2012). Reference genome sequence of the model plant Setaria Nature Biotechnol 30 555-561.

Bokhari, SA., Wan, XY., Yang, YW., Zhou, L., Tang, WL., Liu, JY. (2007). Proteomic response of rice seedling leaves to elevated CO2 levels. Journal of Proteome Research, 6, 4624-4633.

Bonthala, VS., Muthamilarasan. M., Roy, R., Prasad, M. (2014). FmTFDb: A foxtail millet transcription factors database for expediting functional genomics in millets. Molecular Biology Reports.

Bray, EA., Bailey-Serres, J., Weretilnyk, E. (2000). Responses to abiotic stresses. In: Biochemistry and Molecular Biology of Plants (Eds: Gruissem W, Buchannan B and Jones R), American Society of Plant Physiologists, Rockville, MD, 1158-1249.

Canovas, F., Dumas-Gaudot, E., Recorbet, G., Jorrin, J., Mock, H-P., Rossignol, M. (2004). Plant proteome analysis. Proteomics, 4, 285-298.

Caruso, G., Cavaliere, C., Foglia, P., Gubbiotti, R., Samperi, R., Laganà, A. (2009). Analysis of drought responsive proteins in wheat (Triticum durum) by 2D-PAGE and MALDITOF mass spectrometry Plant Science, 177, 570-576.

Catassi, C. and Fasano, A. (2008). Celiac disease. In: Gallagher E, editor. Gluten-free cereal products and beverages. Burlington, MA: Elsevier, 1-27.

Ceasar, SA., Ignacimuthu, S. (2008). Efficient somatic embryogenesis and plant regeneration from shoot apex explants of different Indian genotypes of finger millet (Eleusine coracana (L.) Gaertn.). In Vitro Cellular and Developmental Biology-Plant, 44, 427–435.

Challinor, AJ., Koehler, A., Ramirez-Villegas, J. Whitfield, S., Das, B. (2016). Current warming will reduce yields unless maize breeding and seed systems adapt immediately. Nature Climate Change, 6, 954–958.

Chandrasekara, A. and Shahidi, F. (2010). Content of insoluble bound phenolics in millets and their contribution to antioxidant capacity. Journal of Agriculture and Food Chemistry, 58, 6706–6714.

Chandrasekara, A. and Shahidi, F. (2011b). Antioxidant phenolics of millet control lipid peroxidation in human low density lipoproteins cholesterol and food systems. Journal of American Oil Chemists Society, DOI: 10.1007/s11746-011-1918-5.

Chandrasekara, A. and Shahidi, F. (2011c). Anti proliferative potential and DNA scission inhibitory activity of phenolics from whole millet grains. Journal of Functional Foods, 3, 159-170.

Chethan, S., Malleshi, NG. (2007). Finger millet polyphenols: optimization of extraction and the effect of pH on their stability. Food Chemistry, 105(2), 862-870.

Degenkolbe, T., Do, PT., Zuther, E., Repsilber, D., Walther, D., Hincha, DK., Köhl, KI. (2009). Expression profiling of rice cultivars differing in their tolerance to long-term drought stress. Plant Molecular Biology, 69, 133-153.

Devi, P and Sticklen, M. (2002). Culturing shoot-tip clumps of pearl millet [Pennisetum glaucum (L.) R. Br.] and optimal microprojectile bombardment parameters for transient expression. Euphytica, 125, 45–50.

Devi, P.B., Vijayabharathi, R., Sathyabama, S., Malleshi, N.G., Priyadarisini, V.B. (2014). Health benefits of finger millet (Eleusine coracana L.) polyphenols and dietary fiber: A review. Journal of Food Science and Technology, 51, 1021–1040.

Dita, MA., Rispail, N., Prats, E., Rubiales, D., Singh, KB. (2006). Biotechnology approaches to overcome biotic and abiotic stress constraints in legumes. Euphytica, 147, 1-24.

Dwivedi, S., Upadhyaya, H., Senthilvel, S., Hash, C., Fukunaga, K., Diao, X., Santra, D., Baltensperger, D., Prasad., M. (2012). Millets: Genetic and Genomic Resources. In: Plant Breeding Reviews (Ed: Janick J), 35, 247-375, John Wiley & Sons, USA.

Edge, M.S., Jones, J.M., Marquart, L. (2005). A new life for whole grains. Journal of American Dietetic Association, 105(12), 1856-1860.

Fang, FQ., Qian, Z., Guang, MA., Jing, JY. (2007). Co-suppression of Si401, a maize pollen speciWc Zm401 homologous gene, results in aberrant anther development in foxtail millet. Euphytica, 163, 103–111.

FAO (2009). Declaration of the World Food Summit on Food Security. Rome.

FAO (2014). FAOSTAT. Food and Agriculture Organization of the United Nations, Rome, Italy.

FAO (2015). The state of food insecurity in the world 2015. Food Agric Organ UN.

FAO, IFAD, UNICEF, WFP and WHO (2022). The State of Food Security and Nutrition in the World 2022. Repurposing food and agricultural policies to make healthy diets more affordable. Rome.

FAO, IFAD, UNICEF, WFP and WHO (2018). The State of Food Security and Nutrition in the World 2018. Building climate resilience for food security and nutrition.

FAO, IFAD, UNICEF, WFP and WHO (2019). The State of Food Security and Nutrition in the World 2019 - Safeguarding against economic slowdowns and downturns. Rome.

Furbank, RT., and Tester, M. (2011). Phenomics - technologies to relieve the phenotyping bottleneck Trends in Plant Science, 16, 635-644.

Ginzberg, I., Barel, G., Ophir, R., Tzin, E., Tanami, Z., Muddarangappa, T., de Jong, W., Fogelman, E., (2009). Transcriptomic profiling of heat-stress response in potato periderm. Journal of Experimental Botany, 60, 4411-4421.

Girgi, M., Breese, WA., Lorz, H., Oldach, KH. (2006). Rust and downy mildew resistance in pearl millet (Pennisetum glaucum) mediated by heterologous expression of the afp gene from Aspergillus giganteus. Transgenic Research, 15, 313–324.

Girgi, M., O'Kennedy, MM., Morgenstern, A., Smith, G., Lorz, H., Oldach, KH. (2002). Transgenic and herbicide resistant pearl millet (Pennisetum glaucum L.) R.Br. via micro-projectile bombardment of scutellar tissue. Molecular breeding, 10, 243–252.

Goldman, JJ., Hanna, WW., Fleming, G., Ozias-Akins P. (2003). Fertile transgenic pearl millet [Pennisetum glaucum (L.) R. Br.] plants recovered through microprojectile bombardment and phosphinothricin selection of apical meristem-, inflorescence-, and immature embryo-derived embryogenic tissues. Plant Cell Reports, 21, 999–1009.

Gomashe, S.S.(2016). Barnyard millet: Present Status and Futurethrust Areas. In Millets and Sorghum: Biology and Genetic Improvement; John Wiley & Sons: Hoboken, NJ, USA, 184–198.

Gowda, N. A., Siliveru, K., Vara Prasad, P.V., Bhatt, Y., Netravati, B.P., Gurikar, C. (2022). Modern Processing of Indian Millets: A Perspective on Changes in Nutritional Properties. Foods, 11(4), 499.

Grebmer, K., Bernstein, J., Hossain, N., Brown, T., Prasai, N., Yohannes, Y. (2017). Global hunger index: the inequalities of hunger. International Food Policy Research Institute.

Grimmer, HR., Parbhoo, V., McGrath, RM. (1992). Antimutagenicity of polyphenol-rich fractions from Sorghum bicolor grain. Journal of the Science of Food and Agriculture, 59, 251–256.

Guigaz, M. (2002). Memento de l'Agronome. Montpellier: CIRAD-GRET and Ministère des Affaires Étrangères, Montpellier, France.

Gupta, P., Raghuvanshi, S., Tyagi, AK. (2001). Assessment of the efficiency of various gene promoters via biolistics in leaf and regenerating seed callus of millets, Eleusine coracana and Echinochloacrusgalli. Plant Biotechnology, 18, 275–282.

Gupta, S., Kumari, K., Das, J., Lata, C., Puranik, S., Prasad, M. (2011). Development and utilization of novel intron length polymorphic markers in foxtail millet [Setaria italica (L.) P. Beauv.] Genome, 54 586-602.

Gygi, SP., Rochon, Y., Franza, BR., Aebersold, R. (1999). Correlation between protein and mRNA abundance in yeast. Molecular Cell Biology, 19, 1720-1730.

Hegde, PS., Chandrakasan, G., Chandra, TS.(2002). Inhibition of collagen glycation and cross linking in vitro by methanolic extracts of finger millet (Eleusine coracana) and kodo millet (Paspalum scrobiculatum). Journal of Nutritional Biochemistry, 13(9), 517.

Heng, L., Chih, C., Song, C., Chang, K. (2011). Development of simple sequence repeats (SSR) markers in Setaria italica (Poaceae) and cross-amplification in related species. International Journal of Molecular Sciences, 12, 7835-7845.

Hulse, J.H., Laing, E.M., Pearson, O.E. (1980). Sorghum and the Millets: Their Composition and Nutritive Value; Academic Press: Cambridge, MA, USA.

Jain, N., Arora, P., Tomer, R., Mishra, S.V., Bhatia, A., Pathak, H., Chakraborty, D., Kumar, V., Dubey, D., Harit, R. (2016). Greenhouse gases emission from soils under major crops in northwest India. Science of The Total Environment, 542, 551–561.

Jia, X., Zhang, Z., Liu, Y., Zhang, C., Shi, Y., Song, Y., Wang, T., Li, Y. (2009). Development and genetic mapping of SSR markers in foxtail millet [Setaria italica (L.) P. Beauv.] Theoretical and Applied Genetics, 118, 821-829.

Jia, XP., Shi, YS., Song, YC., Wang, YG., Wang, TY., Li, Y. (2007). Development of EST-SSR in foxtail millet (Setaria italica) Genetic Research and Crop Evolution, 54, 233-236.

Kim, JK., Park, S-Y., Yeo, Y., Cho, HS., Kim, YB., Bae, H., Park, CH., Lee, J-H., Park, SU. (2013). Metabolic profiling of millet (Panicum miliaceum) using gas chromatography–time-of flight mass spectrometry (GC-TOFMS) for quality assessment. Plant Omics Journal, 6, 73-78.

Kissoudis, C., Van de Wiel., C. Visser, RGF., Van der Linden, G. (2014). Enhancing crop resilience to combined abiotic and biotic stress through the dissection of physiological and molecular crosstalk Frontiers. Plant Science.

Krishna Kumari, SK., Thayumanavan, B. (1998). Characterization of starches of proso, foxtail, barnyard, kodo, and little millets. Plant Foods for Hum Nutrition, 53(1), 47-56.

Kumar, A., Sharma, N., Panwar, P., Gupta, AK. (2012). Use of SSR, RAPD markers and protein profiles based analysis to differentiate *Eleusine coracana* genotypes differing in their protein content Molecular Biology Reports. 39, 4949-4960.

kumar, L., Naresh, R.K., Tiwari, H., Kataria, SK., Saharan, S., Reddy, B.R., Singh, O., Qidwai, S., Singh, R.P. (2022). Millets for Food and Nutritional Security in the Context of Climate Resilient Agriculture: A Review. International Journal of Plant & Soil Science, 34 (23).

Kumari, K., Muthamilarasan, M., Misra, G., Gupta, S., Subramanian, A., Parida, SK., Chattopadhyay, D., Prasad, M. (2013). Development of eSSR-markers in Setaria italica and their applicability in studying genetic diversity, cross transferability and comparative mapping in millet and non-millet species. PLoS ONE, 8e67742.

Kumari, PL., and Sumathi, S. (2002). Effect of consumption of finger millet on hyperglycemia in non-insulin dependent diabetes mellitus (NIDDM) subjects. Plant Foods for Human Nutrition, 57, 205-213.

Lambe, P., Dinant, M., Deltour, R. (2000). Transgenic pearl millet (Pennisetum glaucum). In: Bajaj YPS (ed) Biotechnology in agriculture and forestry, Transgenic crops, I (46), Springer, Berlin, 84–108.

Lambe, P., Dinant, M., Matagne, R.F (1995). Differential long-term expression and methylation of the hygromycin phosphor-transferase (hph) and b-glucuronidase (GUS) genes in transgenic pearl millet (Pennisetum americanum) callus. Plant Science, 108, 51–62.

Lata, C. (2015). Advances in Omics for Enhancing Abiotic Stress Tolerance in Millets. Proceedings of the Indian National Science Academy, 81, (2), 397-417.

Lata, C., Bhutty, S., Bahadur, RP., Majee, M., Prasad, M. (2011a). Association of an SNP in a novel DREB2-like gene SiDREB2 with stress tolerance in foxtail millet [Setaria italica (L.)]. Joural of Experimental Botany, 62, 3387-3401.

Lata, C., Gupta, S., Prasad., M. (2013). Foxtail millet: a model crop for genetic and genomic studies in bioenergy grasses. Critcal Reviews in Biotechnology, 33, 328-343.

Latha, MA, Rao, KV., Reddy, TP., Reddy, VD. (2006). Development of transgenic pearl millet (Pennisetum glaucum (L.) R. Br.) plants resistant to downy mildew. Plant Cell Reports, 25, 927–935.

Le Thierry d'Ennequin, M., Panaud, O., Toupance, B., Sarr, A. (2000). Assessment of genetic relationship between Setaria italica and its wild relative S. viridis using AFLP markers Theoretical and Applied Genetics, 100,. 1061-1066.

Lee, SH., Chung, IM., Cha, YS., Park, Y (2010). Millet consumption decreased serum concentration of triglyceride and C-reactive protein but not oxidative status in hyperlipidemic rats. Nutrition Research, 30(4), 290-296.

Li, W., Zhi, H., Wang, Y-F., Li, H., Diao, X. (2012). Assessment of genetic relationship of foxtail millet with its wild ancestor and close relatives by ISSR markers Journal of Integrated Agriculture, 11, 556- 566.

Liu, YH., Yu, JJ., Zhao, Q., Ao, GM. (2005). Genetic transformation of millet (Setaria italica) by Agrobacterium-mediated. Agricultural Biotechnology Journal, 13, 32–37.

Lizumi, T., Furuya, J., Shen, Z., Kim, W., Okada, M., Fuzimori, S., Hasegawa, T., and Nishimori, M. (2017). Responses of crop yield growth to global temperature and socioeconomic changes. Scientific Reports, 7, 7800.

López, MA., Bannenberg, G., Castresana., C. (2008). Controlling hormone signaling is a plant and pathogen challenge for growth and survival. Current Opinion in Plant Biology, 11, 420-427.

Macdiarmid, J.I., & Whybrow, S. (2019). Nutrition from a climate change perspective. Conference on 'Getting energy balance right' Symposium 5: Sustainability of food production and dietary recommendations. Proceedings of the Nutrition Society (2019), 78, 380–387. doi:10.1017/S0029665118002896.

Manach, C., Mazur, A., Scalbert, A. (2005). Polyphenols and prevention of cardiovascular diseases. Current Opinion Lipidology, 16, 77-84.

Miller, G. (2001). Whole grain, fiber and antioxidants. In: Spiller, G.A. (ed). Handbook of dietary fiber in Human Nutrition, Boca Raton, FL: CRC Press, 453-460.

Mishra, RN., Reddy, PS., Nair, S., Markandeya, G., Reddy, AR., Sopory, SK., Reddy, MK. (2007). Isolation and characterization of expressed sequence tags (ESTs) from subtracted cDNA libraries of *Pennisetum glaucum* seedlings. Plant Molecular Biology, 64, 713-732.

Muthamilarasan, M., Venkata Suresh, B., Pandey, G., Kumari, K., Parida, SK., Prasad, M. (2014a). Development of 5123 intron-length polymorphic markers for large-scale genotyping applications in foxtail millet DNA. Res, 21, 41- 52.

Muthamilarasan., M and Prasad., M. (2014.) Advances in Setaria genomics for genetic improvement of cereals and bioenergy grasses. Theoretical and Applied Genetics.

Myers, S.S., Zanobetti, A., Kloog, I., Huybers, P., Leakey, A.D.B., Bloom, A.J., Carlisle, E., Dietterich, L.H., Fitzgerald, G.,Hasegawa, T., Holbrook, N.M., Nelson, R.L.,

Ottman, M.J., Raboy, V., Sakai, H., Sartor, K.A., Schwartz, J., Seneweera, S., Tausz, M., Usui, Y. (2014). Increasing CO2 threatens human nutrition. Nature, 510, 139–142.

Nambiar, V.S., Dhaduk, J.J., Sareen, N., Shahu, T., Desai, R. (2011). Potential functional implications of pearl millet (Pennisetum glaucum) in health and disease. Journal of Applied Pharmaceutical Science, 1, 62–67.

O'Kennedy, MM., Burger, JT., Botha, FC. (2004). Pearl millet transformation system using the positive selectable marker gene phosphomannose isomerase. Plant Cell Reports, 22, 684–690.

O'Kennedy, MM., Grootboom, A., Shewry, PR. (2006). Harnessing sorghum and millet biotechnology for food and health. Journal of Cereal Science, 44, 224–235.

Padulosi, S., Mal, B., Bala Ravi, S., Gowda, J., Gowda, K., Shanthakumar, G., Yenagi, N., Dutta, M. (2009). Food security and climate change: Role of plant genetic resources of minor millets. Indian Journal of Plant Genetic Resources, 22, 1.

Pandey, G., Misra, G., Kumari, K., Gupta, S., Parida, SK., Chattopadhyay, D., Prasad, M. (2013). Genome-wide development and use of microsatellite markers for large scale genotyping applications in foxtail millet [Setaria italica (L.)]. DNA Research, 20, 197-207.

Park, KO., Ito, Y., Nagasawa, T., Choi, MR., Nishizawa, N. (2008). Effects of dietary Korean proso-millet protein on plasma adiponectin, HDL cholesterol, insulin levels, and gene expression in obese type 2 diabetic mice. Bioscience Biotechnology and Biochemistry, 72(11), 2918-2925.

Passot, S., Gnacko, F., Moukouanga, D., Lucas, M., Guyomarc'h, S., Ortega, B.M., Atkinson, J.A., Belko, M.N., Bennett, M.J., Gantet, P., Wells, D.M., Guedon, Y., Vigouroux, Y., Verdeil, J.L., Muller, B., Laplaze, L. (2016). Characterization of pearl millet root architecture and anatomy reveals three types of lateral roots. Frontiers in Plant Science, 7, 829.

Prasad and Staggenborg (2009): Growth and production of sorghum and millets. In: *Soils Plant Growth and Crop Production* (Volume 2) EOLSS Publishers Co., Ltd.

Qi, X., Xie, S., Liu, Y., Yi, F., Yu, J. (2013). Genome-wide annotation of genes and noncoding RNAs of foxtail millet in response to simulated drought stress by deep sequencing. Plant Molecular Biology, 83, 459-473.

Rahman, H., Jagadeeshselvam, N., Valarmathi, R., Sachin, B., Sasikala, R., Senthil, N., Sudhakar, D., Robin, S., Muthurajan, R. (2014). Transcriptome analysis of salinity responsiveness in contrasting genotypes of finger millet (*Eleusine coracana* L.) through RNA-sequencing. Plant Molecular Biology, 85, 485–503.

Rajaram, V., Nepolean, T., Senthilvel, S., Varshney, RK., Vadez, V., Srivastava, RK., Shah, TM., Supriya, A., Kumar, S., Kumari, BS., Bhanuprakash, A., Narasu, ML., Riera-Lizarazu, O., Hash, CT. (2013). Pearl millet [Pennisetum glaucum (L.) R. Br.] consensus linkage map constructed using four RIL mapping populations and newly developed EST-SSRs. BMC Genomics, 14, 159.

Rajasekaran, N.S., Hegde, P.S., Chandra, T.S. (2004). Effects of the antioxidant properties of millet species on oxidative stress and glycemic status in alloxan-induced rats. Nutrition Research, 25, 1109-1120.

Reddy O.S.K. (2017). Smart Millet and Human Health, Green Universe Environmental Services Society

Reddy, DS., Bhatnagar-Mathur, P., Vadez, V., Sharma, KK. (2012). Grain legumes (Soybean, Chickpea, and Peanut): Omics approaches to enhance abiotic stress tolerance. In: Improving Crop Resistance to Abiotic Stress (Eds: Tuteja N, Gill SS, Tiburcio AF, Tuteja R,) DOI: 10.1002/ 9783527632930.

Roshevits, R.Y. (1980). Grasses: An Introduction to the Study of Fodder and Cereal Grasses; NTIS: Alexandria, VA,USA.

Saleh, A.S.M., Zhang, Q., Chen, J., Shen. Q. (2013). Millet grains: Nutritional Quality, Processing, and Potential Health Benefits. Comprehensive Reviews in Food Science and Food Safety, 12, 281-295.

Sarita and Singh, Ekta. (2016). Potential of Millets: Nutrients Composition and Health Benefits. Journal Of Scientific and Innovative Research, 5(2), 46-50.

Scalbert,A., Manach, C., Morand, C., Remesy, C., Jimenez, L. (2005). Dietary polyphenols and the prevention of diseases. Critical Reviews in Food Science and Nutrition, 45, 287-306.

Senthilvel, S., Jayashree, B., Mahalakshmi, V., Kumar, PS., Nakka, S., Nepolean, T., Hash, CT. (2008). Development and mapping of simple sequence repeat markers for pearl millet from data mining of expressed sequence tags. BMC Plant Biology, 8(1), 119.

Sharma, KK and Ortiz, R. (2000). Program for the application of genetic transformation for crop improvement in the semi-arid tropics. In Vitro Cellular and Developmental Biology-Plant, 36, 83-92.

Shulaev, V., Cortes, D., Miller, G., Mittler, R. (2008). Metabolomics for plant stress response. Physiologia Plantarum, 132, 199-208.

Singh, UM., Chandra, M., Shankdhar, SC., Kumar, A. (2014). Transcriptome wide identification and validation of calcium sensor gene family in the developing spiles of finger millet genotypes for elucidating its role in grain calcium accumulation. PLoS One, 9 e103963.

Sireesha, Y., Kasetti, R.B., Swapna, S.A.S., Apparao, C. (2011). Anti hyperglycemic and hypolipidemic activities of Setaria italica seeds in STZ diabetic rats. Pathophysiology, 18(2), 159-164.

Sireesha,Y., Kasetti, RB., Nabi, SA., Swapna, S., Apparao, C. (2011). Antihyperglycemic and hypolipidemic activities of Setaria italica seeds in STZ diabetic rats. Pathophysiology, 18(2), 159-164.

Sood, S., Khulbe, RK., Gupta, AK., Agrawal, PK., Upadhyaya, HD., Bhatt JC.(2015). Barnyard millet–a potential food and feed crop of future. Plant Breeding, 134(2), 135-147.

Suresh, BV., Muthamilarasan, M., Mishra, G., Prasad, M. (2013). FmMDb: A versatile database of foxtail millet markers for millets and bioenergy grasses research. PLoS ONE, 8e71418.

Taylor, J.R.N. and Schüssler, L. (1986). The protein compositions of the different anatomical parts of sorghum grain. Journal of Cereal Science, 4, 361-369.

Taylor, J.R.N., Emmambux, M.N. (2008). Gluten-free foods and beverages from millets. In: Gallagher E, editor. Gluten-free cereal products and beverages, Burlington, MA, Elsevier, 1-27.

Taylor, MG., Vasil, V,. Vasil, IK. (1991). Histology of, and physical factors affecting, transient GUS expression in pearl millet (Pennisetum glaucum (L.) R. Br.) embryos following microprojectile bombardment. Plant Cell Reports, 10, 120–125.

Taylor, MG., Vasil, V., Vasil, IK. (1993). Enhanced GUS gene expression in cereal/grass cell suspensions and immature embryos using the maize ubiquitin-based plasmid pAHC25. Plant Cell Reports, 12, 491–495.

Thompson, T. (2009). The nutritional quality of gluten-free foods. In: Gallagher E, editor. Gluten-free food science and technology, Oxford, UK: John Wiley and Sons, Ltd. 42–51.

Ugare, R., Chimmad, B., Naik, R., Bharati, P., Itagi, S. (2011). Glycemic index and significance of barnyard millet (Echinochloafrumentacae) in type II diabetics. Journal of Food Science and Technology, 51(2), 392-395.

United Nations (2015a). The Millennium Development Goals Report 2015. New York.

United Nations (2015b). Transforming Our World: The 2030 Agenda for Sustainable Development. Resolution adopted by the General Assembly on 25 September 2015. New York.

Upadhyaya, H., Reddy, V.G., Sastry, D. (2008). Regeneration Guidelines Finger Millet; CGIAR System-Wide Genetic Resource Programme, Rome, Italy.

Vadez, V., Hash, T., Bidinger, FR., Kholova, J. (2012). Phenotyping pearl millet for adaptation to drought. Frontiers in Physiology, 3, 386.

Van Rensburg, S.J. (1981). Epidemiological and dietary evidence for a specific nutritional predisposition to esophageal cancer. Journal of the National Cancer Institute, 67,243-251.

Veeranagamallaiah, G., Jyothsnakumari, G., Thippeswamy, M., Reddy, PCO., Surabhi, G-K., Sriranganayakulu, G., Mahesh, Y., Rajasekhar, B., Madhurarekha, C., Sudhakar,.C. (2008). Proteomic analysis of salt stress responses in foxtail millet (*Setaria italica* L. cv. Prasad) seedlings. Plant Science, 175, 631- 641.

Vetriventhan, M., Upadhyaya, H., Anandakumar, C., Senthilvel, S., Parzies, H., Bharathi, A., Varshney, R., Gowda, C. (2012). Assessing genetic diversity, allelic richness and genetic relationship among races in icrisat foxtail millet core collection. Plant Genetic Resources, 10, 214–223.

Wallace, J.G., Upadhyaya, H.D., Vetriventhan, M., Buckler, E.S., Tom Hash, C., Ramu, P. (2015). The genetic makeup of a global barnyard millet germplasm collection. Plant Genome, 8.

Wang, C., Jia, G., Zhi, H., Niu, Z., Chai, Y., Li, W., Wang, Y., Li, H., Lu, P., Zhao, B., Diao, X. (2012). Genetic diversity and population structure of Chinese foxtail millet [Setaria italica (L.) Beauv.] landraces G3 (Bethesda), 2 ,769-777.

Wang, ZM., Devos, KM., Liu, CJ., Wang, RQ., Gale, MD. (1998). Construction of RFLP-based maps of foxtail millet, Setaria italica (L.) P. Beauv. Theoretical and Applied Genetics, 96, 31-36.

Watkinson, JI., Hendricks, L., Sioson, AA., Heath, LS., Bohnert, HJ., Grene, R. (2008). Tuber development phenotypes in adapted and acclimated, drought-stressed Solanum tuberosum ssp. andigena have distinct expression profiles of genes associated with carbon metabolism. Plant Physiology and Biochemistry, 46, 34-45.

Xu, J., Li, Y., Ma, X., Ding, J., Wang, K., Wang, S., Tian, Y., Zhang, H., Zhu, XG. (2013). Whole transcriptome analysis using next generation sequencing of model species Setaria viridis to support C4 photosynthesis research. Plant Molecular Biology, 83, 77- 87.

Yabuno, T. (1987). Japanese barnyard millet (Echinochloa Utilis, Poaceae) in Japan. Economic Botany, 41, 484–493.

Yadav, CB., Muthamilarasan, M., Pandey, G., Khan, Y,. Prasad, M., (2014b). Development of novel microRNA-based genetic markers in foxtail millet for genotyping applications in related grass species. Molecular Breeding.

Yang, W., Duan, L., Chen, G., Xiong, L., Liu, Q. (2013). Plant phenomics and high-throughput phenotyping: accelerating rice functional genomics using multidisciplinary technologies. Current Opinion in Plant Biology, 16, 180-187.

Yin, H., Yu, Q., Dai, Y., An, L., Li, W. (2014). Transcript profiling of foxtail millet seedlings under drought condition and discovery of a new drought- tolerant gene In: 1st International Setaria Genetics Conference, pp 24.

Zarnkow, M., Keßler, M., Back, W., Arendt, E.K., Gastl, M. (2010). Optimisation of the mashing procedure for 100% malted proso millet (Panicum miliaceum L.) as a raw material for gluten-free beverages and beers. Journal of the Institute of Brewing, 116, 141–150.

Zeller, G., Henz, SR., Widmer, CK., Sachsenberg, T., Rätsch, G., Weigel, D., Laubinger, S. (2009). Stress-induced changes in the Arabidopsis thaliana transcriptome analyzed using whole genome tiling arrays. Plant Journal, 58, 1068-1082.

Zhang, G., Liu, X., Quan, Z., Cheng, S., Xu, X., Pan, S., Xie, M., Zeng, P., Yue, Z., Wang, W., Tao, Y., Bian, C., Han, C., Xia, Q., Peng, X., Cao, R., Yang, X., Zhan, D., Hu, J., Zhang, Y., Li, H., Li, H., Li, N., Wang, J., Wang, C,. Wang, R., Guo, T., Cai, Y., Liu, C., Xiang, H., Shi, Q., Huang, P., Chen, Q., Li, Y., Wang, J., Zhao, Z., Wang., J. (2012). Genome sequence of foxtail millet (Setaria italica) provides insights into grass evolution and biofuel potential. Nature Biotechnology, 30, 549-554.

Zhang, J., Liu, T., Fu, J., Zhu, Y., Jia, J., Zheng, J., Zhao, Y., Zhang, Y., Wang, G. (2007). Construction and application of EST library from *Setaria italica* in response to dehydration stress. Genomics, 90, 121-131.

Zhang, L., Liu, R., Niu, W. (2014). Phytochemical and antiproliferative activity of proso millet. PLoS ONE, 9.

Zhang, S., Tang, C., Zhao, Q., Li, J., Yang, L., Qie, L., Fan, X., Li, L., Zhang, N., Zhao, M., Liu, X., Chai, Y., Zhang, X., Wang, H., Li, Y., Li, W., Zhi, H., Jia, G., Diao, X. (2014). Development of highly polymorphic simple sequence repeat markers using genome-wide microsatellite variant analysis in foxtail millet [Setaria italica (L.) P. Beauv]. BMC Genomics, 2, 15.

# 9

# Finger Millet: A Sustainable Approach for Nutritional Security and its Biofortification

Pratikshya Mishra[1*] and Smruti Ranjan Padhan[2]

[1] Department of Plant Breeding and Genetics, Odisha University of Agriculture and Technology, Bhubaneswar - 751003, India

[2] Division of Agronomy, ICAR-Indian Agricultural Research Institute, Pusa campus, New Delhi- 110012.

**ABSTRACT**

Finger millet (*Eleusine coracana*) with its high nutritional value, drought tolerance, and ability to grow in a range of agro-ecological conditions, finger millet has emerged as a promising crop for addressing the pressing challenges of food security and malnutrition by encompassing an excellent source of protein, dietary fibre, and essential micronutrients such as iron, calcium, and zinc. It is also gluten-free, making it an ideal food for people with celiac disease or gluten intolerance. Biofortified finger millet can offer a range of potential benefits, from improving cognitive development and reducing stunting in children, to enhancing immune function and reducing the incidence of anemia in adults.However, there are several challenges that must be overcome to fully realize the potential of finger millet as a sustainable crop for nutritional security. These include improving agronomic practices, addressing the issue of low yields, promoting market access for small-scale farmers, and mitigating the effects of climate change. This chapter explores the potential of finger millet as a sustainable crop for addressing the challenges of food security and malnutrition and concludes by highlighting promising areas for future research on finger millet, such as exploring the use of finger millet in innovative food products and investigating the potential of finger millet as a source of bioactive compounds with potential health benefits.

*Keywords*: Finger millet, bio-fortification, agronomic practices, sustainable approaches.

## Introduction

Finger millet (*Eleusine coracana* L.) is one of the ancient cereal crops in the world and is believed to have been domesticated in East Africa around 5000 years ago. It is one of the important source of food crop in many countries, particularly in Africa and Asia, where it is commonly grown by smallholder farmers for subsistence

* Corresponding author.

and as a cash crop. It is known by many local names such as ragi in India, wimbi in East Africa, and coracan in South Africa. Finger millet is a highly nutritious crop that is rich in protein, dietary fiber, minerals, and vitamins. It is also gluten-free, making it an important food source for people with celiac disease or gluten intolerance. The grain has a low glycemic index, which means it releases sugar into the bloodstream slowly, making it an ideal food for people with diabetes. In addition, finger millet is a hardy crop that can tolerate drought, pests, and diseases, making it well-suited to smallholder farming in marginal environments. Despite its nutritional and agronomic advantages, finger millet has been largely neglected by policymakers, researchers, and development agencies. Due to which production has deteriorated in many countries, and the crop is often seen as a "poor man's food" with low market value. This has led to a perception that finger millet is an inferior crop, which has further hindered its adoption and promotion.

However, there is growing recognition of the importance of finger millet in addressing food and nutrition security in many parts of the world. Several studies have highlighted the nutritional benefits of finger millet, and efforts are underway to promote its consumption and production. For example, ICRISAT has developed high-yielding, disease-resistant varieties of finger millet that are well-suited to smallholder farming systems. In addition, several NGOs and government programs are working to promote the crop and develop value chains that can increase its market value and provide income opportunities for farmers.

## Nutritional profile of finger millet with reference to other crops

Finger milletis a staple crop grown in many parts of the world, particularly in Africa and Asia. It is an ancient grain that has been cultivated for thousands of years and has come to the spotlight in the last few decades due to its nutritional value. Finger millet is a good source of carbohydrates (complex forms of carbohydrates) and dietary fiber, which helps to regulate blood sugar levels and maintain a healthy digestive system. It is also rich in essential minerals like calcium, iron, and potassium, which are important for maintaining healthy bones, red blood cells, and electrolyte balance (Shwetha and Jamuna 2016). Furthermore, finger millet is an excellent source of protein since it contains all the important amino acids that the body needs. Also, it is gluten-free, making it a great replacement for those who have celiac disease or gluten intolerance. With respect to other cereal crops, finger millet has a higher nutritional value. For instance, it contains more iron than rice, wheat, or maize, making it an ideal crop for people with iron-deficiency anemia (Adnan *et al.,* 2021). It also has a lower glycemic index than other grains, which means it releases sugar into the bloodstream at a slower rate, making it a suitable crop for people with diabetes. As compared to other cereals like wheat, finger millet has a higher fiber content, which helps to regulate bowel movements and promote digestive health (Table 1).

**Table 1 :** Nutrient profile of finger millet with comparison to other major crops (Alvarado-Raya *et al.,* 2021)

| Nutrient (per 100 g) | Finger Millet | Wheat | Rice | Maize | Sorghum |
|---|---|---|---|---|---|
| Calories | 378 | 329 | 130 | 365 | 329 |
| Protein (g) | 7.3 | 12.6 | 2.7 | 9.4 | 11.3 |
| Fat (g) | 1.3 | 1.5 | 0.3 | 4.7 | 3.3 |
| Carbohydrates (g) | 72.9 | 71.2 | 28.7 | 76.0 | 72.1 |
| Fiber (g) | 3.6 | 12.2 | 0.3 | 7.3 | 6.3 |
| Calcium (mg) | 344 | 34 | 10 | 7 | 28 |
| Iron (mg) | 3.9 | 3.9 | 0.7 | 0.5 | 4.4 |
| Magnesium (mg) | 114 | 138 | 35 | 127 | 0 |
| Phosphorus (mg) | 283 | 288 | 115 | 210 | 287 |
| Potassium (mg) | 408 | 363 | 115 | 287 | 350 |
| Zinc (mg) | 2.7 | 2.7 | 1.0 | 2.7 | 0.9 |
| Vitamin B1 (mg) | 0.33 | 0.4 | 0.1 | 0.4 | 0.4 |
| Vitamin B2 (mg) | 0.19 | 0.1 | 0.0 | 0.1 | 0.1 |
| Vitamin B3 (mg) | 1.1 | 5.5 | 1.6 | 3.6 | 2.1 |
| Vitamin B6 (mg) | 0.35 | 0.3 | 0.2 | 0.1 | 0.3 |
| Folate (mcg) | 44 | 44 | 8 | 42 | 21 |
| Vitamin E (mg) | 0.05 | 0.1 | 0.1 | 0.1 | 0.1 |
| Vitamin K (mcg) | 0.9 | 0.2 | 1.9 | 0.3 | 0.0 |

(g, gram; mg, milligram; mcg, microgram)

It also contains a higher amount of antioxidants, which helps to neutralize free radicals in the body and prevent cell damage (Bello *et al.,* 2021). In terms of protein content, finger millet contains more protein than rice and maize, making it a suitable crop for vegetarians and vegans (Birol *et al.,* 2014). It also contains a higher amount of essential amino acids like methionine and lysine, which are often lacking in plant-based diets. In comparison to other cereals like wheat and rice, finger millet has a higher calcium concentration. Because of this, it is the perfect crop for those who cannot consume dairy products or have a lactose allergy. As a result of its excellent nutritional content, finger millet is a nutritive and adaptable crop that has grown in popularity recently.It is rich in complex carbohydrates, dietary fiber, essential minerals, and protein, making it a suitable crop for people with various dietary requirements. Compared to other cereals, finger millet has a higher nutritional value and is an excellent alternative for people with iron-deficiency anaemia, diabetes, lactose intolerance, or gluten intolerance (Sood *et al.,* 2017).

## Agronomic practices for finger millet cultivation

Agronomic practices play a vital role in the cultivation of finger millet, also known as ragi. Proper cultivation practices can ensure a good yield, increase the efficiency of resources, and reduce the negative impact on the environment. Table 2 summarizes the key agronomic practices for finger millet cultivation. In conclusion, proper agronomic practices are crucial for successful finger millet cultivation. By following the above practices, farmers can ensure a good yield, reduce the negative impact on the environment, and increase the efficiency of resources (Table 2).

**Table 2 :** Agronomic practices for the cultivation of finger millet.

| **Agronomic Practice** | **Description** |
|---|---|
| Land Preparation | Clear the field of all debris, remove weeds, and plough the land to a depth of 10-15 cm. |
| Seed Selection | Select healthy and vigorous seeds that are free from pests and diseases. Use certified seeds to ensure better yield and quality. |
| Seed Rate | Sow the seeds at a rate of 10-12 kg per hectare. |
| Time of Sowing | Sow the seeds during the onset of the monsoon season or in June-July. |
| Spacing | 22.5-30 cm from row to rows and 7.5-15 cm in between plants. |
| Fertilizer Application | Apply well-decomposed farmyard manure (FYM) at a rate of 10-12 tons per hectare or 2-3 tons of compost. |
| Nutrient Management | Apply 50 kg N, 25 kg $P_2O_5$, and 25 kg $K_2O$ per hectare as a basal dose. Apply another 25 kg N per hectare after 30 days of sowing. |
| Irrigation | Provide adequate irrigation to the crop during the growing period. Irrigate the field at 10-15 days interval during the dry season. |
| Weed Management | Control weeds by hand weeding, mechanical weeding, or use of herbicides. |
| Pest and Disease Management | Control pests and diseases by<br>• cultural practices<br>• chemical control<br>• using resistant varieties<br>• biological control |
| Harvesting | Harvest the crop when the grain turns golden brown and the earhead starts to droop. |
| Post-Harvest Handling | Dry the harvested crop in the sun for 2-3 days and thresh it using a thresher. Clean the grain and store it in a dry and cool place. |

## Challenges in finger millet cultivation

Finger millet, despite its many nutritional benefits and the potential for high yields, finger millet cultivation is faced with several challenges that limit its production and profitability. In this article, we will explore some of the major challenges facing finger millet cultivation.

- **Low yield:** One of the major challenges facing finger millet cultivation is low yield. The average yield of finger millet is often low, compared to other cereal crops such as maize and wheat. This is due to several factors, including poor soil fertility, limited access to quality seeds, and inadequate agronomic practices.
- **Pests and diseases:** Finger millet is susceptible to various pests and diseases that can cause significant yield losses. Some of the common pests that attack finger millet include stem borers, shoot fly, and aphids, while diseases such as head smut, blast, and rust can also cause significant damage. Controlling these pests and diseases can be difficult, especially for smallholder farmers who may lack the knowledge and resources to manage them effectively.
- **Climate change:** Climate change is having a significant impact on finger millet cultivation, with changes in rainfall patterns and increased temperatures affecting crop growth and yield. Erratic rainfall, prolonged dry spells, and rising temperatures can all lead to reduced yields and increased pest and disease incidence.
- **Lack of access to markets:** Finger millet farmers often face challenges in accessing markets for their produce. The lack of established markets and reliable market information can result in low prices and reduced profitability. This, in turn, can discourage farmers from investing in finger millet cultivation.
- **Limited processing facilities:** Finger millet is a highly nutritious crop that has the potential for value addition through processing. However, the lack of processing facilities, especially at the smallholder level, limits the potential for value addition and market diversification. This can result in low prices for the raw product and reduced profitability for farmers.
- **Limited research and development:** There have been limited research and development in finger millet cultivation, with most resources directed towards more popular crops such as maize and wheat. This has limited the development of new varieties, agronomic practices, and processing technologies that could help to improve yields and profitability.
- **Limited policy support:** The lack of policy support for finger millet cultivation has also contributed to the challenges facing the sector. The absence of policies that promote finger millet production, processing, and marketing limits the potential for investment and growth in the sector.

- Albeit, finger millet cultivation faces several challenges that limit its potential for growth and profitability, addressing these challenges will require a concerted effort by various stakeholders, including governments, researchers, extension agents, farmers, and private sector actors. By investing in research and development, improving access to markets, and providing policy support, it is possible to overcome these challenges and unlock the full potential of finger millet cultivation.

## Biofortification of finger millet

Biofortification is the process of increasing the nutritional value of crops through plant breeding techniques (Shukla *et al.,* 2017). Finger milletis a nutritious cereal crop that is particularly rich in iron and calcium. However, the bioavailability of these nutrients in finger millet can be low due to the presence of antinutrients, which bind to minerals and reduce their absorption. Biofortification of finger millet offers a promising solution to improve the bioavailability of nutrients and address micronutrient deficiencies (Lakshmi and Sreeramulu *et al.,* 2014). There are several approaches to biofortification of finger millet, including conventional breeding, genetic engineering, and agronomic practices.

Conventional breeding: Conventional breeding involves selecting and breeding plants with desirable traits, such as high nutrient content. The presence of variability in a crop species the first basis of selection and undertaking any crop improvement programme. Finger millet is still a less explored plant and has ample number of variations present in them (Chebii and Kimaru, 2020). This approach has been used to develop finger millet varieties with higher iron and calcium content (Gao *et al.,* 2019). For example, the finger millet variety Kalukombu 2 has been developed through conventional breeding and has been shown to have a higher iron content than traditional varieties (Ekesa *et al.,* 2017).

Genetic engineering: Genetic engineering involves introducing specific genes into plants to enhance their nutritional content. This approach has been used to develop finger millet varieties with enhanced iron and zinc content (Devi and Prabhakaran 2018). For example, the finger millet variety IR68144 has been genetically engineered to express a gene from the common bean that enhances iron and zinc absorption. Agronomic practices: Practices such as crop rotation, intercropping, and fertilization can also influence the nutrient content of finger millet.

For example, intercropping finger millet with legumes such as cowpea can increase the nitrogen content of the soil, which can lead to higher yields and increased nutrient content. Similarly, the application of fertilizers can increase the nutrient content of finger millet (Antil *et al.,* 2019). Biofortification of finger millet has several benefits and is in a huge demand. This increasing demand is studied in details by Meenakshi *et al.,* 2013 and these are as follows:

Firstly, it can help to address micronutrient deficiencies, which are a major public health concern, particularly in developing countries. Iron and calcium deficiencies, in particular, are widespread, and biofortified finger millet can provide a low-cost, sustainable solution to this problem (Sankaran *et al.,* 2017).

Secondly, biofortified finger millet can improve the economic prospects of smallholder farmers. Biofortified crops often command higher prices in the market, as they are perceived to be of higher quality and have a higher nutritional value. This can lead to increased income for farmers and improved food security for their families (Pushpavalli *et al.,* 2018).

The biofortification of finger millet can help to promote sustainable agriculture. By improving the nutritional content of crops, farmers can reduce their reliance on synthetic fertilizers and pesticides, which can be harmful to the environment and human health. Biofortified finger millet is also more resilient to climate change, as it can tolerate drought and other environmental stresses. Despite the potential benefits of biofortification, there are also challenges to its implementation. Firstly, the cost of developing and distributing biofortified seeds can be high, which may limit the uptake of these varieties by smallholder farmers. Secondly, there may be resistance to the adoption of genetically engineered varieties due to concerns about their safety and potential impacts on the environment. Finally, there may be cultural barriers to the adoption of biofortified foods, as people may prefer traditional varieties or be hesitant to consume foods that are perceived to be genetically modified. In conclusion, biofortification of finger millet offers a promising solution to address micronutrient deficiencies and promote sustainable agriculture. Conventional breeding, genetic engineering, and agronomic practices can all be used to improve the nutritional content of finger millet. While there are challenges to the implementation of biofortification, its potential benefits for public health, smallholder farmers, and the environment make it a promising avenue for future research and development.

## Sustainable approaches for finger millet cultivation

Being a hardy crop finger millet can tolerate drought and other environmental stresses, making it a valuable crop for smallholder farmers in developing countries. Sustainable approaches for finger millet cultivation can help to reduce these impacts and promote long-term food security.There are several sustainable approaches for finger millet cultivation, including conservation agriculture, agroforestry, and organic farming.

Conservation agriculture: A sustainable farming method called "conservation agriculture" seeks to lessen soil erosion, boost soil fertility, and boost crop yields. The three key practises used in this strategy are limited tillage, crop rotation, and soil cover. Less soil disturbance during planting and harvesting through the use of minimum tillage contributes to the preservation of soil structure and the control of erosion. To increase soil fertility and lower pest and disease pressure, crop rotation entails alternating various crops on the same piece of land. To prevent soil erosion and increase soil fertility, soil cover entails leaving agricultural remains on the soil's surface. It has been demonstrated that conservation agriculture can increase finger millet production and quality while minimising negative environmental effects.

Agroforestry: It involves integrating trees and shrubs into agricultural landscapes to provide a range of ecological and economic benefits. For finger millet cultivation, agroforestry can help to improve soil fertility, reduce erosion, and provide shade for the crop. The use of nitrogen-fixing trees and shrubs can also reduce the need for synthetic fertilizers. In addition, agroforestry can provide a source of income and food for smallholder farmers, as they can sell the fruits, nuts, and other products of the trees and shrubs.

Organic farming: Organic farming is a sustainable farming approach that avoids the use of synthetic fertilizers and pesticides, and instead relies on natural inputs such as compost and cover crops. Organic farming can improve soil fertility, reduce water pollution, and promote biodiversity. For finger millet cultivation, organic farming can help to reduce the environmental impacts of cultivation, while also producing a high-quality, nutritious crop that can command a premium price in the market (Subramanian *et al.,* 2020).

Sustainable approaches for finger millet cultivation have several benefits. Firstly, they can help to improve soil fertility and reduce soil erosion, which can improve the long-term productivity of the land. Secondly, they can reduce the environmental impacts of cultivation, such as water pollution and biodiversity loss. Thirdly, sustainable approaches can help to promote food security by improving the yield and quality of finger millet, which is an important staple crop for many smallholder farmers in developing countries (Elanchezhian and Abdul Jaleel 2020).

However, there are also challenges to the adoption of sustainable approaches for finger millet cultivation. Firstly, there may be a lack of knowledge and resources among smallholder farmers to implement these practices. Secondly, there may be resistance to the adoption of these practices due to cultural or economic reasons. For example, farmers may be reluctant to switch to organic farming if they perceive it as less profitable than conventional farming. Finally, there may be a lack of policy support for sustainable agriculture, such as subsidies or extension services.

In conclusion, sustainable approaches for finger millet cultivation can help to improve the long-term productivity of the land, reduce environmental impacts, and promote food security (Rai *et al.*, 2019). Conservation agriculture, agroforestry, and organic farming are all viable options for smallholder farmers, but their adoption may be influenced by factors such as knowledge, resources, and policy support. To promote sustainable finger millet cultivation, there is a need for continued research, education, and policy support to overcome these challenges and promote the adoption of these practices (Table 3).

**Table 3 :** Finger millet-based cropping systems.

| Cropping system | Crop combination | Advantages |
|---|---|---|
| Finger millet-maize cropping system | Finger millet and maize | • Drought-tolerant crops<br>• Efficient use of land and water resources<br>• Reduced pest and disease incidence |
| Finger millet-legume intercropping system | Finger millet and cowpea, groundnut, or pigeon pea | • Improved soil fertility and nitrogen fixation<br>• Enhanced yield of both crops<br>• Complementary nutritional benefits |

## Finger millet-based food products

It is a versatile crop that can be used to produce a range of food products, from traditional dishes to modern convenience foods. Finger millet-based food products are gaining popularity due to their nutritional benefits and versatility (Ghatak *et al.*, 2020). Some popular finger millet-based food products are:

Porridge: Finger millet porridge is a traditional breakfast dish in many parts of Africa and Asia. It is made by cooking finger millet flour with water or milk and sweetening it with sugar or honey. Finger millet porridge is a nutritious and filling breakfast option, as it is high in fibre, protein, and minerals.

Flatbreads: Finger millet flour can be used to make flatbreads, such as roti, chapati, and dosa. These flatbreads are a staple in many Indian and African diets and are often served with curries or other side dishes. Finger millet flatbreads are a healthy alternative to wheat-based bread, as they are gluten-free and high in fibre (Sawicka and Szczyglowska *et al.*, 2016).

Baked goods: Finger millet flour can also be used to make a variety of baked goods, such as cakes, cookies, and muffins. Finger millet baked goods are a nutritious alternative to traditional baked goods, as they are high in fibre, protein, and minerals (Anil Kumar *et al.*, 2015). They are also a good option for people with gluten sensitivities.

Snacks: Finger millet-based snacks are becoming increasingly popular, as they are a healthy alternative to traditional snack foods. Some popular finger millet snacks include roasted finger millet, finger millet chips, and finger millet-based granola bars. These snacks are high in fibre, protein, and minerals, making them a nutritious option for on-the-go snacking.

Beverages: Finger millet can also be used to produce a variety of beverages, such as beer, smoothies, and energy drinks. Finger millet-based beverages are a good source of energy and nutrition, as they are high in fibre, protein, and minerals. They are also a good alternative to traditional sugary drinks, as they are often sweetened with natural ingredients like honey or fruit.

Finger millet-based food products have several nutritional benefits. Firstly, finger millet is high in fiber, which can help to promote digestive health and prevent chronic diseases like diabetes and heart disease. Secondly, finger millet is a good source of protein, which is important for building and repairing tissues in the body. Finally, finger millet is rich in minerals like calcium, iron, and zinc, which are essential for bone health, immune function, and overall health (Alamu and Olaniyi, 2018).

In addition to their nutritional benefits, finger millet-based food products are also sustainable. Finger millet is a hardy crop that can grow in a variety of environments, making it an ideal crop for smallholder farmers in developing countries. Finger millet is also drought-resistant, which is important in regions where water is scarce. However, there are also challenges to the production and consumption of finger millet-based food products. Firstly, there may be a lack of knowledge and resources among smallholder farmers to produce finger millet in large quantities. Secondly, finger millet-based food products may not be widely available in supermarkets and grocery stores, which can limit their accessibility to consumers. Finally, there may be a lack of awareness among consumers about the nutritional benefits of finger millet, which can limit demand for these products.

In conclusion, finger millet-based food products are a nutritious and sustainable option for consumers. They are versatile and can be used to produce a range of traditional and modern food products. Finger millet-based food products are high in fibre, protein, and minerals,making them a healthy alternative to many other processed foods (Saleem *et al.,* 2019). However, challenges remain in the production and consumption of finger millet-based food products, including lack of knowledge and resources among farmers, limited availability in stores, and lack of awareness among consumers. Addressing these challenges will be key to promoting finger millet-based food products as a viable and sustainable food source for the future.

## Future prospects

Finger millet (*Eleusine coracana*) is a hardy, drought-tolerant crop that has been grown for thousands of years in Africa and Asia. It is a staple food for millions of people, particularly in arid and semi-arid regions where other crops struggle to grow. Finger millet is a highly nutritious crop, rich in protein, fiber, and minerals such as calcium, iron, and zinc. It also has a low glycaemic index, making it an ideal food for people with diabetes.

A. **Importance of finger millet for nutritional security:** Finger millet plays an important role in ensuring nutritional security, particularly in developing countries where malnutrition is a major problem. It is a rich source of essential nutrients, and studies have shown that it can help to prevent malnutrition, especially in women and children. In many regions, finger millet is also used as a weaning food for infants, as it is easy to digest and provides a range of essential nutrients.
B. **Role of biofortification in enhancing the nutritional value of finger millet:** Biofortification is a promising approach for enhancing the nutritional value of finger millet. Researchers have been working on developing finger millet varieties that are high in iron and zinc, two essential minerals that are often lacking in the diets of people in developing countries. By biofortifying finger millet, we can increase its nutritional value, making it an even more valuable food source for consumers.
C. **Sustainable approaches for promoting finger millet cultivation:** Sustainable approaches are essential for promoting finger millet cultivation and ensuring its long-term viability as a food crop. One such approach is agroforestry, which involves the integration of trees into farming systems to improve soil health, increase crop productivity, and promote biodiversity. By incorporating trees like moringa, neem, and acacia into finger millet farming systems, we can improve soil fertility, conserve water, and provide additional sources of income for farmers.Another sustainable approach is the use of conservation agriculture techniques such as minimum tillage, intercropping, and crop rotation. These techniques help to improve soil health, reduce soil erosion, and conserve water, leading to better crop yields and increased sustainability (Abrokwah *et al.,* 2017).
D. **Future research directions:** There are several areas of research that hold promise for the future of finger millet cultivation. One such area is the development of improved finger millet varieties that are more resistant to pests and diseases, as well as more drought-tolerant. This will help to ensure that finger millet remains a viable crop in the face of changing climate conditions.

Another area of research is the development of finger millet-based functional foods, which can help to address specific nutritional deficiencies and health problems. For example, finger millet-based products could be developed to address iron and zinc deficiencies, or to help manage diabetes.

## Finger millet in different cropping system

Finger millet is an important cereal crop that has been cultivated for thousands of years and is well adapted to low-input and subsistence farming systems, making it an ideal crop for smallholder farmers. In addition, finger millet has a number of agronomic and nutritional benefits, making it a valuable addition to cropping systems around the world.

**Role of Finger Millet in Cropping Systems:** Finger millet is a versatile crop that can be grown in a widespreadarea of agroecological zones. It is a resilient and drought-tolerant crop that can endure a range of stressful environments, thus making it suitable to be grown on marginal lands. In addition, finger millet has a short growing season, ranging from 90 to 120 days, which allows farmers to grow it as a second crop in the same field after the main crop has been harvested.Finger millet is often grown as a subsistence crop by smallholder farmers in developing countries. It is typically intercropped with other crops such as legumes, pulses, and vegetables, which helps to improve soil fertility and reduce pest and disease pressures. Intercropping also provides farmers with a diversified source of income and food security, as they can sell the surplus of the intercropped crops in the market. Finger millet can also be grown as a cash crop in commercial farming systems. In India, for example, finger millet is grown on a large scale in the semi-arid regions of the country. It is typically grown as a sole crop or intercropped with legumes, and is used for the production of a range of food products such as flour, porridge, and snacks.

**Agronomic Benefits of Finger millet:** It has a number of agronomic benefits that make it a valuable addition to cropping systems. Firstly, finger millet is a low-input crop, which means that it requires minimal inputs such as pesticides, insecticides, weedicides and fertilizers. This makes it a cost-effective crop for small farm holders who cannot afford expensive inputs (Singh *et al.,* 2018).Secondly, finger millet has a high-water use efficiency, which means that it can produce high yields with minimal water. This makes it an ideal crop for regions with low rainfall and limited access to irrigation (Siddalinga and Reddy, 2016). Thirdly, finger millet has a deep root system that can penetrate the soil to a depth of up to 2 meters. This makes it an effective crop for improving soil fertility and structure, as it can break up compacted soil layers and improve water infiltration (Singh *et al.,* 2017).

Some important cropping systems involving finger-millet are as follows:

**Finger millet-groundnut:** Finger millet and groundnut are important crops that are widely grown in India, particularly in the states of Karnataka, Andhra Pradesh, and Tamil Nadu. The finger millet-groundnut cropping system is a popular intercrop system in these regions. In this system, finger millet is sown in rows and groundnut is sown in between the rows. The finger millet provides a good support system for the groundnut, which grows as a trailing crop. This system not only provides a good yield of both crops, but also helps to reduce soil erosion and improve soil fertility.

**Finger millet-pigeon pea:** The finger millet-pigeon pea cropping system is another popular intercrop system in India. Pigeon pea is an important legume crop that is grown for its high protein content and nitrogen-fixing ability. In this system, finger millet and pigeon pea are grown together in the same field. The finger millet provides a good support system for the pigeon pea, which grows as a trailing crop.

**Finger millet-sorghum:** Finger millet and sorghum are both important cereal crops that are widely grown in Africa. In the finger millet-sorghum cropping system, the two crops are grown together in the same field. This system helps to lessen soil erosion and improve soil fertility.

**Finger millet-cowpea:** Cowpea is a prime legume crop that is widely grown in Africa. In the finger millet-cowpea cropping system, the two crops are grown together in the same field. This system helps to improve soil fertility and reduce soil erosion.

Another example of a finger millet-based cropping system is intercropping with legumes. Legumes, such as cowpea, groundnut, or pigeon pea, can be planted in between finger millet rows. This helps in fixing atmospheric nitrogen in the soil, thus improving the soil productivity and increasing the yield of both crops (Ogweno *et al.,* 2014). Moreover, legumes are also known to be excellent sources of protein, which can complement the nutritional value of finger millet. This cropping system has been found to be successful in regions of sub-Saharan Africa, where both finger millet and legumes are important crops.

## Finger millet & the International Year of Millets

India has already celebrated the National Year of Milletsin 2018 (Agriculture and Farmers' Welfare 2018; ICAR 2019) and the year 2023 has been declared as the International Year of Millets by the United Nations, recognizing the importance of millets in promoting food security, nutrition, and sustainability (Malhotra, 2023). India, as one of the leading producers and consumers of millets, has a substantial role to play in this initiative. *Eleusine coracana* is one of the majorly grown millets in India, and it has the potential to play a major role in achieving the goals of the International Year of Millets.Despite its many nutritional and health benefits, the consumption of finger millet has declined in India in recent years, mainly due to the availability of cheaper and more convenient alternatives such as rice and wheat. The International Year of Millets provides an opportunity to promote the consumption of all major and minor millets including finger millet as a part of a healthy and sustainable diet.

One of the key strategies for promoting finger millet in the International Year of Millets is to increase awareness about its nutritional and health benefits. This can be done through various awareness campaigns, including social media campaigns, radio and television programs, and seminars and workshops. The government can also work with private sector companies to promote the production and consumption of finger millet-based products, such as biscuits, bread, and snacks. Another important strategy is to promote the cultivation of finger millet among farmers. The government can provide subsidies and incentives to farmers who grow finger millet, and promote the use of modern farming techniques such as precision farming, which can drastically help save the crop from crop failure and substantially increase the produce of the crop. The government can also work with private sector companies to provide market linkages and ensure that farmers get a fair price for their produce.Research and development can help promote the cultivation and consumption of finger millet. Research can be conducted to develop new finger millet varieties that are more resilient to pests and diseases, and can withstand harsh climatic conditions. Research can also be conducted to develop new finger millet-based products that are more palatable and appealing to consumers. The International Year of Millets provides an opportunity to promote the consumption and cultivation of finger millet in India. Finger millet has the potential to promoting food security, nutrition, and sustainability, and the government and private sector should work together to promote its cultivation and consumption. With the right strategies in place, finger millet can become a key component of India's food security and nutrition strategy in the years to come

## Conclusion

In conclusion, finger millet has emerged as a promising crop for addressing the pressing challenges of food security and malnutrition. With its high nutritional value, drought tolerance, and ability to grow in a range of agro-ecological conditions, finger millet is well-suited to promoting sustainable agriculture and improving nutrition outcomes. One of the most promising avenues for enhancing the nutritive value of finger millet is biofortification, which involves breeding crops with higher levels of key micronutrients such as iron and zinc. Biofortified finger millet can offer a range of potential benefits, from improving cognitive development and reducing stunting in children, to enhancing immune function and reducing the incidence of anaemia in adults. However, there are several challenges that must be overcome to fully realize the potential of finger millet as a sustainable crop for nutritional security. These include improving agronomic practices, addressing the issue of low yields, promoting market access for small-scale farmers, and mitigating the effects of climate change.To address these challenges, a range of sustainable approaches to finger millet cultivation have been developed, including intercropping, crop rotation, and conservation agriculture. By adopting these approaches, farmers can improve the resilience of their crops to environmental stressors, enhance soil fertility, and improve their livelihoods. In addition to biofortification and sustainable cultivation practices, there are also several other promising areas for future research on finger millet. These include exploring the use of finger millet in innovative food products, such as biscuits, pastas and gluten-free alternatives, as well as investigating the potential of finger millet as a source of bioactive compounds with potential health benefits. Overall, finger millet offers tremendous potential as a sustainable crop for promoting nutritional security and enhancing the well-being of communities around the world. By embracing sustainable cultivation practices, investing in biofortification, and exploring new avenues for innovation, we can unlock the full potential of this valuable crop and build a more equitable and sustainable food system for all.

## References

Abrokwah, C., Wiredu-Ankrah, E.,Akromah, E. O., and Salifu, F. K. (2017). Participatory variety selection for improving yield, adaptability and quality of finger millet (Eleusine coracana) in the drylands of Ghana. African Journal of Agricultural Research, 12 (6), 416-424.

Adnan, M., Tahir, M., Hussain, M., Afzal, I., and Shahid, M. (2021). Prospects of finger millet (Eleusine coracana L.) as a novel food crop. Journal of Food Science and Technology, 58 (1), 22-34.

Agriculture and Farmers' Welfare. (2018). Government of India launches National Year of Millets. Retrieved from https://pib.gov.in/newsite/PrintRelease.aspx?relid=177731

Alamu, E. O., and Olaniyi, J. O. (2018). Finger millet (Eleusine coracana L.): a review of its nutritional and health benefits. Journal of Food Research, 7 (2), 1-12.

Alvarado-Raya, C., Reyes-Pérez, J. J., Torres-Pacheco, I., and Guevara-Gonzalez, R. G. (2021). Advances and perspectives of the use of biostimulants in the production of maize, wheat, and millet: A review. Agronomy, 11 (3), 474.

Anil Kumar, P., and Kavi Kishor, P. B. (2015). Exploitation of finger millet as a functional food ingredient: a review. Journal of food science and technology, 52 (3), 1856-1865.

Antil, N. S., Gupta, V., Kaur, S., and Singh, K. (2019). Effect of agronomic practices on nutrient content and mineral uptake of finger millet (Eleusine coracana). International Journal of Chemical Studies, 7 (6), 1036-1040.

Bello, A. U., Fagbemi, T. N., and Gbadamosi, S. O. (2021). Phytochemical, Nutritional and Antioxidant Potentials of Finger Millet (Eleusine coracana) Grains Grown in Nigeria. Journal of Food Science and Nutrition Therapy, 7 (1), 24-31.

Birol, L. R., Meenakshi, A., Oparinde, V., Perez, M., and Zeller, D. (2014). What is the scope for fortification of maize flour and maize meal in Africa? Annals of the New York Academy of Sciences, 1312 (1), 26-38.

Chebii, S. K., and Kimaru, A. G. (2020). Variability in morphological traits among finger millet (Eleusine coracana (L.) Gaertn) varieties in Kenya. Journal of Plant Sciences, 8 (1), 1-7.

Devi, G. R., and Prabhakaran, A. J. (2018). Biofortification of finger millet (Eleusine coracana) with iron and zinc: a review. Journal of Food Science and Technology, 55 (3), 771-776.

Ekesa, N., Opondo, A., and Oduor, G. (2017). An Overview of the Nutritional and Health Benefits of Millets: A Comprehensive Literature Review. In Millets and Sorghum: Biology and Genetic Improvement (pp. 301-320). Springer, Cham.

Elanchezhian, R., and Abdul Jaleel, C. (2020). Sustainable cultivation of finger millet (Eleusine coracana L.) under changing climatic scenario: A review. Journal of King Saud University-Science, 32 (6), 3485-3491.

Gao, F., Wu, X., Song, H., Su, Y., Chen, S., and Sun, G. (2019). Genetic diversity and population structure of global finger millet (Eleusine coracana (L.) Gaertn.) germplasm collection based on microsatellite markers. PLoS One, 14 (12), e0226787.

Ghatak, A., Das, A., Saha, S., Bhattacharya, S., and Jana, B. B. (2020). Production and Nutritional Properties of Finger Millet (Eleusine coracana L.) Based Value-Added Foods: A Comprehensive Review. Food Reviews International, 36 (7), 654-679

ICAR. (2019). ICAR celebrates the National Year of Millets. Indian Council of Agricultural Research.Retrieved from https://www.icar.org.in/content/icar-celebrates-national-year-millets

Lakshmi, S. S. V. S. and Sreeramulu, R. (2014). Nutritional composition and antinutritional factors of malted finger millet (Eleusine coracana) flour as influenced by various domestic processing methods. Journal of Food Science and Technology, 51 (7), 1533-1539.

Malhotra, S. K. (2023). International Year of Millets – 2023, proposal from India – Application to UN adoption. Indian Farming, 73 (1), 10–15. Retrieved from https://epubs.icar.org.in/index.php/IndFarm/article/view/132560

Meenakshi, A., Banerji, N., Kumar, A., and Chauhan, N. (2013). Generating demand for biofortified foods: A review of drivers and challenges. Food Policy, 42, 176-189.

Ogweno, M. O., Wawire, C. W.,Aguyoh, J. N., and Rono, F. K. (2014). Effect of integrated nitrogen and phosphorus management practices on productivity and profitability of finger millet (Eleusine coracana) in Kenya. Agricultural Sciences, 5 (14), 1414-1424.

Pushpavalli, P. N., Sreedhar, K. S., and Babu, S. S. (2018). Finger millet for food and nutritional security: Realizing the neglected potential. Journal of the Science of Food and Agriculture, 98 (5), 1558-1568.

Rai, K. N., Bhattacharya, S., andVadez, V. (2019). Millets for food security in the context of climate change: A review. Agronomy for Sustainable Development, 39 (4), 28.

Saleem, M. F., Akram, M., Anjum, F. M., Khan, M. I., Zulfiqar, B., and Hussain, S. (2019). Effect of Cooking Methods on Bioactive Components of Finger Millet (Eleusine coracana L.) Flour. Journal of Food Processing and Preservation, 43 (11), e14291.

Sankaran, M., Khan, A. A., and Gupta, S. (2017). Nutrition, Health Benefits, and Industrial Uses of Finger Millet (Eleusine coracana L.): A Review. International Journal of Food Properties, 20 (sup2), S3160-S3173.

Sawicka, B., andSzczyglowska, M. (2016). The potential of cereals and pseudo-cereals for the production of gluten-free pasta. Critical Reviews in Food Science and Nutrition, 56 (1), 135-145.

Shukla, S., Bhargava, A., and Chatterjee, A. (2017). Biofortification of staple crops: Progress and prospects. Journal of Agricultural and Food Chemistry, 65 (36), 7831-7848.

Shwetha, C. B., and Jamuna, M. Y. (2016). Finger millet (Eleusine coracana L.): A review of its nutritional properties, processing, and plausible health benefits. Food Science and Human Wellness, 5 (3), 149-157.

Siddalinga, R. S. and Reddy, M. P. (2016). Improving the productivity of finger millet (Eleusine coracana) in the dryland systems of India. International Journal of Agricultural Sustainability, 14 (1), 81-94.

Singh, M. P., Deshmukh, R. K., Lal, S. K., Singh, R. B., and Singh, P. K. (2017). Effect of integrated nutrient management on yield and nutrient uptake of finger millet (Eleusine coracana) under rainfed condition. Indian Journal of Agricultural Sciences, 87 (9), 1219-1222.

Singh, R. B., Singh, M. P., and Singh, P. K. (2018). Effect of Integrated Nutrient Management on Soil Fertility and Productivity of Finger Millet (Eleusine coracana) under Rainfed Condition. International Journal of Current Microbiology and Applied Sciences, 7 (3), 1388-1395.

Sood, S., Kumar, R., and Gupta, A. K. (2017). A review on multifarious properties of finger millet (Eleusine coracana) and its potential for nutraceuticals and food formulations. Journal of Food Science and Technology, 54 (12), 3739-3752.

Subramanian, V., Duhan, J. S., Kumar, A., and Kumar, V. (2020). Organic Farming for Millets: An Overview. In Organic Farming for Sustainable and Resilient Agriculture (pp. 209-230). Springer.

# 10

# Foxtail Millet: Origin, Production, Nutritional Benefits and Medicinal Use

Itishree Nayak[1,2*], Bijayalaxmi Sahoo[1], Parameswaran C[1]

[1] Crop Improvement Division, ICAR-National Rice Research Institute, Cuttack-753006, Odisha, India

[2] Department of Botany, Utkal University, Vanivihar, Bhubaneswar -751004, Odisha, India

**ABSTRACT**

Millets are a type of small grained annual cereal that belongs to family poaceae (grass family) is widely cultivated and used in various parts of the world. Millet is a small, round grain and usually yellow or pale in colour. There are various types of millets including pearl millet, foxtail, proso, finger, kodo,barnyard, guinea, browntop, fonio, adlay and little millet.Out of all millets one nutritional powerhouse is the foxtail millet. This foxtail millets has the right amounts of all essential nutrients. It is Asia's most popular millet species and the second most extensively planted millet species overall.It contains protein, calcium, carbohydrates, iron, dietaryfibres and provides a good source of antioxidants. The vitamin B12 included in foxtail millet is important for maintaining a healthy heart, ensuring that the neurological system is running smoothly, and generally promoting the growth of skin and hair. In Type-2 diabetes patients, a diet including Foxtail Millet may enhance glycemic management and lower insulin, cholesterol, and fasting glucose levels to control diabetes. Besides it helps to decrease high blood pressure, slowing down muscle degradation, aids in sleep, treats coronary artery disorder and celiac disease, reduce risk of colon cancer, helps in weight loss and also relieving menstural cramps. Thus foxtail millets are appropriate for addressing food and nutrition security due to its yielding potential in regions with drought and limited resources, as well as due to its capacity to produce food products with notable health benefits.

*Keywords*: Foxtail millets, essential nutrients, dietary fibres, antioxidants, diabetes, weight loss.

## Introduction

Millets are a type of small grained annual cereal that belongs to family poaceae, commonly known as grass family is widely cultivated and utilized throughout the world. Millet is a small, round grain and usually yellow or pale in colour. There are

* Corresponding author.

various types of millets including pearl millet, foxtail millet, proso millet, finger millet, kodo millet, little millet, guinea millet, browntop millet, fonio millet, adlay millet and barnyard millet. It tastes slightly sweet and nutty flavoured. Millets have diversed method of consumption. These can be boiled, fried, roasted or grinded into flour.Millets are a common food source and an important component of many cultures' traditional dishes. Millets are grown both for food and fooder in all over the world now. It is cultivated mainly in Asia and Africa. The highest millet producing country is India, produce 10910,000 tonnes followed by Nigeria, 5000,000 tonnes followed by Niger produce 2955,000 tonnes of millets. In present days millets took attention because of its high nutritional value and dietary fibres. They contain 65-75% carbohydrates, 2-5% fat, 7–12% proteins, and 15-20% dietary fibre. Its protein contain higher essential amino acid content as compared to some major. Small millets are also used for iron and phosphorous because it has a good amount of these nutrients.

Millets are also rich in phenolic compounds like catechins and ferulic acid which acts as antioxidants and saves our body from damaging oxidative stress. The darker colour millets contain higher antioxidants than the lighter ones (5). The ferulic acid have anti-inflammatory properties as well as protects skin and also helps in early recovery of wounds (Zduńska *et al.,* 2018; Liu *et al.,* 2017). To prevent metal poisoning catechins binds to heavy metals in our blood streams (Chandrasekara and Shahidi, 2010; Bernatoniene and Kopustinkiene, 2018)). Fiber and non-starchy polysaccharides, two forms of indigestible carbohydrates that regulate blood sugar level, are abundant in millets (Devi *et al.,* 2014; Kam *et al.,* 2016). Millets has a low glycemic index that is, it will not spike your blood sugar level thus is a very good grain for diabetic people (Dias-Martins *et al.,* 2018; Narayanan *et al.,* 2016).

Glycemic index ranks carbohydrates on the basis of their raising capacity of blood sugar level. Foods with a lower GI value digest more slowly and cause blood sugar levels to rise more gradually. However, foods with a higher GI rating digest more quickly, which can swiftly elevate blood sugar levels. The range of the GI is 0 to 100. Many varieties of millet have low to medium GI values, allowing us to eat them more frequently without significantly influencing blood sugar levels. Soluble fibre in millets causes our gut to generate a viscous material. This ultimately traps lipids and lowers cholesterol levels (Devi *et al.,* 2014). The proteins in the millets are also useful in reducing cholesterol level.Millets are a great choice for people with celiac disease or who are on a gluten-free diet because they are gluten-free (Dias-Martins *et al.,* 2018; Narayanan *et al.,* 2016; Niro *et al.,* 2019).Cereals like wheat, barley, and rye naturally contain gluten, a protein.

Gluten must be avoided by those who have celiac disease or non-celiac gluten sensitivity since it can induce harmful digestive symptoms like diarrhoea and nutritional malabsorption (Gujral *et al.,* 2012). Out of all millets one nutritional powerhouse is the foxtail millet. This foxtail millets has the right amounts of all essential nutrients. It is a cereal that is suitable for addressing food and nutrition security because it has the potential to yield in areas with drought and limited resources and because it can produce food products with notable health benefits (Sharma and Niranjan 2018).

## Foxtail millet

Foxtail millets (*Setaria italic)* is an annual grass belongs to family poaceae. It is Asia's most popular millet species and the second most extensively planted millet species overall. The earliest indication of foxtail millet cultivation was discovered in Cishan, China, along the historic Yellow River route, and it was carbon dated to be from roughly 8 thousand years ago (Houyuan Lu; *et al.,* 2009; Ian S Hornsey, 2012; Purugganan, 2009). Since ancient times, India has also grown foxtail millet. Foxtail millets is also known as foxtail bristle grass, green foxtail millet, Italian millet, dwarf setaria, giant setaria, Hungarian millet and German millet. This millets is cultivated in almost all over the world and is called as different names in different languages (Table 1). Foxtail millet is a diploid plant with nine chromosomes (2n = 18) (Baltensperger and Cai 2004). However, it shares a close relationship with Setaria species that are tetraploid and polyploidy (Benabdelmouna *et al.,* 2001). Additionally, in order to create fertile hybrids, cultivated foxtail millet crosses with its wild relative Setariaitalica subsp. viridis (green foxtail) (Prasad Rao *et al.,* 1987). Its genome is only about 423 Mbp in size (Taylor, 2019). Three or four races of foxtail millet can be distinguished: maxima, moharia, indica (Taylor, 2019), and nana (Taylor, 2019) (Table 1).

## Origin of foxtail millet

The central Chinese highlands were thought to be where cultivated foxtail millet first appeared (*Setarica italica*). China, India, Manchuria, Afghanistan, Georgia, Korea, and Central Asiaare among the world's major production areas. In Japan, it is also one of the speciality crops. It is primarily grown in Asia for human use. It was just made available in the US for hay and silage. It was presumably introduced to Europe during the Stone Age because of its quick growing cycle, which makes it an excellent crop for nomads (Vilas *et al.,* 2015).It is crucial to know that Setariaviridis, that is inter-fertile with foxtail millet, has been definitively identified as the plant that gave rise to foxtail millet in the wild. Weedy or wild varieties of the foxtail millets also exist. The biology of seed dispersal is the main distinction between the wild and domesticated versions (Zohary and Hopf 2000). While cultivars hold onto the seeds, weedy and wild types scatter them. The Peiligang civilization of China were also cultivated proso millet, provides the earliest evidence of the cultivation of this grain.The Cishan civilization in China is credited with having domesticated foxtail millet first, somewhere between 6500 and 5500 BC (Stevens *et al.,* 2016). The earliest known instance of foxtail millet farming outside of its native range is found at Chengtoushan in the Middle Yangtze River region, which dates to roughly 4000 BC (Castillo, 2010). Genetic analysis has proven that Setaria viridis is Setaria italica's ancestor (Diao and Guanqing, 2017).

**Table 1 :** Names of Foxtail millets in different languages where it cultivated

| languages | Foxtail millet names | languages | Foxtail millet names |
|---|---|---|---|
| Assamese | Konidhaan | Malay | Sekoi |
| Bengali | Kaon dana | Malayalam | Thina |
| Hindi | Kangni | Mandarin Chinese | Su |
| Georgian | Ghomi | Marathi | Kang / Rala |
| German | Hirse | Nepali | Kaguno |
| Gujarati | Kang | Odia | Kangu/Tangana |
| Gurung | Tohro | Punjabi | Kangni |
| Hungarian | Mohar/koles | Russian | Mogara/Chumiza |
| Japanese | Awa | Sanskrit | Priyangu/Kangu |
| Javanese | Jawawut | Sinhala | Thana haal |
| Kannada | Navane/Navanakkl | Tamil | Thinai |
| Korean | Jo | Telugu | Korralu/Korra |

## Spread

Foxtail millet travelled through southern China and eventually arrived in the Chengdu Plain around 2700 BC and Gantuoyan, close to the Vietnamese border, approximately 3000 BC (Castillo, 2010). Foxtail millet also arrived in Taiwan (Nankuanli, Dapenkeng civilization) and the Tibetan Plateau (Karuo) in the vicinity of 2800 BC and 3000 BC, respectively. Numerous pathways are probably used by Setaricaitalica to go to Southeast Asia. The earliest indications of the emergence of foxtail millet in Southeast Asia comes from a number of sites in central Thailand, notably Khao Wong Prachan Valley and the site at Non Pa Wai, both of which point to an early date of about 2300 BC (Weber, 2010). The oldest proof of the foxtail millet's origins in East Siberia was discovered at the archaeological site at Krounovka in PrimorskyKrai, dated to roughly 3620-3370 BC (Diao and Guanqing, 2017).The oldest direct evidence of foxtail millet in Korea dates to the 3360 BC period at the Dongsam-dong Shell Midden, a Jeulmun site in southern Korea (Crawford and Lee 2015).

## Production

### *Soil and Climate*

Foxtail millet may thrive on a variety of soil types, including sandy and heavy clay soils, although it requires a moderately fertile, well-drained soil for high yields.

500–700 mm of rainfall per year is ideal for localised growth. Extreme drought or water logging conditions are intolerable to it.

## Sowing

Foxtail millets can be grown both in kharif and rabi season. In kharif season it is cultivated in Karnataka during July-August. In Tamilnadu, Andhra Pradesh it is cultivated during the month of July and in Maharashtra during the 2nd -3rd week of July. Foxtail millets are cultivated as a rabi crop during August to September in Tamilnadu.8-10 kg/ha foxtail millet seeds were sown and for broadcasting 15kg/ha seeds were sown in the field of spacing 25-30 cm from row to row and 8 – 10 cm from plant to plant. The seed should be planted 2-3 cm in depth.

## Manure and Fertilizers

A month before sowing, apply 5–10 tonnes/ha of compost or farmyard manure. 40 kg of nitrogen, 20 kg of $P_2O_5$, and 20 kg of potassium per hectare are typically the recommended fertilizers for healthy crops. Application of fertilizers based on soil testing is advised. Apply the full amount of $P_2O_5$ and 50% of the nitrogen at the time of sowing, then the other 5% of the nitrogen 30 days later.

## Weeding and Intercultural operation

In a crop that was seeded in lines, two inter cultivations and one hand weeding are advised. When the crop is 30 days old, intercultural operation employing a tyne-harrow should be done. In a broadcast crop, the first weed 15 to 20 days following seedling emergence and to weed again 15 to 20 days afterwards.

## Irrigation

Crops grown in the Kharif season need little or no irrigation. It is mostly cultivated as a rainfed crop. If the dry spell lasts for a longer time, 1-2 irrigations should be supplied. Depending on the kind of soil and the weather, summer crops need anywhere from two to five irrigations.

## Inter Cropping

Growing two or more crops next to one another isreferred to as intercropping. The main goal of intercropping is to increase yield by making use of resources or biological processes that would otherwise be unused by a single crop on a specific piece of land.In India also inter cropping is done using Foxtail millet with other crops. In Andhra Pradesh foxtail millets and pigeon Peas are grown in 5:1 ratio and with groundnut in 2:1 ratio. Inter cropping of Foxtail millet with Cotton (5:1) and with Pigeon Pea (5:1) were cultivated in Karnataka.

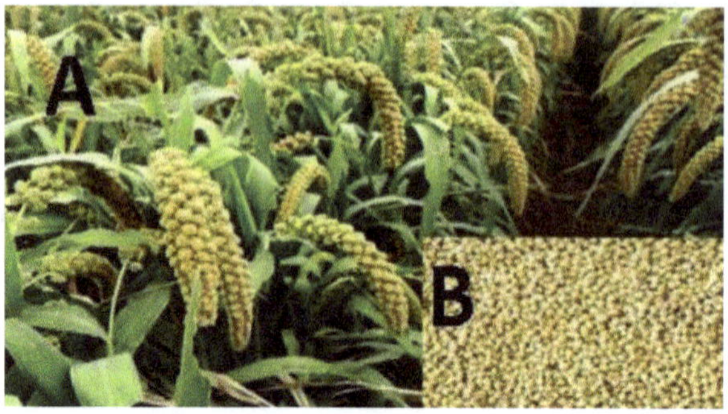


**Figure 1 :** Foxtail millet cultivation in field

## Nutritional Benefits and Medicinal Uses

Foxtail millets include a wealth of vitamins, minerals, dietary fibre, and protein. Contrary to popular thought, millets are enjoyable to chew and can be incorporated into delicious meals. Foxtail millet is a versatile cereal that could be included in our breakfast, lunch, and supper meals. It is high in proteins, carbohydrates, good fats, vitamin E, iron, zinc, phosphorus and magnesium, which assist the brain's brain abilities. As foxtail millets contain various type of nutritional elements it can be used to achieve health benefits as well, following are some areas where foxtail millet can be used as a boon (Figure 2; Figure 3).

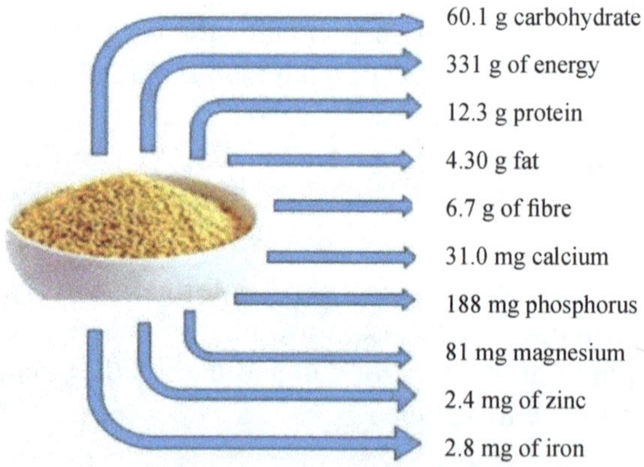


**Figure 2 :** Nutritional content of Foxtail Millet

## Maintain cardiac health

The protein rich and gluten free foxtail millet aids in the synthesis of the neurotransmitter acetylcholine. It facilitates the communication between muscles and nerves. By assisting in blood pressure control, it lessens the likelihood of a heart blockage. Foxtail millet protect our heart from various ailments and keep it healthy.

## Diabetes control

Being a food with a low (50.8) glycaemic index, foxtail millet is the best option for lowering blood sugar and glycosylated haemoglobin. Foxtail millet is an excellent alternative to rice since it keeps you fuller for longer. To minimise mid-afternoon hunger pangs and a sharp rise in blood sugar, the secret is to eat cooked foxtail millet rather than rice.

## Aids in sleep

The tryptophan in foxtail millet increases the body's serotonin level, which aids in lowering stress. Every night, a cup of millet porridge can aid in peaceful sleep.

## Weight loss

Our food is becoming less diverse, which has led to an increase in obesity and overweight people. More refined cereals and packaged foods that are heavy in salt, sugar, and fats are what we want. Compared to the rural population, the urban population is more affected by the obesity or overweight problem. Foxtail millet's high dietary fibre content aids with weight management. Additionally, it includes tryptophan, which slows down digestion and keeps us from absorbing additional calories. We might claim that it provides us a feeling of fullness in our stomachs and keeps us from overeating.

## Strengthen nervous system

Due to its high vitamin B1 content, foxtail millet can help prevent a number of neurological conditions.This nourishing cereal's iron content slows the progression of Alzheimer's and Parkinson's disease and increases brain oxygenation.

## Bone strength

Iron and calcium-rich foxtail millets support the health of bones and muscles. It aids in supplying the body with the calcium and phosphorus requirements for preventing brittle bones, swelling, osteoporosis, arthritis, and spondylitis.

## Boost immunity

Foxtail millet is a nutritional powerhouse that helps you stay healthy, maintain your stamina, and strengthen your immunity so you can fight off any lingering diseases. Include this strength-boosting millet in your regular diet to aid in the battle against illnesses and regain your strength.

## Brain growth

The iron content of foxtail millet is 2.8 mg per 100 g, and iron is necessary for brain oxygenation and the prevention of Alzheimer's disease.

## Skin care

The amino acids in foxtail millet stimulate the production of collagen and aid in delaying the onset of wrinkles on the skin. As a result, it gives us skin that is healthy, young, and wrinkle-free.

## Digestion

Foxtail millet has 6.7 grams of fiber, which keeps us healthy and stops constipation.

## Good for celiac patient

For celiac sufferers, foxtail millet is the best option because it is gluten-free. In the USA, there is an 8–10% adoption rate for the gluten-free trends.

## Relieving menstrual cramps

Foxtail millet is an excellent food for women who experience excruciating agony and cramps throughout their menstrual cycle because of its magnesium content.

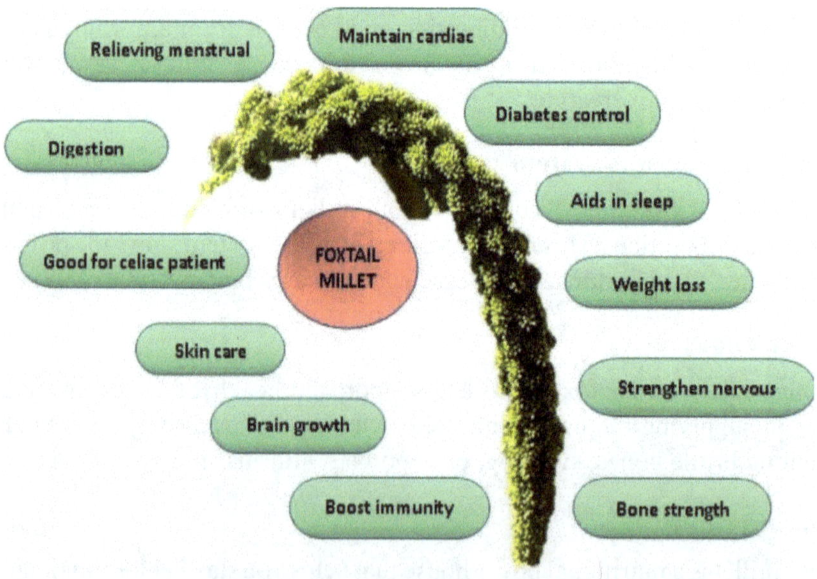


**Figure 3.** Benefits of Foxtail millet

## Foxtail millet based products

Foxtail millet, which can be eaten in a variety of ways including porridge, ready-to-eat snacks, and beverages, is becoming more and more popular outside of Asia and Africa. Utilizable components are concentrated during the milling of foxtail millet and can then be used in the mass production of goods like baby foods, snack foods, wholesome foods, and classic sweets (Subramanian *et al.,* 2007). Additionally, you can use this gluten-free flour in place of some wheat flour when making food (Devisetti *et al.,* 2014). The food industry is concentrating on underused ingredients like foxtail millet as a result of the growing difficulty in producing foods that promote health (Sharma and Niranjan 2018) (Figure 4).

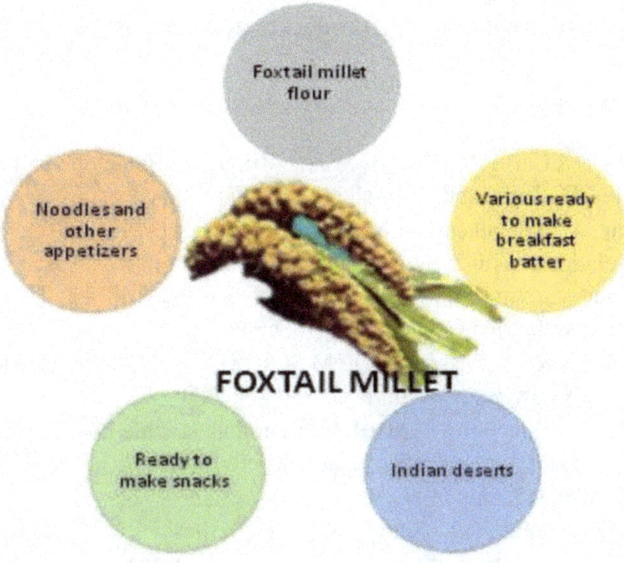


**Figure 4 :** Foxtail millet based products for commercial use

## Genetic studies

Through a crop breeding programme, the focus has recently shifted to millet quality studies. Since there are currently few good quality foxtail millet germplasm resources, advances in quality breeding are severely constrained by this low genetic variety. The nutritional profile of foxtail millet has not been extensively studied. More thorough study is required, particularly on the impacts of agronomic practises and growing conditions on nutrient quality. New superior quality foxtail millet varieties with high yield potential, stress resistance, and stability are needed to stabilise millet production and foster the growth of the millet industry.

## Conclusion

Because of its ability to produce food with significant health benefits and its yielding capacity in drought and low-resource environments, foxtail millet is a cereal grain that is suitable for addressing food and nutrition security. Despite being widely used as a bird and animal feed in wealthy countries, the potential of foxtail millet is still unrealized. Whole grains can produce food that is more nutritious than decorticated grains when they are processed using techniques like roasting, drying, germination, and fermentation. A few examples of foods that can be made with processed whole grain flours include breads, biscuits, and porridge.The foxtail millet properties and potential applications are adequately understood by the literature that has been published to date, but more research and development is necessary to fully realise its potential, particularly on improving the sustainability and efficiency of foxtail millet processing methods, establishing clear relationships between processing conditions and product quality, and assessing the health effects of the products.

## References

Baltensperger, D., &Cai, Y. Z. (2004). Minor Millets In Encyclopedia of Grain Science, CW Wrigley, H. Corke and CE Walker,(eds.), Vol. 2, p.

Benabdelmouna, A., Abirached-Darmency, M., &Darmency, H. (2001). Phylogenetic and genomic relationships in Setariaitalica and its close relatives based on the molecular diversity and chromosomal organization of 5S and 18S-5.8 S-25S rDNA genes. *Theoretical and Applied Genetics*, *103*(5), 668-677.

Bernatoniene, J., &Kopustinskiene, D. M. (2018). The role of catechins in cellular responses to oxidative stress. *Molecules*, *23*(4), 965.

Chandrasekara, A., &Shahidi, F. (2010). Content of insoluble bound phenolics in millets and their contribution to antioxidant capacity. *Journal of agricultural and food chemistry*, *58*(11), 6706-6714.

Devi, P. B., Vijayabharathi, R., Sathyabama, S., Malleshi, N. G., &Priyadarisini, V. B. (2014). Health benefits of finger millet (Eleusinecoracana L.) polyphenols and dietary fiber: a review. *Journal of food science and technology*, *51*(6), 1021-1040.

Devi, P. B., Vijayabharathi, R., Sathyabama, S., Malleshi, N. G., &Priyadarisini, V. B. (2014). Health benefits of finger millet (Eleusinecoracana L.) polyphenols and dietary fiber: a review. *Journal of food science and technology*, *51*(6), 1021-1040.

Devi, P. B., Vijayabharathi, R., Sathyabama, S., Malleshi, N. G., &Priyadarisini, V. B. (2014). Health benefits of finger millet (Eleusinecoracana L.) polyphenols and dietary fiber: a review. *Journal of food science and technology*, *51*(6), 1021-1040.

Devisetti, R., Yadahally, S. N., & Bhattacharya, S. (2014). Nutrients and antinutrients in foxtail and proso millet milled fractions: Evaluation of their flour functionality. *LWT-Food Science and Technology*, *59*(2), 889-895.

Dias-Martins, A. M., Pessanha, K. L. F., Pacheco, S., Rodrigues, J. A. S., &Carvalho, C. W. P. (2018). Potential use of pearl millet (Pennisetumglaucum (L.) R. Br.) in Brazil: Food security, processing, health benefits and nutritional products. *Food research international*, *109*, 175-186.

Dias-Martins, A. M., Pessanha, K. L. F., Pacheco, S., Rodrigues, J. A. S., &Carvalho, C. W. P. (2018). Potential use of pearl millet (Pennisetumglaucum (L.) R. Br.) in Brazil: Food security, processing, health benefits and nutritional products. *Food research international*, *109*, 175-186.

Gujral, N., Freeman, H. J., & Thomson, A. B. (2012). Celiac disease: prevalence, diagnosis, pathogenesis and treatment. *World journal of gastroenterology: WJG*, *18*(42), 6036.

Houyuan Lu; *et al.* (2009), Earliest domestication of common millet (Panicummiliaceum) in East Asia extended to 10,000 years ago, Proceedings of the National Academy of Sciences of the United States of America, Our analytical results of both phytoliths and biomolecular components have established that the earliest cereal remains stored in the Cishan Neolithic sites, during ca. 10,300–8,700 calyr BP, are not foxtail millet, but only common millet. After 8,700 calyr BP, the grain crops gradually contained 0.4–2.8% foxtail millet .

*Ian S Hornsey (2012). Alcohol and its Role in the Evolution of Human Society. pp. 254–256 (chapter 4.7.3).*

Kam, J., Puranik, S., Yadav, R., Manwaring, H. R., Pierre, S., Srivastava, R. K., & Yadav, R. S. (2016). Dietary interventions for type 2 diabetes: how millet comes to help. *Frontiers in plant science*, *7*, 1454.

Kumari, D., Madhujith, T., &Chandrasekara, A. (2017). Comparison of phenolic content and antioxidant activities of millet varieties grown in different locations in Sri Lanka. *Food science & nutrition*, *5*(3), 474-485.

Liu, Y. M., Shen, J. D., Xu, L. P., Li, H. B., Li, Y. C., & Yi, L. T. (2017). Ferulic acid inhibits neuro-inflammation in mice exposed to chronic unpredictable mild stress. *International Immunopharmacology*, *45*, 128-134.

Narayanan, J., Sanjeevi, V., Rohini, U., Trueman, P., & Viswanathan, V. (2016). Postprandial glycaemic response of foxtail millet dosa in comparison to a rice dosa in patients with type 2 diabetes. *The Indian journal of medical research*, *144*(5), 712.

Niro, S., D'Agostino, A., Fratianni, A., Cinquanta, L., &Panfili, G. (2019). Gluten-free alternative grains: Nutritional evaluation and bioactive compounds. *Foods*, *8*(6), 208.

Prasada Rao, K. S., Chetty, S. C., &Desaiah, D. (1987). Effects of tricyclohexylhydroxytin on the kinetics of adenosine triphosphatase system and protection by thiol reagents. *Journal of Biochemical Toxicology*, *2*(2), 125-140.

Purugganan, Michael D.; Fuller, Dorian Q. (2009). "The nature of selection during plant domestication". Nature. Nature Research. **457** (7231): 843–848. Bibcode: 2009 Natur. 457.. 843P. doi:10.1038/nature07895. ISSN 0028-0836. *PMID 19212403. S2CID 205216444*

Sharma, N., & Niranjan, K. (2018). Foxtail millet: Properties, processing, health benefits, and uses. *Food reviews international*, *34*(4), 329-363.

Sharma, N., &Niranjan, K. (2018). Foxtail millet: Properties, processing, health benefits, and uses. *Food reviews international*, *34*(4), 329-363.

Subramanian, S.; Viswanathan, R. Bulk density and friction coefficients of selected millet grains and flours. J. Food Eng. 2007, 81, 118–126.

Taylor, J. R. (2019). Sorghum and millets: Taxonomy, history, distribution, and production. In *Sorghum and millets* (pp. 1-21). AACC International Press.

Zduńska, K., Dana, A., Kolodziejczak, A., &Rotsztejn, H. (2018). Antioxidant properties of ferulic acid and its possible application. *Skin pharmacology and physiology*, *31*(6), 332-336.

# 11

# Kodo Millet (*Paspalum scrobiculatum*) - A Nutri-rich Millet Crop: Nutritional Composition, Health Benefits and Food Product Developments

Rashmi Mishra*, Neela Satheesh*

Department of Food Nutrition and Dietetics, Faculty of Agriculture, Sri Sri University, Cuttack, Odisha,

**ABSTRACT**

Kodo millet (*Paspalum scrobiculatum*), is a cereal grain. It is called "Kodra" in Gujarati,"Kodo" in Bengali, "Kodon" in Hindi, "Harka" in Kannada, "Kodua" in Oriya, "Varagu" in Tamil, and "Arikelu (Arika)" in Telugu, among other regional names. It is one of the earliest domesticated cereals in the world, coming from India. It is typically grown in semi-arid and desert areas of Africa and several Asian countries. Kodo millet is mostly grown in the Deccan region of India, while it is also grown in the foothills of the Himalayas. It contains a higher amounts of minerals like iron, dietary fibres,and other antioxidants. Kodo millet has the highest antioxidant potential of any millet and the lowest phosphorus content of any millet.Processing techniques like parboiling and debranning influence the mineral content and fibre. Kodo millet can be used to make a variety of traditional Indian dishes, or it can be combined with other cereal and legume flours to enhance their flavour.In this book chapter information about kodo millet production trends, distribution, agricultural practices and varietal information, physico-chemical compositions and nutritional aspects, health benefits and applications in food product developments.

*Keywords*: Kodo Millet, Nutrients, Post-harvest processing, Anti-Nutritional Factors, Traditional Food products.

## Introduction

Since long ago, cereal grains have made significant contributions to the advancement of human civilization. They also play a significant part in the daily diets of many people worldwide as staple foods. However, due to a number of issues, including soil nutrient depletion, crop failure due to unpredictable or changeable weather that causes flood and draught conditions, production of the primary cereal crops has been progressively declining in recent years. Millets are major source of basic food for millions of people, particularly those who live in hot, dry conditions,

* Corresponding author.

similar to grains. Millets, which are small-seeded annual grains, are used for food, feed, forage, and fuel (Kothari *et al.,* 2005). Because millets were cultivated at the start of human civilization thousands of years ago, they are regarded as ancient grains. Evidence suggests that millets were first cultivated around 4000 years ago (Shahidi and Chandrasekara 2013). The most draught-resistant crops, millets are widely farmed across Asia, Africa, and the Indian subcontinent and are a vital source of nutrition for those lives in rural areas. As more people become aware of the nutritional and health benefits of the underutilised millet grains, the production of millet, which had been dropping since cereal crops like rice and wheat had received much of the attention, is now on the rise. Global agriculture and food security are also under threat from other socioeconomic causes, including the growing world population, rising food prices and the cost of critical commodities. Particularly those in resource-constrained desert and sub-arid locations can feel the effects (Saleh *et al.,* 2013). Researchers and scientists that study the manufacturing, processing, storage, and nutritional aspects of food now face a significant difficulty. Millet output has been falling as cereal crops like rice and wheat have received much of the attention, but growing knowledge of the nutritional and health benefits of the underutilised millet grains opens the door for an increase in millet production.

## Types of Millets and their Production around the word and India

Millets are traditional grains usually grown and being consumed in the Indian subcontinent since more than 5000 years. These are small grained warm-weather nutricereals belong to grass family. They require less rainfall for grow and are highly drought tolerant crops. Millets come in two varieties: major millets (such as sorghum, pearl millet, and finger millet) and minor millets (Foxtail millet, Kodo millet, little millet, Proso millet and Barnyard millet) (Figure1). The millet production usually distributed in the Asian and African countries around the world. Figure 2 shows the volume share of different countries in the global market in terms of millet production. It is clearly visible that India is the largest producer (41%) and cultivation of millets as compared to other countries. Similarly, the volume of millet market shares in India also higher and on par with the production. The production of the millet in India since three years are constantly increased from 2019 to 2021. In year 2021, the total 13210000 tonnes are produced. Out of all the produced millets, pearl millet possesses around 60% share and followed by the sorghum (27%), finger millet (11%) and minor millets has only 2% of share (Figure 3B). Rajasthan is producing the 39% of the total millets produced in India, followed by Uttar Pradesh (20%), Haryana (12%), Gujarat (11%), Madhya Pradesh (9%) are the top 5 millet producing states in year 2021 and 22.

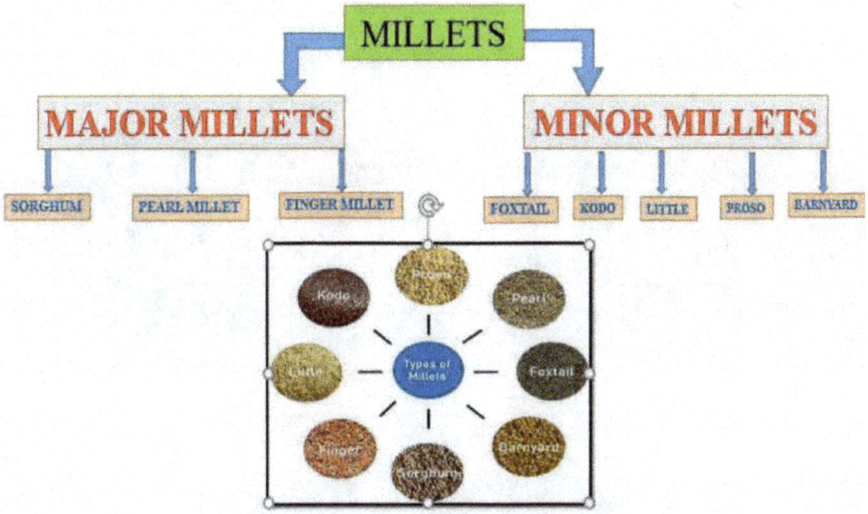


**Figure 1 :** The classification of the millets.

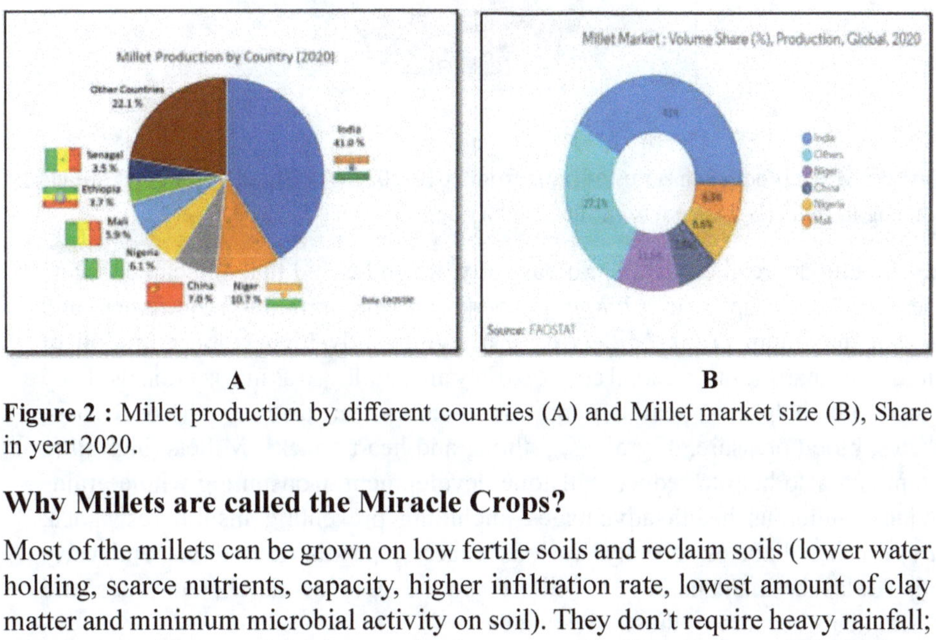


A B

**Figure 2 :** Millet production by different countries (A) and Millet market size (B), Share in year 2020.

## Why Millets are called the Miracle Crops?

Most of the millets can be grown on low fertile soils and reclaim soils (lower water holding, scarce nutrients, capacity, higher infiltration rate, lowest amount of clay matter and minimum microbial activity on soil). They don't require heavy rainfall; chemical fertilizers and they can resist the pest attack. Farmers can cultivate these crops by using domestically prepared manure and even on dry land conditions. These crops are rich in various nutrients especially micro nutrients like vitamins and minerals so they can be used for eradication of various nutrient deficiency diseases from the community, as they are gluten free and low sugar containing crops, so they can be a very good option for celiac disease and diabetes.

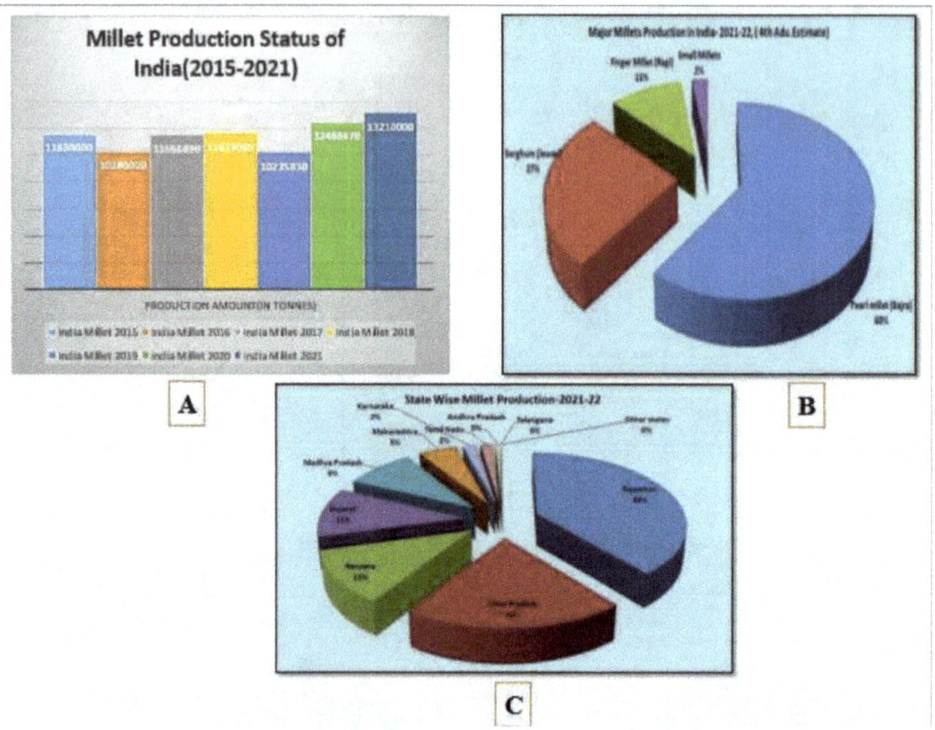


**Figure 3 :** Millet production status of India from 2015-2021 (A); Share of different millets producing in India (B); State wise millet production in Indian (C).

They are climate resilient crops. So basically, it can be said that one can cultivate these nutridense crops with minimum expenditure and minimum requirement and can gain maximum profit. Millets have a significantly higher concentration of antioxidants than the other cereal crops, so they are employed as nutraceuticals. They are said to be helpful in treating conditions such as heart disease, atherosclerosis, diabetes, blood pressure, migraines, asthma, and heart attacks. Millets' high fibre content can also help to reduce gallstone development. Consuming whole grains provides numerous health advantages, including preventing insulin resistance, heart disease, diabetes, obesity, various cancers, paediatric asthma, and early death (Balasubramanian, 2013). Millets can be used as functional foods and nutraceuticals because of these advantages.

## Production and Cultivation of Kodo Millet in India and World

*Paspalum scrobiculatum* is the official scientific name for kodo millet. It is an annual grain that is typically grown in India, although it is also grown in other nations like the Philippines, Indonesia, Vietnam, and Thailand, as well as its true home of West Africa. Kodo millet is one of the most important minor millets because of its distinctive ability to withstand drought and high nutritional value. In addition, it is produced in India's Deccan plateau as a major food source. It is grown as a minor crop in the majority of these places. It belongs to the group of minor millets, which are small-seeded plants raised all over the world for food and fodder. In some regions of India, kodo millet is also a well-liked option for fasting. Unquestionably superior to rice, millet is also devoid of gluten and packed with vitamins, minerals, and nutritional fibre. It is mostly grown in Madhya Pradesh, Chhattisgarh, Maharashtra, Tamil Nadu, and Karnataka states in India. It is also grown in Arunachal Pradesh's Jhum farms. It requires less water and thrives in mild rains of 50–60 cm. Typically, gravel, rocky or stony upland low soils to loam soils are used to grow kodo millet. The best soils for agriculture and greater profit are those that are rich in organic matter, such as deep, loamy soils. The kodo millet needs well-drained soils with the right amount of moisture for continuous growth.

In the post-green revolution era, the area planted with kodo millet is seeing a declining trend due to the predominance of major cereals like rice and wheat. Kodo millet is often grown as a pure crop because of its high unit area productivity, high market price, and usefulness as fodder. When compared to other dry land crops, it generates considerable net returns. Kodo millet produces 312 kg per hectare (Anon., 2017). Madhya Pradesh is the leader in this category because it produces the most kodo millet—about 60% of the state's total land area.Tamil Nadu, Chhattisgarh, Maharashtra, Andhra Pradesh, Karnataka, and Gujarat are additional significant states growing kodo millet.

The wild species of *Paspalum scrobiculatum*, which is native to India, is *Paspalum scrobiculatum var. commersonii*. *Paspalum scrobiculatum var. scrobiculatum* is widely farmed as a major food crop in India and other areas of the world. This wild variety is a crucial food crop in tribal areas and is very well-liked by tribal farmers due to their eating habits and occasionally for therapeutic purposes. It is a particularly resilient crop that can withstand droughts and thrive in soils where other plants might not (Heuze *et al.,* 2012). The quantity of genetic variety and the accessibility of various germplasm are the two key factors that determine how much genetic improvement may be achieved using conventional breeding methods.However, various researchers have developed different kinds of kodo millet to provide the higher yield and better performance variants. As a result, several researchers have created distinct types of kodo millets that are acceptable in various states around the nation. These variations are provided in the Table 1. As it is established that, millets are high draught tolerant and require very fewer needs. The marginal soils are also suitable for the growth cultivation of kodo millets. The all-agricultural practices and requirements of the kodo millet are presented in the Table 2.

**Table 1 :** Improved Varieties of Kodo Millets in India

| S. No | States | Varieties developed/ cultivating |
|---|---|---|
| 1 | Madhya Pradesh | JK 439, JK 65, JK 48, JK 13, GPUK 3, DSP9-1, TNAU86, JK 137, JK 106, JK98, RBK 155, RK 390-25 |
| 2 | Tamil Nadu | TNAU 86, GPUK 3, KMV 20, CO 3, RK 390-25 |
| 3 | Karnataka | TNAU86, RBK 155, RK 390-25, GPUK 3 |
| 4 | Gujarat | JK65, JK13, GK 2, GK 1, RK 390-25, GPUK 3 |
| 5 | Andhra Pradesh & Telangana | TNAU 86 & RK 390-25 |
| 6 | Chhattisgarh | JK 439, JK98, Jawahar Kodo137, Indira Kodo1, GPUK 3 JK 65, Chhattisgarh-2, RBK 155, Indira Kodo 48, RK 390-25, TNAU 86 & Chhattisgarh Kodo-2 |

**Table 2 :** Appropriate conditions required for the cultivation of kodo millet in India

| S. No | Name of the Parameters | Appropriate Requirement/Favourable Condition |
|---|---|---|
| 1 | Climate | Warm and Dry Climate |
| 2 | Rainfall | 40/50-60 cm Annual Rainfall |
| 3 | Soil | gravel and rocky or stony upland poor soils to loam soils, soils rich in organic matter like Deep, loamy, fertile soils |
| 4 | Season | Middle of June to End of July |
| 5 | Spacing | 22.5 cm between Rows and 10 cm between plants |
| 6 | Seed Rate | 10kg $Ha^{-1}$ for line sowing<br>15kg $Ha^{-1}$ for Broad casting |
| 7 | Inter Cropping System in MP | Kodo millet+ Pigeon pea (2:1)<br>Kodo millet+ Green Gram/Black gram (2:1)<br>Kodo Millet+ Soyabean (2:1) |
| 8 | Crop Rotation/Sequence in MP | Kodo millet-soyabean-kodo millet<br>Kodo millet-niger-kodo millet |
| 9 | Irrigation Management | During dry weather, 4-7 days.<br>1st irrigation: - 25-30 DAS<br>2nd irrigation: - 40-45 DAS |
| 10 | Weed Control | 2 weeding in the interval of 15 days |
| 11 | Harvesting Period | Kharif season: - September to October<br>Rabi Season: - January to February |
| 12 | Yield | 15 to 18 Quintal grain &30 to 40 Quintal Straw per Hectare |

## Major Pests of Millets

Even though millets are less likely to be attacked by pests, there are still plenty of pests that cause grain damage and reduce output. Shoot flies, stem borers, and ear head midges are primarily regarded as major pests for millets. In some parts of our nation, white grubs are crucial. In certain seasons, serious yield losses are occurring as a result of irregular and frequent attacks by armyworms, grasshoppers, blister beetles, chinch bugs, leaf beetles, head caterpillars, and head bugs. However, due to changes in ecological and cultural activities, small pests can pose a hazard in some areas. The main pest in various millets at various stages needs to be dealt with using a variety of techniques.Malloch is a common insect that attacks pearl millet in several regions, reducing grain yield and dry fodder production. Other crops like maize, ragi, bajra, sorghum, and various grasses are also found to be infested by the insect. Extreme temperatures (high or low) and persistent rain both cause it to become active. Sorghum is one of the deadly group of millets that are attacked by stem borers. In India, *Chiln partellas Swinhoe* and *Sesarnia inferens* predominate among stem borers. In India, *S. inferens* affects finger millet. Figure 4 shows the pest that infests kodo millet.

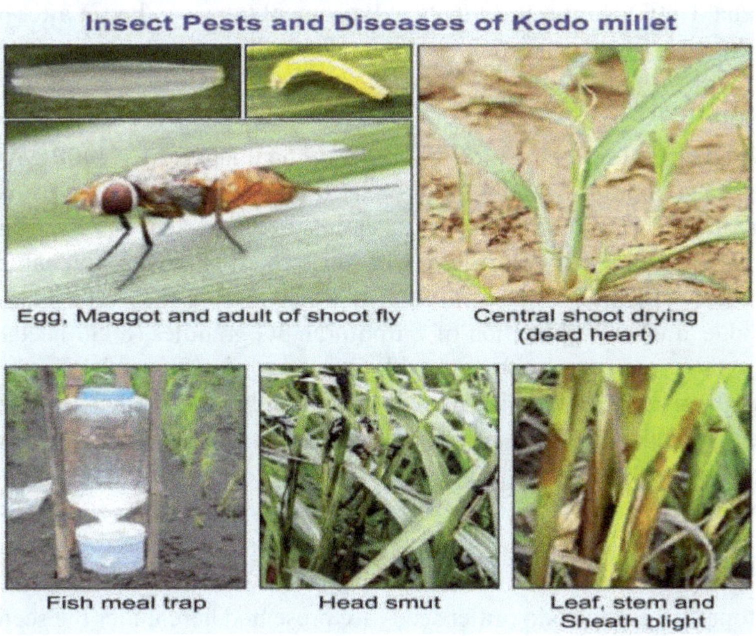


**Figure 4 :** Insect pests and diseases of kodo millet and their management

## Pest Control

In the pest control of the kodo millet, as similar with other millets there are different methods are present. They are summarized here under.

## Cultural methods

Before the start of the monsoon rains, the stubbles can be gathered and burned, and the stalks can then be given to cattle. As a result, midges and stem borers will grow less rapidly. Before planting, a deep plough should be used for a month to expose the various insects' embryonic stages, which can also be used as food by predators. Utilize timely sowings of cultivars with comparable maturities throughout a wide area to lessen the harm that shoot-flies, midges, and other bugs, such as head bugs, might inflict. Sorghum can be intercropped with cowpea and pigeon pea to lessen stem borer damage.Thiamethoxam insecticide can be used to treat seeds to lessen shoot fly damage. It can also aid to some extent minimise steamborer and sucking pest growth, such as phids, leafhoppers, thrips, whiteflies, and other flies, bugs, and mites.

## Mechanical method

Till midnight, light traps can be set up to draw in, watch over, and kill adult grain midges, ear head caterpillars, and stem borer pests. In order to attract male moths of *Hehcwerpa sp.*from flowering to grain hardening, a sex pheromone trap can be set up at 12/ha. Until the crop is 30 days old, fishmeal traps can be set after being impregnated with arpocarb insecticides at a rate of 12/ha.

## Chemical methods

Spraying with Cypermethrin l0 EC (750 ml/ha), Quinalphos 25 EC (400 g/ha), or Carbofuran 3G granules (15 kg/ha) may be used as a base application to reduce the number of dead hearts brought on by shoot flies. For stem borers, you can apply dust or granules in the whorl leaves of the harmed plants, or you can spray Fen valerate or Cypermethrin (0.5 ml/litre of water) across the entire field. For sorghum midge, a whorl application of Carbofuran 3G granules (8 kg/ hectare) is advised. The crop may also be treated with Cypermethrin (0.5 ml/lt of water) at the 50% blooming stage (one midge/panicle).At the end of blooming and when the crop reaches the milk stage, Cypermethrin (0.5 ml/litre of water) may be sprayed on the crop to control head caterpillars (2-4 larvae per panicle) and earhead bugs (1-2 bugs per panicle).

## Kodo millet properties

Different properties of the kodo millet seeds are presented here under the sections. Which include the physical, functional and nutritional properties.

## Physical and function properties of the kodo millet

The whole kodo millet seed before dehulling appears in the dark grey in color. The dehulled raw millet grains possess ellipsoidal in shape and light yellow in colour.

The mean size of the kodo millet of different varieties reported range between 1.58 to 1.89 mm.After dehulling, the seed size is further reduced. However, the reduction in the size depends on the variety of the kodo millet, method of dehulling practiced and the extend of dehulling performed. The thousand kernel weight range between 4.20 to 4.37g and the thousand grain volume ranged from 3.99 to 4.00ml was reported. However, the physical and function values of the kodo millet seed is depends on the variety, geo agricultural conditions and other factors.

## Kodo millet's nutritional profile

Millets stand out among all cereals due to their abundance in vitamins and minerals like calcium, dietary fibre, polyphenols, and protein (Devi *et al.,* 2011). Kodo millet is consider as the good source of the protein in the average range of 8 to 10% and it is considering as the protein source for the tribal populations and other local kodo millet producing arears. Different researchers are reported the variation in the protein content from 6.5 to 10.0%. However, the protein content variation in the kodo millet depends on the genotypic variation, agro geological conditions. In addition, millet protein considers as good quality of the proteins, it contains tryptophan (0.12 to 0.31 g/16 g N) and lysine (2.19 to 2.85 g/16 g N), two important amino acids. Additionally, it is abundantly clear from the research that different millet parts have different amounts of certain amino acids, such as tryptophan, which can range from 25.55 to 33.27 mg/g of protein and lysine, which can range from 135.17 to 179.17 mg/g of protein. Last but not least, kodo millet is regarded as a superior protein source to grains like rice(Ramashia SE *et al.*, 2019).

Kodo millet is considered as the low amount of the fat and reported around mean value of 1.4% of the fat. However, there is a variation in the cultivars as 1.1 to the 3.8%. However, major proportion of the fat (26.6%) is located in the bran portion of the grain. In dehulling process or the preparation practice the oil content reduces drastically. The fat content in kodo millet contains the linoleic acid and oleic acid in similar quantities and they made 70% of the total fatty acids in the lipid fractions.

Kodo millet has a maximum carbohydrate content of 64.3%, although it can also have a minimum carbohydrate content of 58.45%. Similar to this, the researchers reported that the removal of both the fat and protein fractions boosted the starch digestibility and glycaemic index. Decortication thereby eliminates the protein and fat portions (Bhat *et al.,* 2017). The glycaemic index of cooked kodo millet flour was reported to rise from 49.9 to 62.5. Therefore, due to its hypoglycaemic qualities, kodo millet can be taken into account while creating various value-added goods.

Kodo millet is prized for its higher fibre content. The medicinal qualities of kodo millet are responsible for this increased content of fibre. Researchers found that whole millet flour has higher fibre content. However, the amounts of fibre are decreased in milled flours and fractions. Kodo millet has a claimed 9% fibre content, which is significantly higher than the fibre content of rice, a common staple food (0.2%). However, other researchers indicated that the fibre content ranged from 4.06% to 11%. Soluble fibre makes up 4.57% of the total amount of fibre. This characteristic of dietary fibre aids in regulating blood sugar levels in people with diabetes and coronary heart disease. The mineral content of kodo millet is high and includes Fe, Ca, P, and mg. Its ash content serves as a representation. It was noted that the iron level was 3.85 mg/100g, the magnesium value was 147 mg/100g, and the potassium content was 144 mg/100g. Kodo millet reported higher quantities of this minerals than rice and other millets like proso, banyard and little millet. In case of the vitamins, kodo millet is considered as the better source of the B –vitamins especially for the nicotinic acid, folic acid and pyridoxine. However, very limited studies are reported on the quantification on the vitamins in kodo millet.

**Table 3 :** Nutritional composition/Proximate analysis of Kodo millet

| Nutrients | Amount(100gm) |
|---|---|
| Energy | 346 kcal |
| Carbohydrate | 59.2 gm |
| Protein | 10.6 gm |
| Fat | 4.2 gm |
| Calcium | 27 mg |
| Iron | 0.5 mg |
| Moisture | 11.6 gm |
| Ash | 2.95 gm |
| Fibre | 10.2 gm |
| Phosphorous | 188 mg |
| Minerals | 4.4 gm |
| Niacin | 2 mg |
| Riboflavin | 0.09 mg |

*Source*: Hadimani and Malleshi, (1993), Vijay *et al.,* (2013); Devi, *et al.,* (2014)

Studies on areas with increased polyphenol content have demonstrated antioxidant activity (Dykes *et al.*, 2006). The substantial number of nutraceuticals is designated for the millets. Kodo millets are rich in phytates, tannins, and polyphenols. The antioxidant activity is caused by all of these elements. Kodo millet was fed to rats in certain animal trials, and the rats' blood sugar and cholesterol levels were reduced by 42% and 27%, respectively, more than with other millet diets. Kodo millet has a greater polyphenol content than pearl and proso millet, with 368 mg/100g. Comparatively speaking to the other millets, kodo millet had the highest antioxidant activity (70.82 mg AAEAA/100g) (little and proso millet). After germination, the kodo millets' free, bounder, and total phenolic and flavonoid chemicals increased. Additionally, millets are a good provider of phosphorus and magnesium. While phosphorus is a crucial part of adenosine triphosphate (ATP), which is a precursor to energy in the body, magnesium has the potential to help reduce migraines and heart attacks (Badau *et al.,* 2005; Liang *et al.,* 2010; Devi *et al.,* 2011) . Kodo millet is referred to as a "nutria-cereal" because of its abundance in vitamins, minerals, and phytochemicals. It also contains a lot of sulphur-containing amino acids like cysteine and methionine as well as important amino acids like threonine, valine, and lysine. Table 3 displays the general proximate composition of kodo millet. Table 4 displays the availability of the carbs, amylose, and amylo content. Table 5 compares the nutritional makeup of kodo millet with the other millets in more detail.

Usually found in plants, starch is an odourless, colourless polymer that is stored as carbs. The two types of polysaccharide molecules that make up starch are amylose and amylopectin. Amylose, a linear polymer with a lower molecular weight than amylopectin and composed of multiple D-glucose units connected by 1,4-glycosidic linkages, makes up around 20–30% of all starch. Amylase, an enzyme that can hydrolyse amylose into glucose units, is less water soluble than glucose. Starch is transformed into sugars by amylase. Due to the linear structure, the gelling capacity and thickening power are increased.

About 70–80% of the starch is made up of the branching polymer amylopectin, which has four times the molecular weight of amylose. Both α-1,6-glycosidic and α-1,4-glycosidic linkages bind the molecules of amylopectin together. It is either hardly or completely insoluble in water. Due to the branching structure, the gelling capacity and thickening power are reduced. The applications of amylose and amylopectin are directly influenced by their chemical makeup in the starch.

**Table 4 :** Available carbohydrate contents of cereal Vs millets(per 100 gm)

| Grain Name | Available Carbohydrate (g) | Amylose (%) | Amylopectin (%) |
|---|---|---|---|
| Milled Rice | 76.4 | 12-19 | 81-88 |
| Wheat | 59.3 | 25 | 75 |
| Sorghum | 61 | 24 | 76 |
| Pearl Millet | 56 | 21.1 | 78.9 |
| Finger Millet | 62.5 | 16 | 84 |
| Kodo Millet | 66.2 | 24 | 76 |
| Proso Millet | - | 28.2 | 71.8 |
| Foxtail Millet | - | 17.5 | 82.5 |
| Little Millet | 66.4 | - | - |
| Barnyard Millet | - | - | - |

*Source*: Indian Food Composition Tables, 2017, NIN, ICMR

**Table 5 :** Nutritional Composition of Different Millets (per 100 gm)

| Parameters | Protein (g) | Fat (g) | CHO (g) | Minerals (g) | Total Dietary Fiber (g) | Calcium (mg) | Iron (mg) |
|---|---|---|---|---|---|---|---|
| Pearl Millet | 11 | 5.4 | 61.8 | 1.4 | 11.5 | 42 | 8 |
| Sorghum | 10 | 1.7 | 67.7 | 1.4 | 10.2 | 27.6 | 3.95 |
| Finger Millet | 7.2 | 1.9 | 66.8 | 2 | 11.2 | 364 | 4.62 |
| Kodo Millet | 8.9 | 2.6 | 66.2 | 1.7 | 6.4 | 15.27 | 2.34 |
| Proso Millet | 12.5 | 0.52 | 78.2 | 0.6 | 2.81 | 14 | 0.8 |
| Little Millet | 10.4 | 3.9 | 65.6 | 1.3 | 7.7 | 16.06 | 1.26 |
| Foxtail Millet | 12.3 | 4.3 | 60.9 | 3.3 | - | 31 | 2.8 |
| Barnyard Millet | 6.2 | 4.4 | 65.5 | 2.2 | 1.98 | 20 | 5 |

**Source:** Indian Food Composition Tables, (2017); NIN, ICMR and Gopalan *et al*, (2009)

## Effect of processing on nutritional quality of Kodo millet

Kodo millets have significantly more phytic acids, phosphorus, antioxidants, and polyphenols than other millets. These anti-nutrients act as chelating agents, bind to other micronutrients, and impede their usage, which reduces their bioavailability in diet. The tannin and phytate concentrations in kodo millets are decreased using a variety of processing methods, including soaking, heating, and fermentation. This improves the digestibility of protein and carbohydrates and boosts the bioavailability of amino acids and other minerals. The antioxidant activity of kodo millets is considerably reduced during the dehulling and frying operations. Kodo millet has a higher amount of free radical scavenging capacity than other minor millets such finger millet, small millet, foxtail millet, and barnyard millet.Also, it was discovered that fractionating kodo millet's husk and endosperm reduced the grain's antioxidant capacity. Hegde and Chandra (2005) found that whole kodo millet's antioxidant activity decreased from 32.4 to 6.86 in the dehulled version, but only to 6.06 in the dehulled boiling version (Chandrasekara *et al.,* 2012). By using the dehulling method, it is possible to lower the total phosphorus level and phytate content by up to 40% to 50%. (Balasubramanian, 2013). The expected glycaemic index (AGI) of whole Kodo millet starch was discovered to be lower than rice starch (Annor *et al.*, 2013). The Debranning method can improve the bioavailability of minerals and important amino acids like methionine and cysteine that include sulphur, according to research by Amadou *et al.* (2013).

## Effect of Processing Technologies on Kodo Millets

A range of value-added products are made using various processing methods, which can increase millets' nutritional value, sensory appeal, and bioavailability of their numerous micronutrients. These processing methods include heat processing, mechanical processing, fermentation, soaking, malting/germination, and others.

The concentration of anti-nutrients including tannin, oxalate, and phytates is reduced while the bioavailability of some micronutrients is increased.

## Mechanical Processing

The majority of millets and other grains are subjected to mechanical dehulling methods, including hand pounding, hydrothermal treatment, and other techniques. It has been noted that millet's sensory and edible quality are improved by dehulling. Since millets are more difficult to decorticate than other grains, different treatments are employed. The millets' endosperm is made harder by hydrothermal treatment, which also makes it possible for it to decorticate. The millets are also decorticated using other mechanical machines or by pounding them by hand.It has been seen that the decortication method has a negligible impact on millets' levels of fat and protein, but a significant impact on their mineral, phytochemical, antioxidant, and anti-nutritional content.

According to Chandrasekara *et al.* (2012), the uneven distribution of polyphenolics in various layers of the millet grains caused the total phenolic components in kodo millets to significantly decrease following dehulling as compared to whole grain millets. So, millets' nutritional value as a food with functional purposes was decreased. To grind grains into flour, which primarily comprises the endosperm component and removes the bran layer, modern electric and motorised mills are utilised. Historically, non-motorized mills were used to crush millets. The separation of the bran layer has been seen to drastically reduce the nutrients, including minerals, crude fibre, phytochemicals, and other antioxidants and anti-nutrients, while increasing the protein and starch digestibility. Furthermore, it was discovered that the proximate composition declined with rising moisture content and grinding time. As the bran is sieved off of millets, some of their nutritious content is lost.

Even after dehusking, debranned millets appeared to have a total dictary fibre content of 15.9%, with the majority of the bran having a high content. Pulverization has considerably decreased the amount of fat, fibre, and protein in finger millet as well as water-soluble vitamins like thiamine and riboflavin. Because it has all the healthy ingredients, whole grain flour is recommended. In conclusion, millets lose nutrients and anti-nutrients as a result of milling, sieving, and decortication. Thus, food processing businesses need to use practical and cutting-edge technologies in order to produce nutrient-dense millet flour with a maximum yield.

## Bioprocess Technologies

One of the simplest ways to reduce the anti-nutrients in millets is to soak them, which also increases the bioavailability of several minerals. Whole seeds, decorticated seeds, and flour millets have been reported to reduce phytate activity and certain minerals when they are soaked (iron and zinc). Additionally, it was observed that the concentrations of minerals including phosphorus, calcium, and iron decreased as the soaking period increased (Chapke *et al.*, 2020). The polyphenol oxidase enzyme has been reported to cause a reduction in polyphenolic chemicals in finger millet and pearl millet (Naveena *et al.,* 2013). By eliminating anti-nutrients, soaking can help increase the digestion of carbohydrates and proteins (Samuel *et al.*).The biochemical makeup of millets, including their protein, ash, moisture, fat, and fibre content, can vary during fermentation. The partial breakdown of complex proteins into simpler proteins like peptides and amino acids improves protein digestibility in millets, hence the fermentation process is utilised to reduce anti-nutrients and improve protein and starch digestibility. All anti-nutrients, with the exception of tannin, are significantly reduced by fermentation, including trypsin, amylase inhibitors, and phytic acid.

Millets have been fermented using microbial cultures containing Saccharomyces cerevisiae, *Lactobacillus brevis*, *Saccharomyces diastaticus*, and *Lactobacillus fermentum*. The combination of Lactobacilli and yeast will increase the digestion of protein and carbohydrates. Lactic acid fermentation of Pearl millets can reduce their phytate activity. (Stefano *et al.*, 2017). Millets' germination process can increase their free amino acid content and total sugar content while lowering their starch level. Compared to blanching, this procedure can also increase the digestion of protein and carbohydrates. Anti-nutrients including phytic acid, polyphenols, and tannins are also reduced by it. It has been noted that millets' germination has boosted the bio accessibility of minerals like calcium, zinc, and iron (Chauhan *et al.*, 2018).

Probiotic fermentation during germination boosted the levels of many nutrients, including protein, sucrose, soluble dietary fibre, thiamine, niacin, and lysine.When compared to kodo millet that had not been germinated, kodo millet that had been germinated for 35.82 hours had higher levels of phytochemicals (TPC, 83.01 mg GAE/100 g; TFC, 87.53 mg RUE/g) and antioxidant activity of 91.34% of DPPH. Protein level in the germinated kodo millet flour rose from 6.9% to 7.9%, mineral content rose from 232.82 to 251.73 mg/100 g, and dietary fibre content rose from 35.30 to 38.34 g/100 g, whereas phytate and tannin content fell from 1.344 to 0.997 mol/kg and 1.603 to 0.234 mg/100 g, respectively. (Sharma S *et al.*, 2017).

## Kodo-Poisoning and Anti-nutritional factors

Both livestock and humans can become unwell from eating kodo millet. Some deadly fungus is connected to the grain poisoning. The fungi *Aspergillus tamarii*, *Aspergillus flavus*, and *Phomopsis paspalli* can contaminate the crop and cause toxicity by producing cyclopiazonic acid, a mycotoxin (CPA). Which is present in kodo millet and causes "kodua poisoning" (Rao and Husain, 1985; Patwardhan *et al.,* 1974; Antony *et al.,* 2003). Animals with the fungus *Paspalum ergot* experience a variety of difficulties, including poor muscular coordination, anxiety, muscle stiffness, and in severe cases, animal death.

Kodo poisoning in humans can lead to sadness, nausea, vomiting, diarrhoea, stomach pain, and other symptoms like coma (Antony *et al.*, 2003). Additionally, there are issues with the anti-nutritional components of millets. The main anti-nutritional components, such as phytic acid and tannins, are listed in Table 6. Anti-nutrients are substances that bind to the nutrients found in food, lowering their bioavailability to the body. The following is a list of some typical anti-nutrients that can be found in various millets.

## Phytic acid or phytate

It is the main type of phosphorus storage, making up between 1 and 5 percent of foods such grains, legumes, nuts, and oilseeds. It is a by-product of secondary metabolism that serves as a nutritional store for the seed while it ripens (Muahamad *et al.,* 2010 and Gupta *et al.,* 2015). Humans nearly never absorb and hydrolyse this molecule, which makes it less effective at increasing the bioavailability of different minerals. The bioavailability of positively charged mineral ions like Zn, Fe, Ca, and Mg is impacted by the negatively charged ion called phytate (Fekadu *et al.,* 2014). Because phytate levels vary on growth circumstances, processing, harvesting, and even different testing techniques, they are highly variable in nuts, seeds, grains, legumes, and other foods.

## Polyphenols

Polyphenols are regarded as essential for life because they assist in maintaining a healthy body over the course of a person's life. They have anti-mutagenic, anti-inflammatory, antiviral, and anti-carcinogenic properties that can be helpful in reducing and avoiding a variety of disorders (Singh, 2016). Numerous human studies have discovered that certain polyphenols have anti-inflammatory and antioxidant properties, which help prevent and treat a wide range of lifestyle disorders like obesity, cancer, cardiovascular diseases, etc. In addition to reducing the transit of water-soluble vitamins like thiamine and folic acid, polyphenols present in a variety of millets can also change the activity of drugs through a variety of interactions. Iron reserves are low because polyphenols have an inhibiting effect on the absorption of minerals like iron.

## Tannins

After cellulose, hemicellulose, and lignin, tannins are regarded as the fourth most prevalent component of plants and constitute a significant class of antioxidants.

Excessive tannin consumption will harm the digestive system and it may reduce the various mineral status in the body can lead to mineral deficiency diseases like Anaemia (Iron Deficiency), Osteomalacia and Osteoporosis (Calcium Deficiency), Iodine (Goitre, Thyroid), and Lower immunity, Skin insufficiency, etc. Tannin combines with protein and other mineral ions and makes an insoluble complex, lowering their (Zinc Deficiency). As a result, it is advised to consume it in moderation.However, as shown in Table 6, kodo millet has lower levels of the anti-nutritional components (phytic acid and tannin) than do other millet varieties.

**Table 6 :** Anti-Nutritional factors present in different millets (per 100 gm)

| Millets | Phytic Acid (mg/g) | Tannins(mg/g) |
|---|---|---|
| Pearl Millet | 9.2 | 2.2 |
| Finger Millet | 5.54–5.58 | 3.5 |
| Kodo Millet | 1.2–1.4 | 1.0–1.2 |
| Proso Millet | 7.2 | - |
| Little Millet | - | 332.1–336.8 |
| Barnyard Millet | 9.2 | 2.2 |

*Source*: (Sharma. R *et al.*, 2021 and Guha. M *et al.*, 2015).

## Health Benefits of Kodo Millet

Various studies reported the health benefits of kodo millet consumption. This information is summarized here under.

### Kodo millet for diabetes

It has been seen that millet consumption has reduced diabetes incidence rates (Bunkar *et al.*, 2021). Alpha glucosidase and pancreatic amylase, two phenolic substances found in millets, partially prevent the enzymatic degradation of complex carbohydrates, lowering postprandial hyperglycaemia (Post Prandial sugar level). Pre-diabetic and diabetic individuals typically undergo postprandial blood glucose level monitoring to track their blood glucose levels two hours after eating (Shobana *et al.,* 2009). Aldose reductase is one of the inhibitors that prevents sorbitolbuild-up and lowers the risk of cataract illnesses brought on by diabetes (Chethan and Malleshi 2007).

### Millets and aging

The main factor causing the link between diabetes and ageing is non-enzymatic glycosylation, a chemical interaction between the amino group of proteins and the aldehyde reduction group of sugars. The high concentration of antioxidants and other phenolic compounds found in kodo millet, including phytates, phenols, and tannins, among others, may have considerable antioxidant effects that are beneficial for delaying ageing and metabolic syndrome (Hegde *et al.,* 2005).

## Millets against cancer and celiac disease

Millets are full of phenolic substances including phytates, phenols, and tannins, among others, which function as "anti-nutrients." However, these anti-nutrients lower human risk for colon and breast cancer. Kodo millets having the free radical scavenging ability which is very much beneficial for preventing various types of cancers (Hegde, *et al.*, 2005). It contains phenolic chemicals that have been demonstrated to be useful and have the potential to stop the growth of cancer in vitro (Chandrasekara *et al.,* 2010). An autoimmune ailment called celiac disease may be brought on by consuming gluten in one's diet. It is a specific kind of digestive problem that impacts the gastro intestinal system and prevents the body from absorbing nutrients. Millets are gluten-free grains that can be appropriate for those with celiac disease (Taylor, 2006; Ezeogu *et al.,* 2008).

## Millets in protection form cardiovascular disease

The chance of developing various cardio vascular illnesses is increased by obesity, smoking, an inadequate food, an unhealthy lifestyle, and insufficient physical exercise. Cardiovascular disease is on the rise and is prevalent in the majority of nations. Free radical scavenging activity is significantly higher in millets, which may lower the risk of cardiovascular illnesses (Hegde and Chandra 2005).

## Other Health Benefits of Kodo millets include

- It has a high concentration of lecithin, a phospholipid that is great for bolstering the nervous system.
- The vitamin B complex, particularly vitamins B3 (niacin), B6 (pyridoxine), and B9 (folic acid or dietary folate), as well as several minerals like calcium, iron, potassium, magnesium, and zinc, are abundant in this food.
- Its high magnesium content makes it a great choice for people with high blood pressure and other cardiovascular problems.
- Linoleic acid, which has anti-tumor action, is present in it.
- It is beneficial for issues with obesity, diabetes, cardiovascular disease (CVD), and constipation since it is high in dietary fibre, low in sugar, and has the ability to lower LDL cholesterol.

## Value Added Food Products or Traditional Food Products Prepared by using Kodo millets

Kodo millets can be used to make both conventional and experimental cuisines. Unprocessed or processed grains can be boiled whole or decorticated if necessary, and they can also be ground into a powder using manual or automated processes to make flour for pudding. In tribal communities, it is prepared like rice using several recipes that are made with the flour. According to several research, kodo flour is used between 30 and 100 percent while making classic and innovative cuisine items like idli, dosa, chapati, pongal, biscuits, soup, cutlets, cookies, and ladoo (Padma and Rajendran, 2013, Kalpana *et al.,* 2013; Senthamarai *et al.,* 2013, Chakraborty and Kotwaliwale, 2016).

Kodo millet flour and black gram flour can be combined in equal parts to make papad. Cumin seeds, salt, and sodium bicarbonate can also be added for flavour and texture. The hard dough is rolled out into a circle and allowed to dry. Salt, cumin seeds, and kodo millet flour are combined, and then water is added to create a thick batter. After that, this batter is dropped onto oiled plates to dry in the sun (Desai *et al.,* 2010).

It can also be used to make Idli and Dosa by combining it with black gram in a 3:1 ratio. To prepare the batter must first the black gram and kodo millet be soaked before being ground either coarsely for idlis or finely for dosas. To improve the flavour, fenugreek seeds and salt should be added, and the mixture should ferment for an entire night. With this batter, idli can be steamed using idli pots (stands), and dosa can be made using a greased flatten pan or tawa.

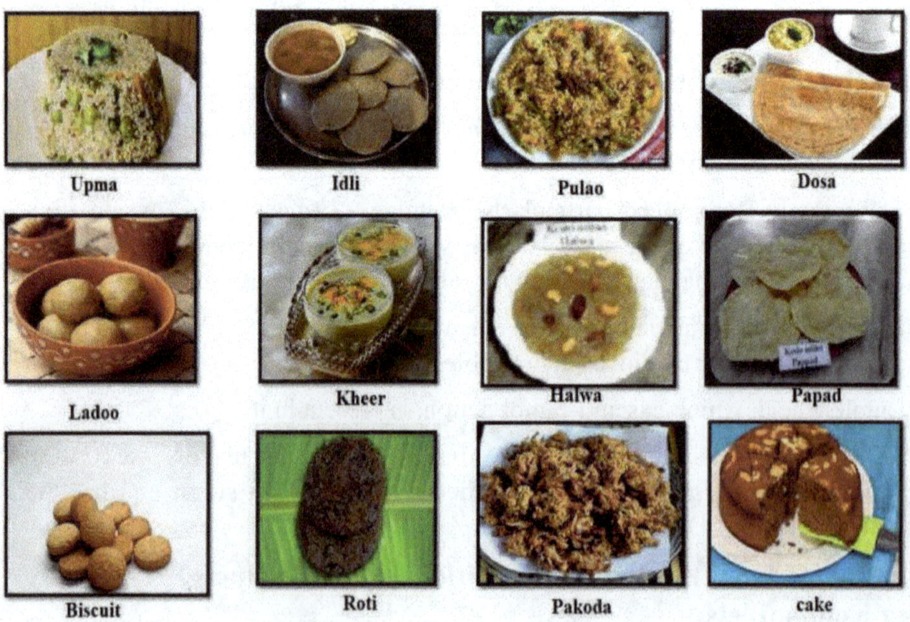


**Figure 5 :** Traditional foods from kodo millets (Source: Malathi *et al*, 2012, Chakraborty and Kotwaliwale, 2016).

In order to achieve a crispy texture, kodo millet flour along with other ingredients like chopped onion, green chilies, coriander or curry leaves, and other necessary spices or condiments must be deep-fried in heated oil. Kodo Pakoda and Kodo Vara are very popular dishes served throughout India. Kodo millet's coarse flour (rawa/ suji) can be used to produce upma. For sputtering or seasoning, chopped onion, green chilies, curry leaves, black gram dhal, bengal gramdhal, mustard seeds, and cumin seeds are used. To prevent any lump formation, water must be added to the seasoning ingredients, cooked, and then the roasted kodo rawa must be added while continuously stirring.To make sweet foods like halwa, coarse kodo (rough-textured) flour and wheat flour in a 2:1 ratio must be toasted with ghee or oil and added to boiling milk. Continuous stirring is required to prevent lumps. After the mixture has solidified, sugar and ghee must be added to give it the necessary consistency and flavour. After that, it can be seasoned or adorned with various dry fruits, such as cashews, raisins, and almonds, among others (Malathi *et al.,* 2012). It might also be a smart idea to use it as animal feed for livestock like chickens, goats, pigs, and lambs. The figure 5 displays many millet products.

## Extruded products

Extruded foods are often cooked at high temperatures for a brief period of time, which causes the starch to gelatinize and the protein to become denaturized. This procedure facilitates the inactivation of anti-nutrient components and enhances the digestibility (Awika and Rooney, 2004). Numerous benefits of the extrusion technique include constant quality, high production, product variety, and increased protein digestion (Dahlin and Lorenz, 1993). The availability of iron in extruded foods is improved by this method (Cisse *et al*, 1998).Using a twin-screw extruder, Kodo millet and chickpea blended flour (70:30) as well as soybean flour, pearl millet, and finger millet mix can be used to make millet-based extruded snack meals (Deshpande *et al.*, 2015, Geetha *et al.*, 2014). In 2012, Balasubramanian *et al.,* investigated the potential of composite millets. To make ready-to-eat extruded products from a mixture of millet powder and maida (50:50), finger millet and pearl millet can be combined to create milk powder (Devi and Narayanaswamy, 2013). Preparationof vermicelli, spaghetti, noodles, macaroni, murukus, vadi, bhujia sev, biscuits, cookies, chips, and other foods by combining different millets can successfully have prepared with the with cutting-edge extrusion techniques (Devi *et al.*, 2014). Figure 6 illustrates how the extruded kodo millet products were processed.

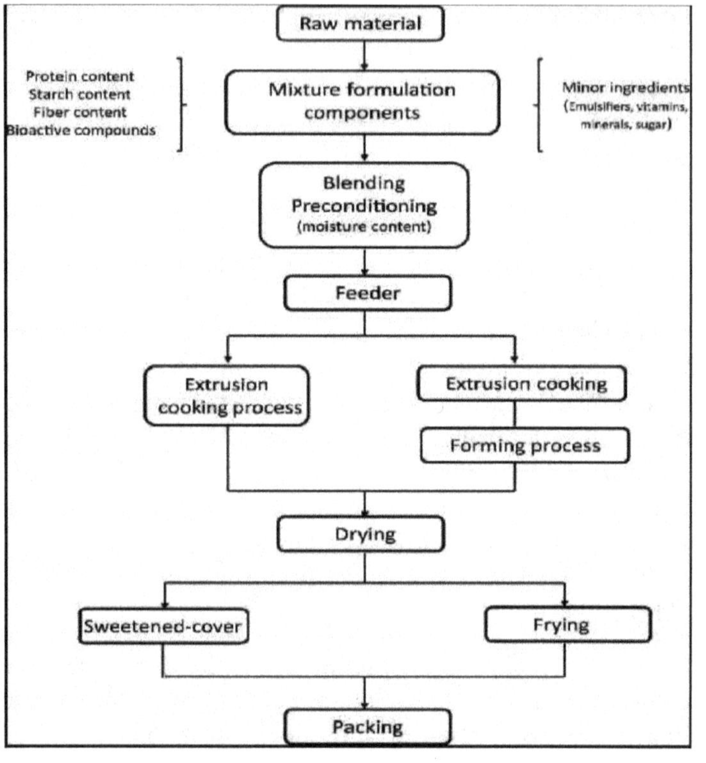


**Figure 6 :** Millet Extrusion Process Flow Chart

## Conclusion

Different types of the millets are the staple food for millions of poor people reside in continents like Asia and Africa. As compared to cereals, millets are highly nutritious in terms of protein and other nutrition content. Millets are a cheaper and nutritious option for low socio-economic people. Due to its low sugar and gluten content, it is beneficial for diabetes and celiac diseases also. Combination of cereals and milletswith pulses and legumes can give complimentary protein as both food group compliment to each other in terms of essential amino acid content in diet. There should be emphasis on the millet consumption in the developed as well as developing countries. More focus should be on millet production and processing to grow the millet industries in India as well as world so that more nutritious value-added millet products can be available for consumption purpose. Though kodo millet has so many potential health benefits but it contains anti-nutritional factors also so proper cooking and other post-harvest mechanisms are necessary to make the grain safe and wholesome for its consumption. Apart from the anti-nutritional factor, it can also cause poisoning due to the presence of toxic fungus so to prevent the toxicity proper handling and storage is very much necessary. Suitable and adequate precautionary measures should be taken by farmers and other stake holder in production, mechanization, cultivation, harvesting and processing areas.

## Acknowledgements

Both the authors are thankful to the authorities, Faculty of Agriculture, Sri Sri University, Cuttack, Odisha for providing the support and required facilities for completion of this book chapter.

## References

Amadou I, Gounga ME and Le GW (2013). Millets: Nutritional composition, some health benefits and processing-A review. *Emirates Journal of Food and Agriculture*, **25**(7): 501.

Annor GA, Marcone M, Bertoft E and Seetharaman K (2013). In-vitro starch digestibility and expected glycemic index of Kodo millet (Paspalum scrobiculatum) as affected by starch-protein-lipid Interactions. *Cereal Chemistry*, **90**(3): 211-217.

Antony M, Shukla Y and Janardhanan KK (2003). Potential risk of acute hepatotoxicity of kodo poisoning due to exposure to cyclopiazonic acid. *Journal of Ethnopharmacology*, **87**(2): 211-214.

Balasubramanian S (2013). Processing of Millets. Paper presented National Seminar on Recent Advances in processing, utilization and nutritional impact of small millets. Madurai Symposium, Thamukkam Grounds, Madurai, 13 September, 2013.

Balasubramanian, S., Singh, K. K., Patil, R. T., and Onkar, K. K. (2012). Quality evaluation of millet-soy blended extrudates formulated through linear programming. *Journal of food science and technology*, **49**(4), 450–458.

Begum, J. M., Vijayakumari, Begum, S., Pandy, A., Shivaleela, H. and Meenakumari (2003). Nutritional composition and sensory profile of baked products from finger millet. In: Recent Trends in Millet Processing and Utilization, *CCS Hisar Agricultural University, Hisar, India*, 82-87.

Bhat, S., Nandini. C., Tippeswamy and Prabhakar (2017). Significance of Small Millets in Nutrition and Health -A Review, AICRP On Small Millets, *Asian Journal of Dairy and Food Research*, **37**(1): 35-40.

Bunkar D.S, Goyal S.K, Meena K.K, Kamalvanshi V (2021). Nutritional, Functional Role of Kodo Millet and its Processing: A Review. *International Journal of Current Microbiology and Applied Sciences*, **10**(01): 1972-1985.

Bunkar, D. S., Jha, A., Mahajan, A. and Unnikrishnan, V. S. (2012). Kinetics of changes in shelf-life parameters during storage of pearl millet kheer mix and development of a shelf-life prediction model. *Journal of Food Sciences and Technology*, **51**(12): 3740-3748.

Chakraborty S and Kotwaliwale N (2016). Development of leavened bread from minor millet flours. Paper presented at 50th ISAE convention at Bhubaneswar, January 19-21, 2016.

Chandrasekara A and Shahidi F (2012). Bio accessibility and antioxidant potential of millet grain phenolics as affected by simulated in vitro digestion and microbial fermentation. *Journal of Functional Foods*, **4**(1): 226- 237.

Chandrasekara A, Naczk M and Shahidi F (2012). Effect of processing on the antioxidant activity of millet grains. *Food Chemistry*, **133**(1): 1-9.

Chandrasekara, A. and Shahidi, F. (2011). Inhibitory activities of soluble and bound millet seed phenolics on free radicals and reactive oxygen species. *Journal of Agricultural and Food Chemistry*, **59**(1), 428-436.

Chandrasekara, A. and Shahidi, F. (2010). Content of Insoluble Bound Phenolics in Millets and Their Contribution to Antioxidant Capacity. *Journal of Agricultural Food Chemistry*, **58**(11): 6706–6714.

Chapke R.R, G. Shyam Prasad, Das I.K, K Hariprasana, Singode A, Kanthisri B.S and Tonapi V.A. (2020). Latest Millet Production and Processing Technologies (Under Farmer First Programme), Indian Institute of Millets Research, Rajendranagar, Hyderabad.

Desai, A. D., Kulkarni, S. S., Sahoo, A. K., Ranveer, R. C., and Dandge, P. B. (2010). Effect of supplementation of malted ragi flour on the nutritional and sensorial quality characteristics of cake. *Advance Journal of Food Science and Technology*, **2**(1), 67-71.

Deshpande S.S, Mohapatra D, Tripathi M.K and Sadvatha R.H (2015). Kodo Millet-Nutritional Value and Utilization in Indian Foods. *Journal of Grain Processing and Storage*, **2**(2):16-23.

Devi, G. S., Palanimuthu, V., and Arun K. P., (2014). Studies on development and storage of Kodo millet based porrdige. *International Journal of Processing and Post Harvest Technology*, **5**(1): 33-40.

Devi, M. P. and Narayanaswamy, S. (2013). Extraction and dehydration of millet milk powder for formulation of extruded product. *IOSR Journal of Environmental Science, Toxicology and Food Technology*, **7**(1): 63-70.

Devi, P. B., Vijayabharathi, R., Sathyabama, S., Malleshi, N. G. and Priyadarisini, V. B. (2011). Health benefits of finger millet (Eleusine coracana L.) polyphenols and dietary fibre: a review. *J. Food Sci. Technol.* DOI: 10.1007/s13197-011-0584-9.

Dykes, L., and Rooney, L. W. (2006). Sorghum and millet phenols and antioxidants. *Journal of cereal science*, **44**(3), 236-251.

Geetha R, Mishra HN, Srivastav, P. P. (2014). Twin screw extrusion of kodo millet chickpea blend: process parameter optimization, physico-chemical and functional properties. *J Food Sci Technol,* **51**(11):3144-53.

Hadimani, Na. and Malleshi, Ng. (1993). Studies on Milling, Physicochemical Properties, Nutrient Composition and Dietary Fiber Content of Millets. *Journal of Food Science and Technology*, **30**:193–198.

Hegde, P. S. and Chandra, T. S. (2005). ESR spectroscopic study reveals higher free radical quenching potential in kodo millet (Paspalum scrobiculatum) compared to other millets. *Food Chemistry*, **92**(1), 177-182.

Hegde, P. S., Rajasekaran, N. S. and Chandra, T. 2005. Effects of antioxidant properties of millet species on oxidative stress and glycemic status in alloxaninduced rats. *Nutrition Research*,**25**(12):1109-1120.

Ramashia SE, Anyasi TA, Gwata ET, Meddows-Taylor S, Jideani IAO. (2019). Processing, nutritional composition and health benefits of finger millet in sub-saharan Africa. *Food Sci. Technol*, **39**(2):253-266.

Rao BL and Husain A (1985). Presence of cyclopiazonic acid in kodo millet (Paspalum scrobiculatum) causing 'kodua poisoning' in man and its production by associated fungi. *Mycopathologia*, **89**(3): 177-180.

Shahidi F and Chandrasekara A (2013). Millet grain phenolics and their role in disease risk reduction and health promotion: a review. *Journal of Functional Foods*, **5**(2): 570-581.

Ushakumari SR, Rashtogi NK, Malleshi NG. (2004). The functional properties of pooped, flaked, extruded and rolled dried foxtail millet (Setaria italic). *Int. J Food Sci. Tech*, **39**:907-915.

# 12

# Millets: Its Diseases and Management

Shiv Kumar Yadav[1*] and Ruchi Kumari[2]

[1] RNB Global University, Jaipur

[2] Nirwan University, Jaipur

**ABSTRACT**

Millets are known as a superfood and are thought to be future crops because they are rich in minerals and can survive harsh environments easily. Millets are a rich source of vitamins and minerals and consist of slowly digestible starch. Since diseases and pests cause significant reductions in crop productivity, it is essential to manage them. Millets are susceptible to a few diseases and pests that are not only economically relevant but have an important place in history.In order to maximize crop productivity, disease management is crucial, yet using pesticides like insecticides, fungicides, and bactericides degrades soil quality.To preserve soil quality and ecological balance, integrated disease management strategies must be adopted.This chapter will cover a variety of millet diseases and how to manage them.

*Keywords*: Disease, integrated disease management, millet, pest, soil quality.

## Introduction

First cereal crops to be cultivated is none other than millet. With variations coming from both Asia and Africa, millet has a wide range of origins. They have grown from the beginning of time. Almost 6,000 different types of millet are grown globally. Millets are said to as "today's nutri-cereals and yesterday's coarse grains."The dry land regions of the world traditionally eat millet as a primary diet. Millets are produced on roughly 17 million acres in India, producing 18 million tonnes annually and making about 10% of the nation's total grain production. These are nutri-cereals, which are known for their high nutritive value and high protein, essential fatty acid, dietary fiber, B-Vitamin, and various mineral contents. They aid in providing health advantages such as lowering blood sugar levels (diabetes), controlling blood pressure, and preventing thyroid, cardiovascular, and celiac disorders. The millet that is commonly farmed is pearl millet, a significant crop in India (Figure 1).

Some important millet apart from pearl millet is finger millet, kodo millet, foxtail millet, etc.Sorghum and millets have long been significant staple foods in the

* Corresponding author.

semi-arid tropical regions of Asia and Africa. Millions of the most vulnerable people in these places still rely primarily on these crops for their supply of energy, protein, vitamins, and minerals. Sorghum and millets are cultivated in arid regions when other crops do not thrive or produce inadequate yields. They are raised by numerous smallholder farmers in numerous nations using scarce water resources and typically without the use of any fertilizers or other inputs. They are frequently referred to as "coarse grain" or "poor people's crops" since they are mostly consumed by underprivileged communities.

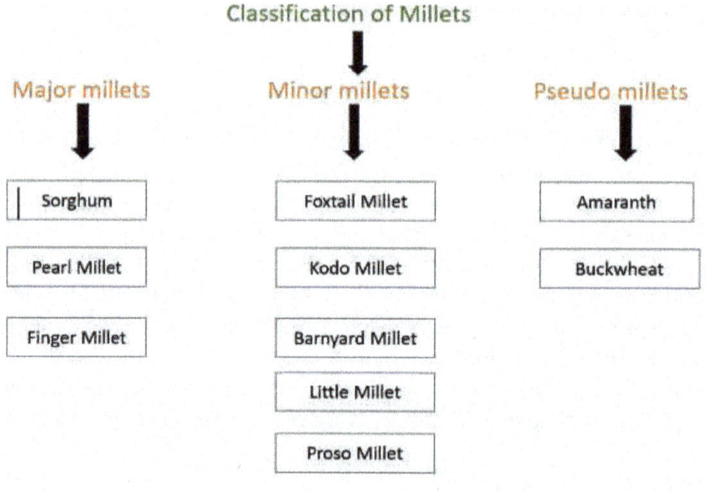


**Figure 1 :** Classification of millets

## Nutritive Value of Millets

Millets contain 6-8% protein, 1-1.7% fat, 65-75% starch, 2-2.5% minerals and 18-20% dietary fiber (Chethan and Malleshi 2007). They are very effective sources of phytochemicals with nutraceutical properties (Table 1).

## Health Benefits of Millets

Millets have many health advantages. Consuming millet lowers the risk of heart disease, protects against diabetes, improves the digestive system, lowers the risk of cancer, detoxifies the body, boosts immunity and respiratory health, increases energy levels, and strengthens the muscular and neurological systems (Table 2).

## Diabetes

By enzymatically hydrolyzing complex carbohydrates in hyperglycemia. The aldose reductase enzyme aids in reducing sorbitol build-up and lowers the chance of developing diabetes.Millets also aid in regulating blood sugar levels and slow the healing process after wounds (Rajesh Keran *et al.,* 2004).

**Table 1 :** Proximate and dietary fiber content of millets and major cereals (per 100 g)

| Millets and Cereals | | Moisture (g) | Protein (g) | Ash (g) Total | Total Fat (g) Insoluble | Dietary Fibre (g) | | | Carbohydrates (g) | Energy (KJ) |
|---|---|---|---|---|---|---|---|---|---|---|
| | | | | | | Soluble | | | | |
| Bajra (Pennisetum glaucum) | | 08.97 ± 0.60 | 10.96 ± 0.26 | 1.37 ± 0.17 | 5.43 ± 0.64 | 11.49 ± 0.62 | 9.14 ± 0.58 | 2.34 ± 0.42 | 61.78 ± 0.85 | 1456 ± 18 |
| Sorghum (Sorghum vulgare) | | 09.01 ± 0.77 | 09.97 ± 0.43 | 1.39 ± 0.34 | 1.73 -0.31 | 10.22 ± 0.49 | 8.49 ± 0.40 | 1.73 ± 0.40 | 67.68 ± 1.03 | 1398 ± 13 |
| Ragi (Eleusine coracana) | | 10.89 ± 0.61 | 07.16 ± 0.63 | 2.04 ± 0.34 | 1.92 ± 0.14 | 11.18 ± 1.14 | 9.51 ± 0.65 | 1.67 ± 0.55 | 66.82 ± 0.73 | 1342 ± 10 |
| Little Millet (Panicum miliare) | | 14.23 ± 0.45 | 08.92 ± 1.09 | 1.72 ± 0.27 | 2.55 0.13 | 06.39 ± 0.60 | 5.45 ± 0.48 | 2.27 ± 0.52 | 65.55 ± 1.29 | 1449 ± 19 |
| Kodo Millet (Setaria italica) | | 14.23 ± 0.45 | 08.92 ± 1.09 | 1.72 ± 0.27 | 2.55 ± 0.13 | 06.39 ± 0.60 | 4.29 ± 0.82 | 2.11 ± 0.34 | 66.19 ± 1.19 | 1388 ± 10 |
| Foxtail Millet* | | 11.20 | 12.30 | - | 4.30 | - | - | - | 60.09 | 331 |
| Barnyard Millet* | | 11.90 | 06.20 | - | 2.20 | - | - | - | 65.55 | 307 |
| Proso Millet* | | 11.90 | 12.50 | - | 1.10 | - | - | - | 70.04 | 341 |
| Wheat | Whole | 10.58 ± 1.11 | 10.59 ± 0.60 | 1,42 ± 0.19 | 1.47 ± 0.05 | 11.23 ± 0.77 | 9.63 £ 0.19 | 1.60 ± 075 | 64.72 ± 1.74 | 1347 ± 23 |
| | Refined flour | 11.34 ± 0.93 | 10.36 ± 0.29 | 0.51 ± 0.07 | 0.76 0.07 | 02.76 ± 0.29 | 2.14 ± 0.30 | 0.62 ± 0.14 | 74.27 ± 0.92 | 1472 ± 16 |
| | Atita | 11.10 ± 0.35 | 10.57 ± 0.37 | 1.28 ± 0.19 | 1.53 ± 0.12 | 11.36 ± 0.29 | 9.73 ± 0.47 | 1.63 ± 0.64 | 64.17 ± 0.32 | 1340 ± 07 |
| | Semolina | 08.94 ± 0.68 | 11.38 ± 0.37 | 0.80 ± 0.17 | 0.74 ± 0.10 | 09.72 ± 0.74 | 8.16 ± 0.58 | 1.55 ± 0.18 | 68.43 ± 0.99 | 1396 ± 18 |
| Rice | Raw brown | 09.33 ± 0.39 | 09.16 ± 0.75 | 1.04 ± 0.18 | 1.24 I 0.08 | 04.43 ± 0.54 | 3.60 ± 0.55 | 0.82 ± 0.15 | 74.80 ± 0.85 | 1480 ± 10 |
| | Raw milled | 09.93 ± 0.75 | 07.94 ± 0.58 | 0.56 ± 0.08 | 0.52 ± 0.05 | 02.81 ± 0.42 | 1.99 ± 0.39 | 0.82 ± 0.22 | 78.24 ± 0.68 | 1491 ± 15 |
| | Parboiled | 10.09 0.43 | 07.89 ± 0.63 | 0.65 0.8 | 0.55 ± 0.08 | 03.74 ± 0.36 | 2.98 ± 0.35 | 0.76 ± 0.09 | 77.16 ± 0.76 | 1471 ± 8 |
| Quinoa (Chenopodium quinoa) | | 10.43 | 13.11 | 02.65 | 5.50 | 14.66 | 10.21 | 4.46 | 53.65 | 1374 |
| Ama-ranth Seed | Black | 09.89 | 14.59 | 02.78 | 5.74 | 07.02 | 5.76 | 1.26 | 59.98 | 1490 |
| | Pale brown | 09.20 ± 0.40 | 13.27 ± 0.34 | 3.05 ± 0.30 | 5.56 ± 0.3 | 07.47 ± 0.09 | 5.80 ± 0.17 | 1.67 ± 0.21 | 61.46 ± 0.60 | 1489 ± 10 |
| Maize | Dry | 09.26 ± 0.55 | 08.80 ± 0.49 | 1.17 0.16 | 3.77 ± 0.48 | 12.24 ± 0.93 | 11.29 ± 0.85 | 0.94 ± 0.18 | 64.77 ± 1.58 | 1398 ± 25 |

**Table 2 :** Health Benefits of Millets

| Types of Millets | Health Benefits |
|---|---|
| Finger millet | Inhibit cataract eye lens, Lower plasma glucose level, Antimicrobial activity against Bacillus cereus and Aspergillus, flavus |
| Foxtail millet | Anti hyperglycemic activity |
| Proso millet | Improved HDL, Lower triglycerides, Prevent cardiovascular disease |
| Kodo millet | Inhibit glycation and cross linking of collagen leads to inhibition of aging |
| Pearl millets | Inhibiting the growth of the phytopathogenic fungi |
| Barnyard millets | Improved the levels of HDL |
| Little millet | Inhibitory effects on lipid peroxidation |

## Heart diseases

Magnesium, which is found in millet, helps to lower the risk of a heart attack. Millets are abundant in phytochemicals that decrease cholesterol and assist to avoid heart disease (Lee *et al.,* 2010).

Plant diseases are known from a long time ago, even from the era when we didn't have had any written record. According to fossil evidence, the disease began to harm plants 250 million years ago. Since the beginning of recorded history, diseases have caused faminelike rusts, mildews, and blights and other severe disruptions in the economies of nations, according to the Bible and other ancient sources.Diseases are among top most reasons responsible for loss of yield in crops. In developing nations like India disease cause a lot of loss in yield of crops which ultimately leads to hunger and starvation. There are many examples of famine occurs due to diseases that was caused due to various plant diseases, among which Irish famine, Bengal famine are well known for its devastation. Some diseases of millets are also responsible for causing a lot of havoc in the history that includes erogitism, dancing plague, St Anthony's Fire, etc.

A plant is said to be diseased when its metabolism is affected which in turn affect its structure growth function or other activities by any pathogen.

## Conditions Necessary for Disease

There are basic three factors that are required to cause a disease which includes-Pathogen, Host, and Environment. These three factors together form a disease triangle (Figure 2).

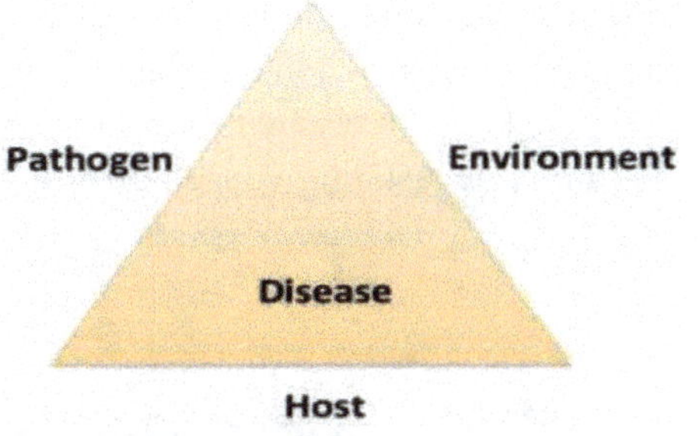


**Figure 2 :** Disease Triangle

Three prerequisites must be fulfilled for the disease to exist. A susceptible host plant must be present first. Only a few viruses tcan infect each species of plant. Also, the plant needs to be in a developmental stage where it can be infected by the disease agent. The existence of an active pathogen is the second prerequisite.There cannot be a disease if a pathogen is present. The pathogen must also be in a stage of development that makes it easy for it to infect or have an impact on the host plant. A pathogen-friendly environment is the third prerequisite for a plant to get ill. The relationship between the host, pathogen, and environment is occasionally illustrated by a triangle.If any one of the three legs is missing, the "disease triangle" cannot be built. There is no disease if one of the triangle's legs is broken. Breaking one leg of the triangle can serve as the basis for disease prevention measures.

One of the main issues of the modern era is food security. The average annual global carryover stock of grain was 107 days' worth of consumption from 1986 to 2001; however, from 2002 to 2011, as the world's population grew, the stock fell to 74 days' worth of consumption. By 2050, the globe must produce 50% more food to meet the demands of 9 billion people.Millets were referred to be "orphan crops" by Dr. M. S. Swaminathan, the pioneer of the Indian Green Revolution. Before the first green revolution, millets made up 40% of the cultivated grains; after 1965, that percentage fell to roughly 50%. (Rawat *et al.,* 2021). Identifying conventional or native plants that are particularly adapted to the local environment, have high nutrient costs, and can effectively withstand biotic and/or abiotic challenges and increase their production is one workable alternative.

Wheat, maize, and rice only give food security, whereas millets account for a number of security factors, including grain, fodder, fiber, nutrition, health, environment, and livelihood at low cost, providing excellent potential for food and nutrition security (Gupta *et al.,* 2017).The primary factors causing significant yield losses in agricultural production around the world are mainly biotic factors like bacteria, fungi, phanerogamic plants, and other pests. The degree to which biotic stressors are felt varies with the weather, cropping system, cultivation techniques, kind of crops, and crop varieties in relation to their level of resistance. The crop is typically prone to these pressures due to hot, humid conditions, extensive production, and inadequate crop management techniques. When compared to other crops, millets, and pseudocereals are less affected negatively by biotic stressors because they are climate-resilient. One of the most devastating causes of millet's low output and field damage is a fungus.

## Ergot

A significant barrier in the generation of hybrid seeds is ergot. Sorghum (c.o. *Claviceps sorghi* & *C. africana*) and pearl millet are frequently affected by the disease (c.o. *Claviceps fusiformis*). The first observable symptom is the exudation of droplets resembling honeydew from infected florets. The thin, sticky, or viscous droplets have a pin-pinkish-to-brownish colorand a sweet taste. An infected floret gradually develops a wart-like fungal growth termed a sclerotium in place of the grain. The sclerotia grow and release ascospores, which spread via the air and infect the floret (Figure 3).

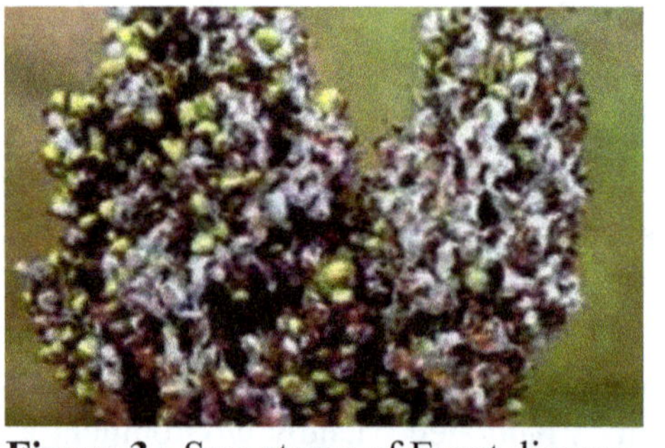

**Figure 3 :** Symptoms of Ergot disease

### *Management*

- Spray any fungicides Mancozeb 2 kg/haat the emergence of ear head (5-10 percent flowering stage) followed by a spray at 50 percent flowering and repeat the spray after a week, if necessary.
- Change in date of sowing to avoid the chances of disease.

## Downy mildew

There have been reports of downy mildew on finger millet (c.o. *Sclerophthora-macrospora*), foxtail millet (c.o. *Sclerospora graminicola*), and sorghum (c.o. *Peronosclero sporasorghi*). The infection begins at the seedling stage and lasts until the plant dies. The bottom portion of the leaf blade on sorghum, foxtail, and pearl millet displays a white, downy growth made up of conidia and conidiophores of the pathogen that later migrate upward. Finger millet does not exhibit this type of downy growth, which gives the plant's top a bush-like look while still exhibiting the classic "green ear" symptom. Foxtail and pearl millet both frequently exhibit the symptoms of green ears (Figure 4).

*Management*

- Crop rotation should be adopted.
- Metalaxyl @ 6g/kg should be used for seed treatment.
- Spray Metalaxyl 500 g or Mancozeb 2 kg or Ziram 1 kg or Zineb 1kg/ha.
- Rouging out of infected plants control the spread of disease.

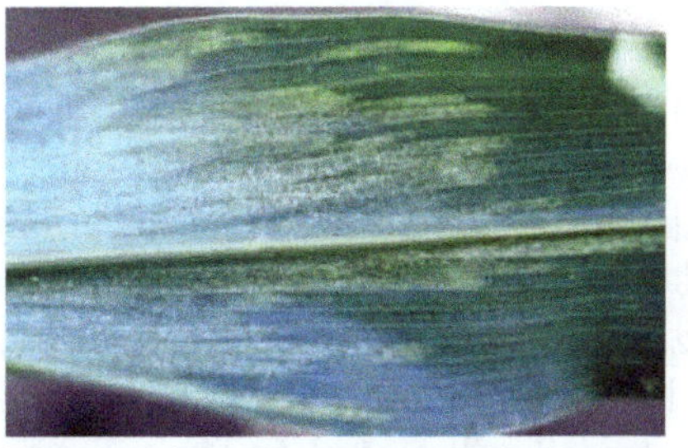

**Figure 4 :** Symptoms of Downy Mildew,source, http://eagri.org/eagri50/PATH272/lecture 02/006.html

## Smut

There are four different kinds of smut that are usually seen in millets and these are head smut, covered smut, loose smut and long smut. Sorghum is infected by all four types of smuts namely, head smut (c.o. *Sporisorium reilianum*), covered smut (c.o. *Sporisorium sorghi*), loose smut (c.o.*Sporisorium cruenta*), and long smut (c.o. *Tolyposporium ehrenbergii*). The ear might become completely or partially infected with Smut disease.The majority of the infected ear's grains are replaced by the sori in the covered smut, which has a fungal structure that resembles a membrane (Figure 5).

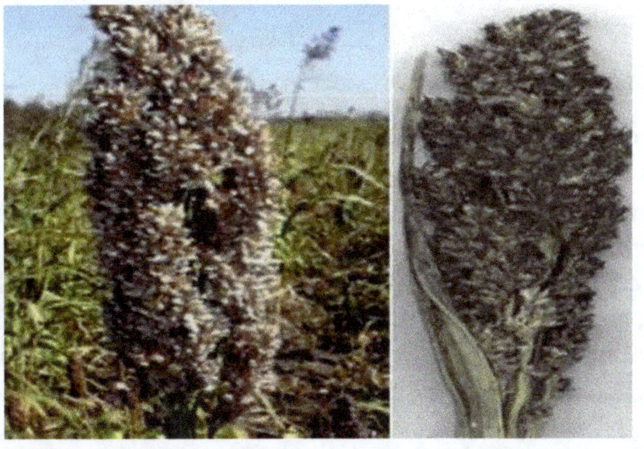

**Figure 5 :** Symptoms of smut, source, http://eagri.org/eagri50/PATH272/lecture02/006.html

*Management*

- Seed treatment with Thiram @4 g/kg is considered good for the management of smut disease.
- The residue of diseased parts should be bury in the soil

## Rust

On both of the lower leaves' surfaces, rust symptoms take the form of reddish-brown pustules. The infection in the top part is more serious than in the bottom half. The infection spreads to the younger leaves as the condition worsens.Almost all the millets are infected by rust, but pathogens are different for different millets viz., *Puccinia purpurea* (on sorghum),*Puccinia substriata* var. indicia (on pearl millet), *Puccinia substriata*(on finger and kodo millets), *Uromyces setariaeitalica* (on foxtail millet), and *Uromyces eragrostidis* (on little millet) (Figure 6).

### *Management*

- Mancozeb @ 2kg/ha is considered for the management of disease.

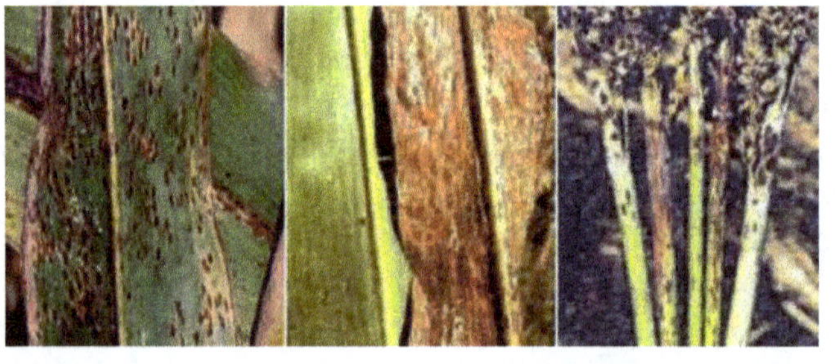

**Figure 6 :** Symptoms of Rust, source, http://eagri.org/eagri50/PATH272/lecture02/005.html

## Conclusion

Millets are regarded as a superfood and the crops of the future because of their mineral richness and ease of surviving severe settings. Millets provide slowly absorbed carbohydrates and are a good source of vitamins and minerals. It is crucial to handle diseases and pests since they significantly lower agricultural output. A few diseases and pests that are not only significant commercially but also have a significant historical impact might affect millets. Disease control is essential for maximizing crop output, however employing pesticides like insecticides, fungicides, and bactericides decreases the quality of the soil.Integrated disease control measures must be used in order to maintain soil quality and ecological balance.

## References

Chethan, S., and Malleshi, N.G. (2007). Finger Millet Polyphenols: Optimization of extraction and the effect of pH on their stability, Food chemistry. **105**: 862-872.

Chandrasekara, A. and Shahidi, F. (2012). Bioaccessibility and antioxidant potential of millet grain phenolics as affected by simulated in vitro digestion and microbial fermentation. Journal of Functional Foods.**4**: 226-237.

ChandrasekaraA, Shahidi F. 2011. Antioxidant phenolics of millet control lipid peroxidation in human LDL cholesterol and food systems. J Am Oil ChemSoci DOI: 10.1007/s11746- 011-1918-5. Available from Springer [http://www.springerlink.com]. Posted August 20, 2012

Geervani, P. and Eggum, B.O., (1989). Nutrient composition and protein quality of Minor millets, Plant Foods for Human Nutrition, Dordrecht, Netherlands, **39**: 201 -208.

Gupta SM, Arora S, Mirza N, Pande A, Lata C, Puranik S, Kumar A(2017) Finger millet: a "certain" crop for an "uncertain"future and a solution to food insecurity and hidden hunger under stressful environments. Front Plant Sci **8**: 643.

India: Health of the Nation's States. The India State-Level Disease Burden Initiative, Indian Council of Medical Research, Public Health Foundation of India, Institute for Health Metrics and Evaluation, November, 2017.

Kumar B (2016) Status of small millet diseases in Uttarakhand. Int JPlant Protec **9**(1): 256-263.

Krishnakumari, S., and Thayumanavan, B. (1995). Content of starch and sugars and in vitro digestion of starch by α-amylase in five minor millets. Plant Foods for Human Nutrition, **48**(4), 327-333.

Lee, S. H.; Chung, I M. Cha, Y S. and Parka, Y. (2010). Millet consumption decreased serum concentration of triglyceride and C reactive protein but not oxidative status in hyperlipidemic rats. Nutr Res. **30**: 290– 296.

Manach, C., Mazur, A. and Scalbert, A. (2005). Polyphenols and prevention of cardiovascular diseases. Current Opinion Lipidology. **16**: 77-84.

Nagaraja A., Bijendra Kumar, Jain A.K., Patro T.S.S.K., Nageswar Rao T.G. 2016. Diseases of small millets. Diseases of field crops and their management. Indian Phytopathological Society. New Delhi. 295-371.

Rawat L, Bisht TS, Kukreti A (2021) Potential of seed biopriming with Trichoderma in ameliorating salinity stress and providing resistance against leaf blast disease in finger millet (Eleusinecoracana L.). Indian Phytopath **75**:147-164.

Rajasekaran, N. S., Nithya, M., Rose, C. and Chandra, T. S. (2004). The effect of finger millet feeding on the early responses during the process of wound healing in diabetic rats. BiochimBiophysActa **1689** (3–4): 190– 201

Scalbert, A., Manach, C., Morand, C., Remesy, C. and Jimenez, L. (2005) Dietary polyphenols and the prevention of diseases. Critical Reviews in Food Science and Nutrition. **45**: 287-306.

Verma, Veenu and Patel, S. (2012), Nutritional security and value added products from finger millets (ragi), Journal of Applicable Chemistry, **1** (4):485-489

# 13

# Economic Importance of Major Millet Pests and their Management Techniques

S. Sen[1*], S. Borkataki[2], C. A. Reddy[3] and P. S. Saranya[2]

[1] Department of Agricultural Entomology, Bidhan Chandra KrishiViswavidyalaya, Mohanpur, West Bengal-741252

[2] Department of Entomology, Assam Agricultural University, Jorhat, Assam-785013

[3] Department of Entomology, College of Post Graduate Studies in Agricultural Sciences, Central Agricultural University, Imphal, Megahalaya-795004

**ABSTRACT**

Millet grains have been used for long as staple food in few rural parts of China, India, and sub-Saharan Africa. Additionally, millet is fed to livestock and poultry in the United States, while in India, the leaves have been utilized as cattle fodder. At least 150 insect pests cause the crop harm as it grows and develops.Millets are attacked in the field and while being stored. Some are widespread in millet-growing regions. Grain midges and stem borers are frequent occurrences. White grubs and spike worms become significant in India and West Africa respectively. During the rainy season, storage bugs are more common. The strategies of millets pest management vary depending on the agro-ecosystem and the pest complex. However, it has been found that a mix of societal norms and resistant cultivars works best. To manage pests in millets, the pest complex, and the agro-ecosystem, an interdisciplinary approach might be provided by the exchange of genetic material and research data. By small and resource-constrained farmers, different IPM solutions have been followed with the increasing use of modern crop production techniques. In order to decrease the usage of insecticides, which are frequently used in highly pest infested areas, multiple pest resistance techniques have become more crucial. However, it has been found that a mix of societal norms and resistant cultivars works best.

*Keywords*: Millet, fodder, agro-ecosystem, insecticides, resistant, IPM

## Introduction

Chinese, Sub-Saharan African, and Indian subcontinent diets all heavily rely on the millet cereal. It is also used in the United States as part of the feed for poultry and cattle. Cattle are fed millet leaves in India. The estimated yearly millet

* Corresponding author.

production for the entire world is 28.4 mt, of which Africa produces 8.3 mt and India 10.3 mt (FAO, 2017). The year 2019 is considered as the "national year of millets" in response to an increased emphasis on nutritional security by the Indian government (Gahukar and Reddy, 2019). Around the world, eight millet species are grown. Pearl millet, *Pennisetum glaucum* (L.) is the most predominant one; the rest are little millets grown for domestic use. Nevertheless, there is no information on the ground beneath each millet (*Eragrostistef* Trotter) and african finger millet (*Eleusine coracana* Gaertner) are both routinely grown in Ethiopia and India, respectively. Other small millets include common or proso millet (*Panicum miliaceum* L.), foxtail or Italian millet (*Setariaitalica* L.), little millet (*Panicum sumatrense*), ditch or kodo millet (*Paspalum scrobiculatum* L.) (Gahukar and Reddy, 2019).

Production of millet has increased recently. For rural residents who are struggling financially, millets offer a sustainable food source. Urban residents also value millets for their high mineral and vitamin content. Farmers are being urged to grow millet either by itself or in intercropping with legumes due to the rising market demand for the grain. In fact, despite the importance of ensuring food security due to a growing global population, millets are underused in emerging nations.Millets are also hardy plants, which makes them suitable for reducing the agricultural consequences of drought and climate change as well as addressing nutritional inadequacies in rural regions. Around 150 different insect species were found to feed on millets, all over the globe (Nwanze and Harris 1992); 116 species of them have been identified in India (Kishore, 1996). All kinds of millet are affected by the majority of the pests (Gahukar, 1989). Short-cycle cultivars (cvs.) which mature within 85-95 days are extensively grown and have undergone more extensive pest management research in comparison to long-cycle cultivars (120-130 days maturity).

Insect feeding on various plant constituents at various plant development phases results in economic loses because it lowers agricultural output, cereal quality, and fodder yield. According to Gahukar and Jotwani, 1980, crop losses caused by millet bug infestations ranged from 10 to 20% (in India) to 50% (in Ghana) (Tanzubil and Yakubu 1997). There is little research on potential control methods, in part because crops are not worth much and different species attack rates, particularly on less common millets.Entomology studies on millet were scarce until recently. Advancements in cultural practises and the irregular rainfall in the tropics led to introduction of new pests or change in the relative proportion of established pest population. While few are widespread in the regions where millets are grown extensively, the economic significance of others varies greatly from season to season. Gahukar and Jotwani in 1980, recorded yield loss of 10–20% in India. The insect situation is investigated in order to contribute to the development of more effective pest control strategies, given the increasing importance of millets in the provision of food in emerging countries. Pests are dealt with in accordance with the state of the produce that was harmed. Here, suggestions for IPM are examined along with changes in insect status over the previous 20 years to make it simpler to create and implement IPM in future research, development, and outreach projects. The goal of this study is to compile the dispersed or fractured literature that is difficult for research organisations and development organisations to access.

## Soil pests

Only minor pests of millets among soil-dwelling insects are termites and cutworms (Gahukar, 1989). White grubs, on the other hand, can seriously harm pearl millet stems by feasting on them in dry and semi-arid regions (Choudhary *et al.*, 2018). *Holotrichia consanguinea* Blanch, is a significant, pervasive root feeding insect of millet in India. Patches of dead seedlings can easily be seen in the field because grubs eat on the roots of millet seedlings, causing withering and ultimately die. The seedlings are cut at ground level by crickets, cutworms and root beetles, (Rangarajan 1965; Jotwani and Butani 1978), termites like Odontotermes and Microtermes damage roots and gnaw through stems in sandy environments. In early season, if droughts persist, damage is significant. Root infesting bugs, or *Stibaropus minor* Fb., suck sap from the rootlets of millets and thriving in very sandy soils.Imidacloprid 600FS seed treatment at a rate of 10–12 ml/kg has been proven to be the most efficient method of controlling white grubs, which reduces seedling mortality to 2.1% from 28.6% while increase grain output to 27.52 q/ha from 12.30 q/ha (Choudhary *et al.*, 2018). The soil dwelling pests can also be controlled by applying clothianidin 50 WDG at a rate of 10 g/kg (seedling treatment). It was also equally successful to saturate the soil with imidacloprid 17.8SL at a rate of 300 ml/ha, or to combine chlorpyriphos 20EC or quinalphos 25EC with irrigation water at a rate of 4.0 liters/ha three weeks after seedling emergence (WAE). Chlorpyriphos or quinalphos dust used at planting in a 2:3 mixture with farmyard manure (FYM) is also efficient for furrow application. Use of pesticides may be advised in regions with high levels of endemic white grub pressure and during pest outbreaks.

## Seedling pests

Stem flies, grey weevils, and leaf beetles all plague seedlings. All millets are attacked by several species of shoot flies (Diptera: Muscidae) throughout India and Africa (Kalaisekar *et al.*, 2017). Early on in their development, the shoot fly larvae feed the leaf sheath, severing the growth tip, causes the stem to wilt, yellow, and die, a condition called as "dead heart". Immature stages of these insects consume rotting matter just above the wound. It has been found that the pest harm caused by these flies results in pearl millet production losses of 20–50% (Natarajan *et al.*, 1973, Kishore, 1996), 39% in small millet and 36% in common millet (Natarajan *et al.*, 1974). Infestations of the shoot fly (*Atherigona approximate)* of pearl millet are common in India (Selvaraj *et al.*, 1974). The TNAU (2016) suggested a series of management tactics for the pearl millet shoot fly. While cultural methods can be applied with no additional expense and relative ease, synthetic insecticides should only be used as a last resort. Tef yield loss from the shoot fly (*Atherigona hyalinipennis)* of tef has been calculated to be between 9% (Mideksa *et al.*, 2014) and 20% (Bayeh *et al.*, 2008) in two distinct areas of Ethiopia.

This insect attacks at seedling as well as panicle stage. Aleminew and Legas (2015) investigated how fertiliser rates of 50–100 kg/ha and plant spacing of 15–30 X 15 cm, and various broadcast planting techniques interacted to affect the occurrence of shoot flies in eastern Ethiopia in 2012 and 2013. Due to the modest (1.4–3.1%) pest incidence, no significant difference was discovered, and their efficacy is unknown yet. Mideksa *et al.* (2014) tested two distinct botanical pesticides and bug diseases in the field in western Ethiopia. The treatments were administered topically. No matter the sowing technique, a water extract of powdered Nicotiana sp. leaves (3 kg in 500 litres of water/ha) demonstrated the highest insect mortality of 80–83%. Neem seed kernal extract of 3 kg in 500 litres of water/ha was applied after this treatment, and the larval mortality rate was 78%.

*Metarhizium anisopliae* and *Beauveria bassiana*, two entomopathogenic fungi, proved ineffectual in suppressing pest attack. During the peak of pest occurrence in August-September, a hymenopteran wasp called *Neotrichoporoides nyemitawus* (Eulophidae) where eastern Ethiopian caterpillars were 7–19% parasitized. (Sileshi, 1997). These days, an effective IPM programme for such insect pests should include planting in time, intercropping, treating seeds with imidacloprid, and using botanical pesticides. Synthetic pesticides can be used as a last resort in cases of serious damage.

## Foliage pests

### *1. Stem borer*

The frequency and significance of lepidopteran stem borers attacking millets varies by region. Finger millet stem borer (*Sesamia inferens*) (Noctuidae), sorghum stem borer (*Chilo partellus*) (Pyralidae), and white stem borer (*Saluria inficita*) (Pyralidae) are significant species in the Indian subcontinent (Kalaisekar*et al.*, 2017). Pearl millet is harmed by the stem borer *Acigon ignefusalis* (Pyralidae), the pink stem borer *Sesamia calamistis* (Noctuidae), the sugarcane borer *Eldana sacchaina* (Pyralidae). In Senegal, often constituting 92% of the entire population of larval stem borer, *A. ignefusalis* is a significant pest of pearl millet, however in the Ivory Coast, *Eldana sacchaina* and *Sesamia calamistis* are the dominating species (Bekoye and Dadie 2015). According to recent research, there have been modified in the species makeup of pest populations in Senegal, whereas *S. calamistis* emerged as most dominant pest (making up 31–72 percent of the population of borer larvae), followed by *A. ignefusalis* (16–53 percent) (Goudiaby *et al.*, 2018). By comparing the grain yield of treated and untreated fields, as well as fields treated with Thioral (heptachlor + thiram) seed treatment with carbofuran granules applied to the soil and granules placed in leaf whorls, the loss was calculated. These are the borers which attack plants that age in between 30 days until grain maturity. Early instar larvae feed on soft tissues by invading the leaf whorl; the harmed leaves unfold with pinhole damage. Larvae later create tunnels packed with frass by boring through stems. The DH condition is brought on by the core shoot or growth point drying out or withering at the early (vegetative) stage.

i) **Pink borer:** The pink borer, *S. inferens*, is a major pest of finger millet in South India where the cereal is cultivated in the winter. (Sasmal, 2018). All types of millets are also infrequently attacked by the borer. Despite the borer's economic significance, nothing is known about how to control it. Little study has been done since crop returns and market demand are poor. Sasmal (2015) assessed 33 submissions by determining the percentage of plants with Dead Heart infestations 45 days after planting. On CV GPV-93, an infestation of up to 20.0% was recorded, but none were found on the 18 other entries. Farmers already engage in cultural activities which are useful to decrease insect numbers at different immature phases, such as removing and destroying Dead Hearts, stubble burning, fields ploughing after harvest, and harvesting crops closely to ground (Sasmal, 2018). If plant damage is severe, early therapy with granular pesticide formulations is possible because doing so does not impede the activity of nearby natural foes, primarily egg parasitoids and entomopathogenic fungi (Sasmal, 2018). Generally, the Integrated Pest Management strategy against borers should include treatment of seed, early transplanting, the use of cultivars that are tolerant of or resistant to borers, clean cultivation, and the preservation of native parasitoids.

*2. Defoliators*

i) **Grasshopper:** African millets are currently susceptible to grasshopper infestations on a regular basis and frequently seen at dry and semi-arid regions. Coop and Craft in 1993, reported that two grasshopper species (*Kraussaria angulifera* and *Oedaleus senegalensis*); (Orthoptera: Acridiidae) resulted in a 56 percentage yield reduction in pearl millet, and in another, it resulted in a 90% yield loss (Maiga *et al.*, 2008). Passerini (1991) graded *K. angulifera* leaf damage during field tests on pearl millet in Mali on a scale of 1 to 5, with 1 denoting no damage and 5 denoting severe damage. Pearl millet intercropped with cowpea or fields treated with fertiliser received a greater damage rating (3.01–3.18), but delayed plantings, high plant densities, and a comprehensive survey of typical farmer's fields received a lower damage rating of 2.07–2.70. Synthetic chemicals or pesticides which have no significant importance to prevent hopper population by the researchers, nevertheless, because of the potential harm to the ecosystem and the low return from millet crop (Jago *et al*., 1993). Farmers frequently disregard field sanitation procedures such weeding, vigorous tillage, flooding fields with water, and covering millet heads with paper bags because they believe these methods are impractical and farmers prefer pesticides because of their quick-acting nature (Maiga *et al*., 2008).

ii) **Blister beetle:** West Africa is home to 97 different blister beetle species (Coleoptera: Meloidae) (Gahukar, 1991). Each nation has a different geographic distribution of them and a different economic impact on pearl millet. Adults of blister beetle feed on pollen, stigmas, or complete flowers that hamper the development of grains. Furthermore typical is feeding on milky grains. According to estimates, *P. fusca* in the Gambia has reduced grain yield by 4–84%. (Zethner and Lawrence, 1988). Millet fields in Mali were damaged by occasional outbreaks, prompting farmers to completely give up growing crops (Gahukar, 1989). According to Lale and Sastawa (2000), in Nigeria, millet planted alone had the maximum yield, but intercropping it with sorghum or cowpea decreased pest infestation, presumably because the production difference may have been made up for by late productive tillers. Millets with a short maturation cycle may be attacked by blister beetles if they are planted too late, whereas long-cycle varieties may be protected by late flowering.

## Sucking pests

i) **Grain midge:** According to Coutin and Harris (1968), the grain midge *Geromyia penniseti* (Diptera: Cecidomyiidae) is a significant millet pest in semi-arid portions of India and savannah regions of Africa (Santharam *et al*., 1976). The tops of the spikelets have attached empty glumes and white pupal casings because the larvae feed on developing grain. The appearance of plants is horrendous. Senegal had reported yield losses of up to 90% by Coutin and Harris (1968). Gahukar (1990) noted midge damage in Senegal's long-maturity cultivars during the 1990s, where floret infestation ranged from 80.4% in the native Sanio to 97.0% in the improved P-5. Since then, there hasn't been any documented insect damage and farmworkers frequently fail to recognise their damage. During peak pest prevalence, the predatory bug *Orius* sp. and the parasitoid wasp *Tetrastichus* sp. are both prevalent (Coutin and Harris 1968). Farmers utilised readily accessible synthetic insecticides in the absence of IPM (Santharam *et al*., 1976 ; Coutin and Harris 1968). Future

IPM formulation for various agro-ecosystems will require pest monitoring, and additional trial observations on existing and novel approaches, notably on pest-resistant cvs.

ii) **Green bug:** *Schizapus graminum*, a green bug that occasionally causes significant damage to pearl millet, is a pest in Pakistan (Akhtar *et al*., 2012). Among the local varietal collection a total of 135 entries were screened in a field experiment on a scale of 0 to 9, with 0 being the most resistant and 9 being the most vulnerable. The entry with the highest level of resistance was cv. C-591, which was subsequently chosen for the multiplication programme. 21 items in that experiment had a rating of 3.0, indicating that they were moderately resistant (Akhtar *et al*., 2012). No other types of management have been examined. Field studies are still neededon all the control measures in order to build an IPM approach.

iii) **Head miner:** The millet head miner *Heliocheilus albipunctalla* de *joannis* (Lepidoptera: Noctuidae), a significant insect of different millet in the regions of Sahelian, West Africa, was the subject of an update by Gahukar and Ba (2019). 20% of pupae perished after fields were ploughed down to a depth of 15 to 25 cm between April and June (Gahukar, 1990). The majority of cultivators do not, however, plough soil since evaporation can become soil moisture to decrease and ploughing can result in soil erosion after significant rain. Also, if none of the local farmers plough their fields, moths may fly in from nearby fields. To avoid moth flying coincident with plant head growth, pearl millet planting should be delayed.Moth pheromone traps were ineffective at controlling pests (Green *et al.,* 2000). In Niger (Guevremont, 1983; Ba, 2017) and Senegal, light traps with 25–250 watts mercury vapour lamps were consequently placed (Bhatnagar, 1983). Light traps have not yet been proven to be a viable pest control strategy or part of a comprehensive pest management programme. Three seasons of consistent resistance have been noted in the cvs. Moro, Souna-3, and PE-08043 (Ba, 2017). Antibiosis and antixenosis, among other traits, have all been linked to resistance to head miners (Guevremont, 1983; Gahukar*et al*., 1986). In other cases, to improve conservation and augmentation of natural enemies, Brevault and Clouvel (2019) and Thiaw *et al.* (2017) explored importance and effectiveness consequences of field characteristics, between cultivated and uncultivated pest ecosystems. Additionally, *Habrobracon hebetor* is hazardous to chemical insecticides (Dastijerdi *et al*., 2009). Single or two applications of insecticides can significantly reduce pest incidence at 75% flowering, the first one at flower initiation and the second one after 5-7 days. Examples include in Sudan, cypermethrin (Hughes and Rhind, 1988) and chlorpyriphos, acephate, trichlorofon, endosulfan and chlordimeform in Senegal as well as Niger (Gahukar *et al*., 1986).

## Storage pests

Some important storage pests of millets are *Corcyra cephalonica*, *Ephestia cautella*, the rice moth, *Tribolium castaneum*, the almond moth, *T. confusum*, the saw-toothed grain beetle, *Oryzaephilus surinamensis*, the khapra beetle, *Trogoderma granarium*, the red flour beetle, and *Acarus* sp. An embiopteran pest, *Oligotomahum bertiana*, during cleaning the stocks and godowns, which coats millet seeds with white silken strands, can occasionally be challenging (Asafali and Subramaniam 1973). The most efficient way to handle pests is to store well-dried grains in hygienic settings. Grain carried in from the fields, transport trucks, gunny bags, etc. should all be checked at entrance locations. India is now providing improved handling and storage facilities as well as government and commercial godowns (Pingale, 1970). Tin bins and silos are useful in small towns. In a few African nations, it has been discovered that airtight store house and the use of aeration technologies when temperature is low, are beneficial (De Lima, 1981). Originally used to preserve seeds, methyl bromide and malathion are now being supplanted by pyrethroids and phosphine gas. In addition, research is being done on various pesticides, including diflubenzuron (Faragalla *et al*., 1985), ash, neem seed powder, and road dust (Jotwani and Butani 1978 ; Lakhani and Patel 1985).

## Conclusion

Compared to others who plant income crops, millet growers face different challenges. With conventional farming practises, millets are a significant source of sustenance, but their production inputs are frequently low and their benefits are insignificant. In India, a typical farmer can't afford the insecticides until production increases and stabilizes (Jotwani and Butani 1978). If governments create appropriate price policies, intensive cultivation offers certain incentives. Several recommendations for integrated pest control have been given based on a rudimentary understanding of pest biology.More research is still required, particularly in the areas of screening technique standardisation, resistance mechanisms, insect rearing, summer diapause termination, yield loss estimation, economic injury levelsestablishment, natural enemiesefficacy, and application in their existing ecosystems. Hybrid plants, in particular, that have recently been introduced, are vulnerable to several species. Hence, multipest resistance should be prioritised.

## References

Akhtar, N., Y. Ahmad, M. Skakeel, W. A. Gillani, J. Khan, T. Yasmin, and I. Begum. 2012. Resistance in pearl millet germplasms to greenbug, *Schizaphis graminum* (Rondani). Pak. J. Agr. Res. 25: 228–232.

Aleminew, A., and A. Legas. 2015. Determination of row spacing and fertilizer rate of transplant planting methods on the growth and yield of tef in eastern Amhara region Ethiopia. Journal of Biology, Agriculture and Healthcare 5: 195–201.

Asafali, K. and subramaniam, T. R., 1973. Severe incidence of the embiid, *Oligotoma-humbertiana* Saus. on stored bajra. *Madras Agricultural Journal* 60, 336.

Ba, M. N. 2017. Suitable large-scale biological control of the millet head miner in the Sahel. ICRISAT Technical Annual Report to McKnight Foundation. ICRISAT Center, Niamey, Niger.

Bayeh, M., J. Tafa, M. Yeshaltela, D. Asmare, and W. Biruk. 2008. Review of research outcomes of insect pests of economic importance to major small cereals, pp. 325–374. *In* A. Tadesse (ed.), Increasing crop production through improving plant protection. Plant Protection Association of Ethiopia, Addis Ababa, Ethiopia.

Bekoye, B. M., and A. Dadie. 2015. Evaluation des pertes en grains de mil dues aux insectes. Eur. Sci. J. 11: 266–275.

Bhatnagar, V. S. 1983. Programme de lute biologique, Projet CILSS de LutteIntegreeNioro du Rip, Senegal. ProjectTechnical Report for the period June-October 1982. Senegalese Institute for Agricultural Research (ISRA), Kaolack, Senegal.

Brevault, T., and P. Clouvel. 2019. Pest management: reconciling farming practices and natural regulations. Crop Prot. 115: 1–6.

Choudhary, S. K., B. L. Tandi, and S. Singh. 2018. Management of white grub, *Holotrichiaconsanguinea*Blanchard in pearl millet. Indian J. Entomol. 80: 619–622.

Coop, L. B., and B. A. Craft. 1993. Pearl millet injury by five grasshopper species (Orthoptera: Acrididae) in Mali. J. Econ. Entomol. 86: 891–898.

Coutin, R., and K. M. Harris. 1968. The taxonomy, distribution, biology and economic importance of the millet grain midge, *Geromyiapenniseti* (Felt.) gen. n. comb. n. (Dipt., Cecidomyiidae). Bull. Entomol. Res. 59: 259–273.

Dastijerdi, H. R., M. J. Hejazi, G. N. Ganbalani, and M. Saber. 2009. Sublethal effects of some conventional and biorational insecticides on ectoparasitoid, *Habrobraconhebetor*(Hymenoptera: Braconidae). J. Entomol. 6: 82–89.

Delima, C. P. F., 1981. Africa: assessment and control of losses in stored food. *Span* 24, 104-107.

FAO. 2017. Statistics, statistical pocketbook. FAO, Rome, Italy.

Gahukar, R. T. 1989. Insect pests of millets and their management: a review Int. J. Pest Manag. 35: 382–391.

Gahukar, R. T. 1990. Sampling techniques, spatial distribution and cultural control of millet spike worm, *Raghuvaalbipunctella*(Noctuidae: Lepidoptera). Ann. Appl. Biol. 117: 45–50.

Gahukar, R. T. 1991. Pest status and control of blister beetles in West Africa. Int. J. Pest Manag. 37: 415–420.

Gahukar, R. T. 1992. Effect of various fertilizers and rates on insect pest/pearl millet relationship in Senegal. Trop. Agric. 69: 149–152.

Gahukar, R. T., & Reddy, G. V. (2019). Management of economically important insect pests of millet. *Journal of Integrated Pest Management*, *10*(1), 28.

Gahukar, R. T., and M. G. Jotwani. 1980. Present status of field pests of sorghum and millets in India. Int. J. Pest Manag. 26: 138–151.

Gahukar, R. T., and M. N. Ba. 2019. An updated review of research on *Heliocheilusalbi punctela* (Lepidoptera: Noctuidae), in Sahelian West Africa. J. Integr. Pest Manag. 10: 3.

Gahukar, R. T., W. S. Bos, V. S. Bhatnagar, E. Dieme, A. R. Bal, and E. Fytizas. 1986. Acquisrecents en entomologie du mil au Senegal. Rapport, Reunion d'evaluation du programme mil-sorgho du 19–21 mars 1986. InstitutSenegalais de RecherchesAgronomiques (ISRA), Bambay, Senegal. pp. 29.

Goudiaby, M. P., I. Sarr, and M. Sembene. 2018. Source of resistance in pearl millet varieties against stem borers and earhead miner. J. Entomol. Zool. Stud. 6: 1702–1708.

Guevremont, H. 1983. Recherchesurl'entomofaune du mil. Rapport Annuel de Recherches pour l'annee 1982. Centre National de RecherchesAgronomiques de Tarna, (CNRAT), Maradi, Niger.

Hughes, D., and D. Rhind. 1988. Control of the millet head worm in the western Sudan. Int. J. Pest Manag. 34: 346–348.

Jago, N. D., R. Kremer, and C. West. 1993. Pesticides on millet in Mali. NRI Bulletin no. 50. University of Greenwich, Chatham Maritime, United Kingdom. pp. 52.

Jotwani, M. G. and butani, D. K., 1978. Crop pests and their control: Pearl millet. *Pesticides* 12, 20-30.

Kalaisekar, A., P. G. Padmaja, V. R. Bhagwat, and J. V. Patil. 2017. Insect pests of millets: systematics, bionomics and management, 1st ed. Elsevier, New York, NY.

Kennedy, C. W. 2002. Phytotoxicity in pearl millet varies among in furrow insecticides. Crop Prot. 21: 799–802.

Kishore, P. 1996. Evolving management strategies for pests of millets in India. J. Entomol. Res. 27: 357–360.

Lakhani, G. K. and patel, N. G., 1985. New insecticidal control of *Ephestiacautella*Walker. *Pesticides* 19, 46-48.

Lale, N. E. S., and B. M. Sastawa. 2000. Evaluation of host plant resistance, sowing date modification and intercropping as methods for the control of *Mylabris*and *Coryna*species (Coleoptera: Meloidae) infesting pearl millet in the Nigerian Sudan savanna. J. Arid Environ. 46: 263–280.

Maiga, I. H., M. Lecoq, and C. Kooyman. 2008. Ecology and management of the Senegalese grasshopper, *Oedaleussenegalensis*(Krauss 1877) (Orthoptera: Acrididae) in West Africa: review and prospects. AnnalesSocieteEntomologique de France 44: 271–288.

Mideksa, A., M. Negeri, and T. Shiberu. 2014. Management of tef shoot fly, *Atherigonahyalinipennis*(Reg.) (Diptera: Muscidae) on tef at Ambo, West Showa of Ethiopia. J. Entomol. Nematol. 6: 134–139.

Natarajan, V. S., S. Selvaraj, and A. Reghupathy. 1974. Assessment of loss in grain yield caused by shoot fly, *Atherigona destructor* M. (Anthomyiidae: Diptera) in certain varieties of Panivarugu, *Panicummiliaceum*. Scientific Culture 40: 502–504.

Natarajan, V. S., V. D. G. Raja, and S. Anavardham. 1973. Extent of damage caused by shoot fly (*Atherigona approximate*) on bajra hybrid. Madras Agric. J. 60: 584–585.

Ni, X., J. P. Wilson, J. A. Rajewski, G. D. Buntin, and I. Dweikat. 2007. Field screening of pearl millet for chinch bug (Heteroptera: Blissidae) resistance. J. Entomol. Sci. 42: 467–480. Nigus, C., and T. Damte. 2018. Id

Nwanze, K. F., and K. M. Harris. 1992. Insect pests of pearl millet in West Africa. Rev. Agric. Entomol. 80: 1132–1185.

Passerini, J. 1991. Field and lab trials in Mali to determine the effects of neem extracts on the millet pests: *Heliocheilusalbipunctella*De Joannis (Lepidoptera: Noctuidae), *Coniestaigneusalis*Hampson (Lepidoptera: Pyralidae) and *Kraussariaangulifera*Krauss (Orthoptera: Acrididae). Department of Entomology, McGill University, Montreal, Canada.

Pingale, S. V., 1970. *Storage Facilities.* Hapur, India: Indian Grain Technologists' Research Association of India.

Rajewski, J. A., X. Ni, J. P. Wilson, and I. Dweikat. 2009. Evaluation of resistance to chinch bug in pearl millet in temperate and subtropical environments. Plant Health Prog. 10: 31

Rangarajan, A. V., 1965. *Arthrodes*sp., a new tenebrionid beetle pest of cumbu (bajra) and its control. *Science and Culture* 31, 41-43.

Santharam, G., M. Mohanasundaram, and S. Jayaraj. 1976. Control of bajra grain midge, *Geromyiapenniseti*Felt. with insecticides. Pesticides 10: 45–46.

Sasmal, A. 2015. Screening of finger millet varieties against major insect pests at Odisha. J. Crop Weed 11: 227–228.

Sasmal, A. 2018. Management of pink stem borer (*Sesamiainferens*Walker) in finger millet (*Elusinecoracana*Gaertn.). J. Entomol. Zool. Stud. 6: 491–495.

Selvaraj, S., V. S. Natarajan, and A. Raghupathy. 1974. On the occurrence of shoot fly and its damage in some varieties of little millet. Indian J. Entomol. 44: 556–557.

Sileshi, G. 1997. Biology of shoot fly, *Atherigonahyalinipennis*van Emden in eastern Ethiopia. Int. J. Trop. Insect Sci. 17: 349–355.

Tanzubil, P. B., and E. A. Yakubu. 1997. Insect pets of millet in northern Ghana.1. Farmers' perceptions and damage potential. Int. J. Pest Manag. 43: 133–136.

Thiaw, I., T. Brevault, N. F. Diallo, A. Sow, D. Ngom, V. Soti, L. Sarr, S. Dorego, M. Diop, M. Cisse, and M. Sembene. 2017. Incidence et regulation naturelle de la chenille mineuse de l'epi de mil, *Heliocheilusalbipunctella*de Joannis (Lepidoptera: Noctuidae) a Bambeydans le bassinarachidier au Senegal. AgronomieAfricaine 29: 83–95.

TNAU. 2016. AgriTech portal. Tamil Nadu Agricultural University, Coimbatore, Tamil Nadu, India.

Wilson, J. P., B. Ouendeba, and W. W. Hanna. 2008. Diallel analysis of chinch bug damage to pearl millet. International Sorghum Millets Newsletter 41:78–79.

Wright, R. J. 2013. Chinch bug management. Institute of Agriculture and Natural Resources, University of Nebraska, Lincoln, NE.

Zethner, O., and A. A. Lawrence. 1988. The economic importance and control of adult blister beetle, *Psalydolyttafusca* Olivier (Coleoptera: Meloidae). Int. J. Pest Manag. 34: 407–412.

# 14

# Insect Pests of Major Millets and Integrated Strategies for their Management

Saraswati Mahato[1] and Bhabani Mahankuda[2*]

[1] Pesticide Residue and Food Quality Analysis Laboratory, University of Agriculture Sciences, Raichur, Karnataka

[2] College of Agriculture, Odisha University of Agriculture and Technology, Bhawanipatna

**ABSTRACT**

India is one of the largest producers of millet and is treasured by urban residents for their high mineral and vitamin content and is regarded as a sustainable food supply for rural populations therefore it is called as 'cereals of poor'. In the field and in storage, millets are attacked by around a hundred insect pests (Gahukar, 1989). Grain midge, stem borers, earhead bug and earhead caterpillar frequently occurred. In some seasons, sporadic infestations by armyworms, grasshoppers, root aphids, mites, termites, chinch bugs and leaf beetles, cause significant yield losses. As a result, every aspect of insect-pest management in millets is mentioned in detail in this chapter covering their biology, identification, the peak period of activity, nature of the damage, damage symptoms and management are described below.

*Keywords*: Millets, insects and pest, management strategies

## Introduction

Millets are annual,small-grained cereals that belongto the family Poaceae (Fahad *et al.,* 2017) They are highly drought-resistant and grown under dry and high-temperature conditions. It is nutritiously rich in protein, vitamins and minerals compared to other cereals *i.e.,*wheat and rice (Fahad *et al.,* 2017). The crop is preferred to grow in the semi-arid tropics of Asia and Africa because of its high yield, low water intake and short growing season, (FAO, 1995; McDonough *et al.,* 2000; Mikulajova *et al.,* 2017). Millets are consumed by humans over the long run and played a crucial and integral role in the development of farming civilizations and multi-crop agriculture (Cherfas, 2015). The major millets grown in India are sorghum (*Sorghum bicolor* (L.) Moench), pearl millet (*Pennisetum glaucum* (L.) R.Br.), finger millet (ragi) (*Eleusine coracana* Gaertn), proso millet (*Panicum miliaceum*), and foxtail millet (*Setaria italica*). Minor millets *viz.,* Indian

* Corresponding author.

barnyard millet (*Echinochloa* spp.), little millet (*Panicum sumatrense*), kodo millet (*Paspalum scrobiculatum*). The main millet-growing states in India are Rajasthan, Maharashtra, Karnataka, Andhra Pradesh, and Madhya Pradesh. In addition to the major millet-producing states, there are also several smaller millet-producing states such as Uttar Pradesh, Bihar, and Madhya Pradesh. The pest attacking these millets have been divided into six groups under this chapter (Prasad *et al.,* 2015) *viz.,* Shoot flies, Stem borers (Ragi stem borer, Spotted stem borer, white stem borer), Foliage pests (red and hairy caterpillar, armyworm, ash weevil, leaf folder and flea beetle), Earhead pests (Grain midge, head caterpillar, gram caterpillar, semilooper, tussock caterpillar, earhead bug), Sucking pests (shoot bug, aphids and spider mites), Soil dwelling insects (white grub and termites). The chapter also includes the most recent recommendations and dosages of insecticides for millet management.

## Major insect pests of Millets and Their damage

### I. Shoot Fly

Shoot fly (*Atherigona sp.*) is one of the most destructive pests attacking to a wide range of millets during an early stage of the crop; causing significant yield loss. Depending upon the host, the species of shoot fly vary from crop to crop and the details of shoot fly species along with their host crop are given below (Table 1).

**Table 1 :** Major insect pests of millets and their host plant

| Host Plant | Name of the shoot fly |
|---|---|
| Sorghum (*S. bicolor)*<br>Ragi (*Eleusine coracana)* | *Atherigona soccata* Rondani |
| Bajra (*Pennisetum glaucam)* | *A. approximata* Malloch |
| Porso Millet (*Panicum miliaceum)*<br>Kodo Millet (*Paspalum scorbiculatum*) | *A. simplex* Thompson |
| Little Millet (*Panicum sumatrense*) | *A. pulla* Wiedmann |
| Barnyard Millet (*Echinochloa esculenta*) | *A. falcate* Thompson |
| Fox Tail Millet (*Setariaitalical)* | *A. atripalpis* Malloch |

The pest attacks several major millets including sorghum, bajra, ragi, and some minor millets (Proso Millet, Kodo Millet, little Millet) and some other crops of the Poaceae family.

## Identification and life cycle

The adult fly resembles a housefly but is smaller and has six dark dots on the female's dorsal abdomen. In contrast, there are only 4 dark dots on the male. One generation takes 17–22 days to complete. Eggs are laid by the adult female on the lower surface of leaves, especially the second to fifth-youngest leaves. Most eggs have a cigar or cylindrical form. Maggots are yellow in color and don't have legs. Pupation occurs inside the central shoot or occasionally in the ground.

### *Damage Symptom*

The damaging stage is the maggot stage. They continuously bore inside the central shoot, weakening it, and making it easy to pull out and generally known as a dead heart. Seven days after germination until less than thirty days after harvest, it prefers to bore inside the immature shoot, which affects the crop establishment as a result. A dead heart can occasionally cause the growth of side shoots or tillers (ETL: 10% dead heart). Its incidence is increased by early winter sowing and late kharif sowing. This pest's activity is influenced by temperature fluctuations, which might be high or low. The prevalence of this pest is further increased during the crop season by persistent rain.

## II. Stem Borers

There are three different types of stem borers *viz.* spotted stem borer, finger millet stem borer, and white stem borers were seen infesting and causing severe damage to the millets. The most predominant species of stem borer reported under Indian conditions are spotted stem borer (*Chilo partellus*) and pink stem borer (*Sesamia inferens*) infesting sorghum and finger millets, respectively. Pearl millets are less attacked by the stem borers during the initial stages of crop growth. Whereas, internode injuries are observed during the later stages of crop growth.

### *i. Spotted Stem borer*

Scientific Name-*Chilo partellus* Swinhoe; Family- Crambidae, Order- Lepidoptera

This pest has been reported from all the major millets including bajra, sorghum, and ragi.

### *Identification and life cycle*

The adult moth has numerous black spots on the apical region of the forewings and straw colored body. It takes 30 to 40 days to complete a single generation. Fecundity rates for adult females range from 400 to 500 eggs per female. On the underside of leaves, close to the midrib, eggs are placed in tiny bunches of 10 to 80. Eggs are flat, scale-like, and stacked on top of one another. Larvae have a dark prothoracic shield and a yellowish-brown body. It takes a larva between 19 and 27 days to get through all the larval instars. Inside the infected stem, larvae pupate before emerging as adults after 7–10 days.

*Damage Symptom*

The harmful stage is the larva. After the second week of germination, the infestation begins and lasts until the crop is harvested. It creates holes and tunnels inside the stem to feed on the interior area of the stem. Over time, this disrupts the supply of nutrients to the growth points, which eventually weakens the center shoot, sometimes known as the "dead heart", damaged stem easily uproots (ETL: 10% dead heart). Tunneling within the peduncle subsequently leads to panicle breakdown or the development of a chaffy panicle. Within a month, it infests the sorghum crop and reduces yields by roughly 25% to 30%. The leaves have several pinholes as a result of pest attacks.

*ii. Finger millet stem borer*

**Scientific Name - *Sesamia inferens* Walker; Family-Noctuidae, Order- Lepidoptera)**

This pest has also been seen infesting major millets like sorghum, ragi, bajra, and some other crops like barley.

*Identification and lifecycle*

Adult moths are small, straw-colored, and possess white wings. The fecundity rate of adult females is 150 eggs/female, and lay eggs on the host plant's stem and leaf sheath. The eggs laid down in rows (batches) by an adult female are creamy white and hemispherical in shape. The incubation period is seven days. The larval body is light pink with a dark head. During summer, the larval stage is completed in 25 days. However, in winter, the life cycle gets prolonged up to 75 days. After 12 days of pupa formation, the larvae emerge as adults. The larvae feed on the stem by creating tunnels. The entire life cycle lasts between 45 and 75 days, and there are typically 4-6 generations every year.

*Damage Symptom*

The attack of this pest on the crop has been reported from the early vegetative stage of the crop and continues till the reproductive stage. The larva enters through the central shoot and then starts feeding on the developing leaves. As a result, the leaves when they come out exhibit five fine pinholes and as the larva grows, it goes deeper (forms tunnels inside) and then cause damage to the growing shoot. In the vegetative stage, the central shoot dies, and it is called as 'Dead heart' symptom. Larvae undergo pupation and pupate inside the infested stem. Adults emergethrough the exit hole. Whereas, infestation during the reproductive stage leads to chaffing of grains, often called 'white earhead'. The damage at the reproductive stage is economic. Both at the vegetative and as well as reproductive stages, it leads to the complete death of the plant.

*iii. White stem borer*

**Scientific Name-*Saluriainficita* Walker; Family-Noctuidae, Order- Lepidoptera)**

This pest has been reported from finger millet.

*Identification and lifecycle*

The eggs resemble the eggs of yellow stem borer. Eggs are laid down by the adult females in a batch of 100 on the tip of leaf blades and covered with greyish silky hairs. Adult moths have medium-sized dark brown color body. The costal margin of the forewings possesses a pale white band and the hind wings are white. Hatching of larvae from eggs takes place after 8 days of oviposition.

*Damage Symptoms*

The pest is reported from ragi plants in the southern parts of India. The larva infestsmostly to the base of tillers in proximity to soil; causing dead hearts. Pupation of the larvae takes place inside the infested stem.

**III. Sucking Pests**

*i. Shoot Bug*

**Scientific Name- *Peregrinus maidis* Ashmead; Family- Delphacidae, Order- Hemiptera**

The pest has been reported from crops likesorghum, other millets, and a few members of Poaceae

*Identification and life cycle*

The adult is small, active, and pale brown with translucent wings. The adult female has a fecundity rate of 97 eggs/bug and laid in small groups of one to four eggs beneath the leaf tissue. Adults usually cover the egg mass with white waxy substances. The incubation period of eggs lasts for a week. The nymphal stage consists of five instars, completed in about 16 days.

*Damage Symptoms*

It is one of the major sucking pests on sorghum, especially on rabi sorghum in southern India. The adult female inserts eggs into the leaf tissues. Both the mature(adult) and immature (nymphs)forms of insect suck sap from central leaf whorls, sometimes from the leaf sheath of tender plants, resulting in leaf yellowing and plant stunting. In case of severe damage, plants dry up. Shoot bugs also act as a vector in transmitting the maize dwarf mosaic virus and freckled yellows. The pest can be easily diagnosed in the field by the presence of ant activities in the central leaf whorls. Under favorable conditions, the pest becomes sporadic producing several generations in a year and complete death of the plant.

*ii. Aphids*

**Green aphid, S.N.- *Rhopalosiphum maidis* Fitch (Family- Aphididae, Order-Homoptera)**

**Ragi aphid, S.N.- *Hysteroneura setariae*Thomas (Family- Aphididae, Order-Homoptera)**

**Ragi root aphid, S.N.-*Tetraneura nigroabdominalis* Sasaki (Family- Aphididae, Order-Homoptera)**

This pest has been reported from sorghum, bajra, and other members of the Poaceae family.

*Green aphid; Rhopalosiphum maidis*

*Identification and life cycle*

The aphids are dark bluish-green, ovate, and coloniesare seen inside the central leaf whorl of the plant. The aphids are minute insects (2mm long) which have a pair of black legs on the thorax,a pair of antennae on the head, and a pair of cornicles on the abdomen. Whereas, the adult aphids during the rabi season are yellow with dark green legs. Two forms of insect *i.e.* both the apterous and alate forms of insect are observed. Females show parthenogenesis and a generation is completed in only seven days or so.

*Damage Symptoms*

Aphids tend to be present in groups and are mostly found on the innersurface of the leaves, panicles, and stems. Sometimes, it is also found deep inside the plant whorl of the middle leaf. Nymphs and adults suck the plant sap, which eventually leads to leaf mottling and marginal necrosis of leaves. The aphid secretes honeydew through its cornicles, which attracts and encourages the growth of sooty mold fungus in panicles and makes it difficult to harvest the plant. The aphid aids in the spread of the maize dwarf mosaic virus.

*Ragi aphid, Hysteroneura setariae*

*Identification and life cycle*

The duration of the life cycle varies in the apterous and alate forms of aphids. The former completes its life cycle in 31-35 days with the emergence of 35-78 nymphs per female. Whereas, the latter completes its life cycle in 39-46 days with approximately 52 nymphs/female.

*Damage Symptom*

Adults and nymphs of this pest cause damage to the plant by sucking the sap from the tender leaves and spikelets, which later spreads to the entire plant. The plant usually loses its vigor and shows stunting. In severely infested crops; the colonization of aphids is seen on earheads.

*Ragi root aphid; Tetraneura nigroabdominalis*

*Identification of the pest*

The adults are globular, and pinkish and undergo a viviparous mode of reproduction. The four instars of the nymphal stage are finished in 7-9 days. The lifespan of an adult is 5–11 days, and they have 10-35 progeny.

*Damage symptoms*

Both the adult as well as the nymph, mainly congregated below the ground level, especially around the root zone, and continuously suck the sap from the root. Both stages are responsible for causing the damage. Because of the continuous sap feeding from the root zone, the plant will show a wilted symptom and ultimately the plant dries up.The Aphid has got a very close association with the ant, especially the black ant, *Camponotus*. And these ants will protect the aphids from their natural enemies and as well as helps in transferring the young ones from one plant to the other plant. First, manage the ants and cut off their association with the aphids. So, drenching insecticide to the base of the affected plant is going to eliminate or control this aphid.

## IV. Foliage Pest

*i. Red hairy caterpillar*

**Scientific Name- *Amsacta albistriga* Walker; Family- Arctiidae, Order- Lepidoptera)**

This pest is polyphagous and has been reported from many crops like sorghum, bajra, ragi, maize, barley, cotton, cowpea, castor, etc.

*Identification of the pest and life cycle and Damage Symptom*

The moths are medium-sized as adults. Both the forewings and the hindwings are white, with the forewing having brown patterns and streaks and the latter having black dots. *A. moorei* has a red band on the head and a red streak along the coastal border of the wing, in contrast to *A. albistriga*, which has a yellow band on the head and a yellow streak along the forewings' coastal line. In batches of 50 to 100, cream or bright yellow eggs are occasionally placed on tender plant parts, soil, or other vegetation. Within two to three days, a single female will lay about 1000 eggs. Larval emergence occurs after 3–4 days, and the entire larval life cycle is completed in 40–50 days. The larval body is covered with black hair and is made up of red bands sandwiched between black bands.

A high infestation of red hairy caterpillars *Amsacta albistriga* has been recorded from the north, south, and western parts of our country. The incidence of this pest is more in red soil and they prefer feeding on young plants. The larvae feed voraciously by scrapping the chlorophyll content from the lower surface of leaves and complete defoliation of millet plants may occur in case of a severe attack of this pest. Feeding on the young seedlings was also reported. The larvae are dark in color during the early instars. Whereas, it turns ashy brown after 10 days and feeds gregariously moving from one plant to another and eventually from one field to other for feeding.

### *ii. Black hairy caterpillar*

**Scientific Name- *Estigmenel actinea* Hubner ; Family- Arctiidae, Order- Lepidoptera)**

This pest is reported from different millets like sorghum, pearl millet, and finger millet.

#### *Identification and Life cycle*

The adult moth has crimson red markings on the head, thorax, and wings and is white. Fecundity in adult females ranges from 100 to 150, which are laid in small groups on the leaf surface. The eggs are creamy white. A 6-7 day incubation period is typical. While the lifespans of larvae, pupae, and adults are respectively 23–25 days, 11 days, and 8–9 days. On soil, the larva pupates.

#### *Damage symptoms*

The caterpillar feeds on the younger leaves by scrapping the chlorophyll; leaving the midribs and veins. Defoliation of leaves is seen in case of severe infestation. They also attack and feed on the panicles.

### *iii. Grasshopper*

**Scientific Name- *Hieroglyphus nigrorepletus* Bolivar, *H. banian* Fabricius, *Colemania spheneroides* Bolivar, Chrotogonus spp.**

**Family: Acrididae, Order: Orthoptera**

This pest has been reported by all millets and other members of Poaceae.

*Identification and life cycle*

The body colors and patterns of the mature grasshopper are distinctively yellowish-green. Adults lack wings, have blue-black antennae, and have purple bands behind their eyes and along the sides of their thorax. Small batches of eggs are placed in soil over October and November at a depth of 6 cm. Grubs begin to emerge right away after receiving monsoon rain.

*Damage symptoms*

The nymph and adult are the damaging stages of the insect. They attack the leaves by causing marginal notching or holes. In case of a severe attack, defoliation of the whole plant takes place giving the field a grazed appearance.

*iv. Ash weevils*

**Scientific Name *Myllocerus maculosus* Desb, *M. viridanus* Fab, *M. subfasciatus* Guerin Meneville & *M. discolor* Boheman;**
**Family- Curculionidae, Order- Coleoptera**

This pest is polyphagous and reported from a wide range of host crops like bajra, maize, sorghum, pulses, groundnut, cotton, guava, etc.

*Identification of the pest and life cycle*

The dorsal surface of the wing of an adult is covered in black dots and is brown or grey. Adults lay pale yellow eggs during the summer at a rate of 360 eggs per female over 24 days. After 3-5 days, eggs begin to hatch; resulting in creamy white grubs, which grow into adult grubs after 1-2 months. In 6 to 8 weeks, the entire life cycle is completed. Pupation occurs in soil and the emergence of adults takes place after ten days.

*Damage symptoms*

Adults cause notching of leaf margins. Grubs and adults of this pest often eat away the roots, resulting in wilting of the plant in patches.

*v. Leaf folder*

**Scientific Name- *Cnaphalocrocis medinalis* Guenee; Family- Pyralidae, Order-Lepidoptera**

The pest is seen attacking a wide variety of crops *viz.,* Rice, Finger millet, Pearl millet, and members of the Poaceae family, etc.

*Identification of the pest and life cycle*

The body of the adult moth is pale yellow or golden yellow, and the anal region of the hind wings is broad. Three oblique, dark-black lines can be seen on the forewings. Each female moth lays 300 whitish-yellow eggs, one on each side of the leaf blade. A 4-6 day incubation period is typical. The eggs hatch into larvae after 15 to 20 days. The pronotum of the larvae has one or two pairs of dots, a black head, and a yellowish-green body. The pupa develops inside the leaves, and after 6 to 10 days of pupation, the adult emerges.

### Damage symptoms

The larval stage of this insect is damaging to the crop and causes damage by the formation of leaf folds and scrapping the chlorophyll; remaining inside the fold. The leaf blades are folded longitudinally and glued with silk strands to form the leaf folding. White patches along the leaf margin are seen as a result of feeding.

*vi. Armyworm*

**Scientific Name: *Mythimna separata*; Family; Noctuidae, Order-Lepidoptera**

This pest is polyphagous.

*Identification and life cycle*

A small group of eggs are laid by the females and are covered with brown hairs. Early instar larvae are dark green, which later turns into greenish brown, nocturnal in habit. Larvae tend to hide inside the central leaf whorl or in the plant debris or sometimes under the stone or clots etc. Pupation occurs in the soil. Adult moths are medium-sized and usually straw-colored.

### Damage symptoms

It is a major defoliator of sorghum . The larval stage is damaging. Larvae feed on the leaf from the margin, leaving only the midrib and stalk of the plant resulting in defoliation of the plant.

*vii. Flea beetle*

**Scientific Name: *Chaetocnema pusaensis* Maulik; Family: Chrysomelidae, Order: Coleoptera**

This pest is reported from finger millet.

*Identification and life cycle*

Dark bluish color adult beetles with an enlarged hind femur and oblong shape

*Damage symptoms:*

Flea beetles can be considered a minor pest of finger millets. Adult beetles damage young plants by biting and making holes in the leaves of young plants. Thereby, affecting plant vigor in both the nursery crop as well as newly transplanted crop.

## V. Soil-dwelling insects

### *i. White grubs*

**Scientific Name- *Holotrichia sp., Anomala sp.*; Family- Melonthidae, Order-Coleoptera**

This pest has been reported from infesting different crops *viz.,*pearl millet, maize, groundnut, sugarcane, etc

#### *Identification and life history*

This pest has been reported from pearl millet causing extensive damage to the crop in India. The beetles are 13-20 mm long, and hatch during November- December, duringfavorable climatic conditions. Unless the pest undergoes hibernation and becomes active during the summer months (May-June) of next year. The egg period, grub period, and pupal period vary from 1-3 weeks, 8-22 weeks, and 1-8 weeks, respectively. The Grubs are C-Shaped or scarabeiform type.

#### *Damage symptoms*

The grubs feed extensively on underground roots resulting in withering and eventually death of the plant. Infested seedlings do not produce seeds and remain stunted. A single plant may get attacked with 3-4 grubs simultaneously. Late sown millets generally escape the damage of this pest.

### *ii. Termites or white ants*

**Scientific Name- *Odontotermes spp., Microtermes spp., Macrotermes spp.;* Family-Termitidae, Order-Isoptera**

Termites are highly polyphagous and attack a wide variety of hosts includingbajra, sorghum, ragi, cereals (maize, wheat) and sugarcane, etc.

#### *Identification and life history*

Severe infestations of termites are seen in dry or semi-dry areas. The females lay the first batch of eggs consisting of 100-130 eggs after 7-10 days of aerial flight. The queen has an ability of 30,000 eggs per day. Hatching of eggs takes place after 40-42 days. Termites are social insects consisting of workers, soldiers, kings, and queen. They mainly feed on the underground plant roots and build an underground nest to live which becomes very difficult to locate.

#### *Damage Symptoms*

Termites infest the plant by feeding on underground roots, which block the translocation of nutrients and water in the vascular system of the plant, which leads to the toppling over of the plant and death ultimately.

## VI. Earhead Pests

### i. *Grain Midge*

**Scientific Name- *Stenodiplosis sorghicola*; Family-Cecidomyiidae, Order-Diptera**

This pest has been reported fromsorghum, pearl millet, and other wild graminaceous crops.

#### *Identification and life cycle*

Adults have long legs and resemble mosquitoes. Transparent wings on the abdomen, which are orange or orange-yellow. Six to ten eggs are laid by the females in each floret as it develops. The number of eggs laid by the mature female varies from 30-35 in 3-4 days. The larval stage of the maggots lasts for around 9 to 11 days and involves three moultings. Behind the glumes, pupation occurs, and three days later, adults start to emerge. Once the adults emerged, white pupal cases were visibly adhering to the spikelets.

#### *Damage Symptoms*

Adult females insert eggs into the floret and hatching maggots feed on the ovary inside the floret, causing chaffy grains or blighted grains. If you press the blighted grains, pinkish fluid comes out from the grains. That indicates the presence of the pest (ETL- 5 blighted grains per ear head or 5 midges per ear head).

### *ii. Earhead bug, Calocoris angustatus; Family- Miridae, Order-Hemiptera*

**Identification and life cycle**

Adults are fragile, have long legs, and are often light green. Female bugs lay about 150–200 blue eggs, cigar-shaped, preferably underneath the glumes or inside the center of florets. Slender green nymphs emerge from the eggs after seven days of oviposition. The nymphal stage lasts 10–14 days. From egg to adult, the entire life cycle takes less than three weeks.

#### *Damage symptom*

In contrast to open-type types, it favors attacking varieties with compact ear heads. It strikes when the crop is in the milky stage. Adults and nymphs are in the destructive stage. At the milky stage of the crop, they suck the juice, causing the grains to become chaffy and shrivel. Even the damaged ear head looks crooked (ETL-10 bugs per ear head).

### *iii. Head Caterpillars Cryptoblabesangus tipennella (Lepidoptera: Pyralidae)*

This pest has been seen infesting different millets like sorghum and bajra.

#### *Identification and life cycle*

The adult moths are tiny, brown in color, and have forewings that are dark brown and light-brown hindwings. A female moth lays one egg on each spikelet. Eggs have a creamy white color and are spherical or conical in shape. The incubation phase lasts 3 to 4 days. The larva's body color is light brown, and it has two black lateral lines. Pupae form inside the silken webs that the larvae weave. Larval and pupal phases last between 9 -10 days and 7 days, respectively. A single generation of the insect is completed in about one month.

#### *Damage Symptom*

The caterpillars are normally found at the grain filling or the milky stage of the grain. They are found between the fingers of the finger millet ear head and continuously feed on the developing grains. The habit of webbing the silken webs around them and being hidden inside these webs, and then feeding on the developing grains. Varieties that have got closed ear head characters are highly susceptible to an attack by ear-head caterpillars. Normally the open-ear heads will have less infestation by the caterpillar.

### iv. *Gram caterpillar*

**Scientific Name-*Helicoverpa armigera*; Family- Noctuidae, Order-Lepidoptera**

This pest is highly polyphagous and has been reported feeding from a diversified group of crops including cotton among fiber crops, Lab lab, and soybean among pulses, tomato, and chili among vegetables, groundnut among oilseeds, maize from cereals and sorghum among millets, etc.

#### *Identification and life cycle*

The forewings of the adult moth have a distinctive "V"-shaped spot, while the borders of the hind wings are dull black. The larval body varies from green to brownand possesses lines on the lateral sides of the body, which are dark grey.

#### *Damage Symptoms*

Larvae feed on the developing grains by concealing inside the ear head. Earheads might become half-eaten and appear chalky in cases of severe infestation. Within the earhead, feces are visible as pallets.

### *v. Semilooper*

**Scientific Name: *Eublemma silicula* Swinhoe; Family-Noctuidae, Order-Lepidoptera**

The pest is reported from different crops likesorghum, bajra, and finger millet

*Identification and life cycle*

Moths are small insects that have red forewings with wavy lines along their borders. Eggs are laid on the grains or spikelets by adult females. Eggs are incubated for four days. The larval stage completes in about two weeks and the larval body is light yellow. Inside the gallery, the larvae go through pupation, which can last up to 12 days.

*Damage Symptoms*

Ear heads are extensively webbed and can be seen with broken grains.

## VI.Tussock Caterpillar

**Scientific Name: *Euproctes subnotata* Walker**
**Family- Noctuidae, Order- Lepidoptera**

This pest has been reported from sorghum, bajra, and finger millet.

*Identification and Life Cycle*

Eggs are clear white and spherical. The larvae have a yellow strip across their dark brown body. The strip of yellow is bordered by an orange-red line. All the larval instars are completed in 15 to 40 days. Pupation takes place underground, and after 25–30 days adults start emerging from the pupa. The front pair of wings in adult moths is dark brown in color, and the hindwing is yellowish. The adult female oviposit insmall clusters of five to twenty eggs, which are covered in orange-yellow hairs.

*Damage Symptoms*

The attack of this pest is observed during the panicle formation stage. They feed on the milking grains and destroy the panicles during the soft dough stage. Webbing of earheads with silken threads is also observed. Frass materials are seen on the panicles. Compact panicles are preferred more by the insect

## Integrated Pest Management strategies for millet

Millet production has increased in recent years, for its rich mineral and vitamin content compared to other cereal crops. But, the insect-pest infestation is a major challenge in millet production.It was estimated that in India, 116 insect species cause varying degrees of damage from sowing to harvest, which decreases crop productivity, grain quality and fodder yield (Kishore, 1996; Bekoye and Dadie 2015; Arun Kumar and Channaveerswami 2015).Therefore, pest management in millets is to be aimed as an integrated approachrather than managing individual pests, which includes cultural, mechanical, biological, host plant resistance, biorational and chemical control.

### *Cultural control*

- As a preventive measure go for synchronized/early sowing in June & avoid late sowing in august to reduce the infestation by grain midge, shoot-flyand head bugs.
- Keep the field clean and the surrounding plants, as the larvae take shelter in the plant debris or sometimes under the stone or clots to reduce the damage of army worm.
- After harvest of the crop, collect the left-over stubbles and chaffy earheads and burn it, this prevents harbour of different insect pest *viz.,* stem borers and midges.
- Young plant showing symptom of dead heart in the early stage of crop, may be pulled out to decrease the damage of shoot-fly and borers.
- Deep ploughing of the field one month before onset of rain will expose immature stages (larva, pupa) of insects to direct sunlight, predatorsand insectivorous birds.
- Wild grasses *i.e.,*Johnnson grass should be removed within and around the field as midge goes through one or two generations on wild grasses.
- Areas where borers and shoot fly damage are regularly observed, increase the seed rate by 20-30% (2 kg seeds extra), which will offset the borer and shoot-fly damage by maintaining optimum field population to get good yield (5-6 kg/ acre).
- Seed treatment with imidacloprid 60FS @ 3g/kg seeds to control shoot-fly, shoot-bug and borers damage.
- Intercropping with legumes *viz.,* cowpea, pigeon pea and lablab reduces the damage by stemborers in sorghum as the pest will take more time to establish on the crop.
- Crop rotation of sorghum and millets with non-cereals (sugarcane, peanuts, cotton and sunflower) to break the pest's life cycle *viz.,* midge, shoot-fly and head bugs.
- Irrigate the field for proper soil moisture maintenance to reduce root aphid in finger millet and other soil dwelling insects *viz.,* white grub.

*Mechanical control*

- Mechanical collection and destruction of egg masses (stem bores, armyworms, cutworm), grown-up larvae *viz.,* head caterpillars, hairy caterpillars, cutworms, and armyworms.
- Install light traps to attract and kill adults of grain midge, stem borers, and earhead caterpillars.
- Install fish meal traps impregnated with insecticides @ 5 traps per acre for mass trapping of adult shoot-flies.
- Set up sex pheromone traps @ 5 per acre to attract male moths (*Helicover paarmigera*) from flowering to grain hardening stage.

*Biological control*

- Spray fungal pathogen like *Metarhizium rileyi* @ 2-5 g/l (2 X $10^8$ CFU/g) of water to control the damage of head caterpillars and armyworm.
- Two applications of Ha NPV @ 100 LE/acre at 10 days interval when *Helicoverpa*damage is serious.
- Spray fungal pathogen like *Lecanicillium lecanii*@ 2-5 g/l (2X$10^8$ CFU/g) of water for control of shoot bug.
- To control ragi cutworm, larvae are infected by *Nomuraea rileyi* fungus and parasitised by *Bracon sp.*
- Conserve the natural enemies such as lady bird beetle *Coccinellaseptum puctata* and *Menochilussex maculatus* to manage shoot bug.

*Host Plant Resistance*

- Select varieties that do not produce side shoots from the base of the plant.
- Use resistant/hybrid varieties: ICSV 197, ICSV 745, ICSV 843, ICSV 88013, ICSV 88032 for control of sorghum midge.
- The pearl millet varieties possess multiple resistance to shoot-fly and spotted stem bores: MP-67, MP-19, Pusa-23, HHB-67, MH-855 and MH-91.
- Varieties resistance to pink stem borer in finger millet were IE 982, 932 and 1037.
- Varieties relatively less damaged by shoot-fly and stem borers: SV 1616, M 35-1, CSV 15, Phule Yashoda.

*Biorational control*

- Spray NSKE @ 5% or commercial neem product containing Azadirachtin 1EC @ of 2ml per liter of water for the control of different pests viz., stem borers, head caterpillars, shoot-fly, midge, hairy caterpillars and sucking pests.

*Chemical control*

- Two whorl application of Cartap hydrochloride 4G or Carbofuran 3G to control borer pests.

  (Apply 5 kg/ha 25-30 days after crop emergenceand secondly, 10 kg/ha at 10-15 days later)
- Spray Flubendamide 48% SC 0.2 ml/l and Chlorantraniliprole 18.5% SC 0.2 ml/l of water at every 20 days interval after germination to controlstem bores damage.
- If root aphid infestation is severe, drench with Dimethoate 50% EC in the root zone.
- Spray Lamda-cyhalothrin 5 EC @ 1ml/l or Chlorantraniliprole18.5SC @ 0.3ml/l or Emamectin benzoate 5SG @ 0.5g/l or Spinetoram 11.7SC @ 0.4ml /l as foliar sprays are recommended to manage head caterpillars, cutworm, armyworm and hairy caterpillars.
- Spray insecticide like imidacloprid 17.8SL @ of 3ml per liter of water, at 12 to 14 days after sowing for the management of shoot-fly.
- Dust with Malathion 5D at 25 kg/ha or Fenvalerate 0.4 DP at 10 kg/ha synchronising during milking stage on 3rd and 18th day after emergence of panicle against earhead bugs (1-2 bugs/panicle).
- To control sorghum midge, spray Cypermethrin 0.5ml/l of water at 50% flowering stage (1 midge/panicle).

## Conclusion

In millets, the major pests that occur frequently arestem borer, shoot-fly, grain midge and white grubs which infest the crop throughout the growing season. The problem of pink stem borer is more in case of finger millet. Research on pest management needs to be intensified to reduce damage and yield loss. Determination of relationship between insect density and crop yield loss for important panicle-feeding insects needs to be established. Areas to be focused and explored for better management of insect pest through biological control such as natural enemies (predators, parasitoids) and host plant resistance (resistant varieties) to reduce the use of chemicals.

## References

AEPED, https://apeda.gov.in/apedawebsite/SubHead_Products/Indian_Millets.htm

Arun Kumar, D.&A. S. Channaveerswami. (2015). Pre and post-emergence control measures for shoot fly incidence and its influence on seed yield of little millet (*Panicum sumatrense*). Journal of Experimental Zoology, 18: 811–814.

Bekoye, B. M.&A. Dadie. (2015). Evaluation des pertesen grains de mil dues aux insectes. European Scientific Journal, 11: 266–275.

Cherfas, J. (2015). Millet: how a trendy ancient grain turned nomads into farmers. National Public Radio. The Salt.

Fahad, S., Bajwa, A.A., Nazir, U., Anjum, S.A., Farooq, A., Zohaib, A., Sadia, S., Nasim, W., Adkins, S., Saud, S.&Ihsan, M.Z. (2017). Crop production under drought and heat stress: plant responses and management options. Frontiers in plant science, p.1147.https://doi.org 10.3389/fpls.2017.01147.

Food and Agriculture Organization of the United Nations. (1995). Archived from the original on 1 October 2018. Retrieved 7 January 2012. Sorghum and millet in human nutrition.

Gahukar, R.T. (1989). Insect pests of millets and their management: a review. International Journal of Pest Management, 35(4): 382-391.

Kishore, P. (1996). Evolving management strategies for pests of millets in India. Journal of Entomological Research, 27: 357–360.

McDonough, C.M., Rooney, L.W. and Serna-Saldivar, S.O. (2000). The Millets: Food Science and Technology. Handbook of Cereal Science and Technology. CRC Press, New York, 99 2nd ed:177-210.

Mikulajova, A., Sediva, D., Certik, P.G., Nemeth, K.&Hybenova, E. (2017). Genotypic variation in nutritive and bioactive composition of foxtail millet. Cereal Research Communication, 45(3): 442-455.https://doi.org/10.1556/0806.45.2017.018

Prasad, S., Bhagwan, V.R.&Srinivasa, B. (2015). Insect pests of millets and their management. Indian farming, 65(4): 46-49

A. Pink stem borer, *Sesamia inferense* (Lepidoptera: Noctuidae)

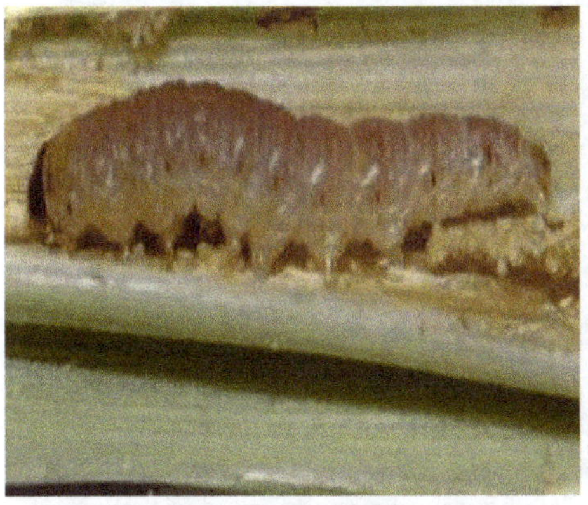

Pink colour Larva

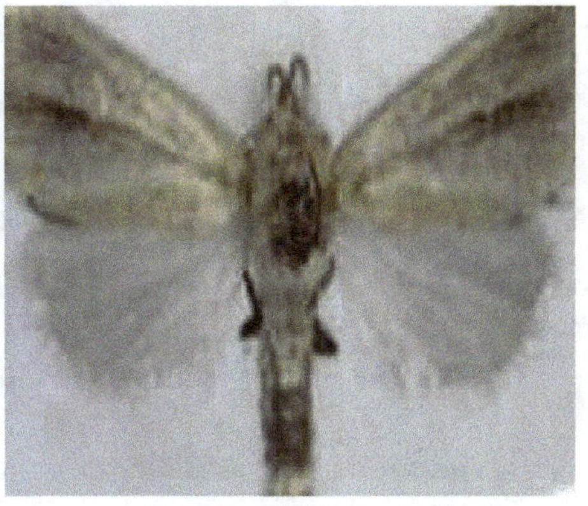

Adult

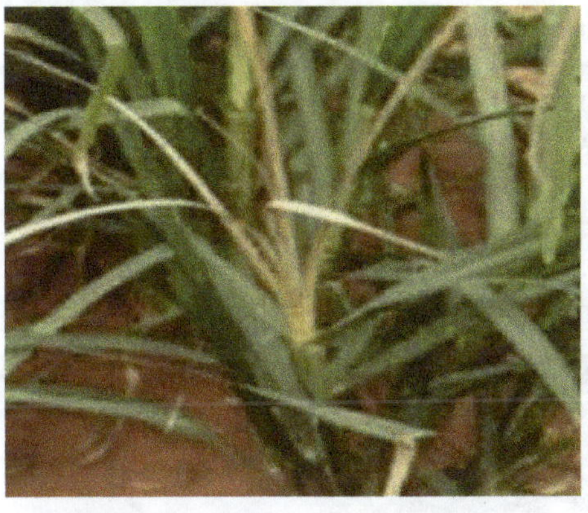

**"Dead heart"** at vegetative stage

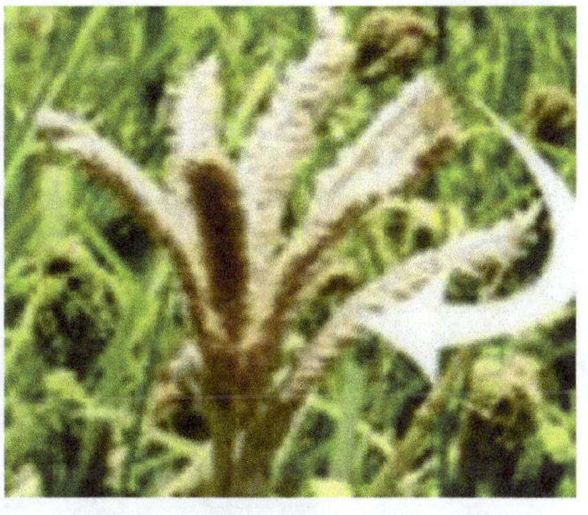

**"White ear"** at reproductive stage

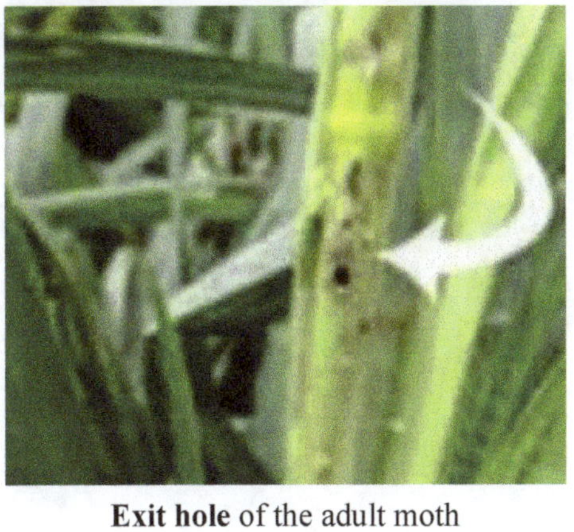

**Exit hole** of the adult moth

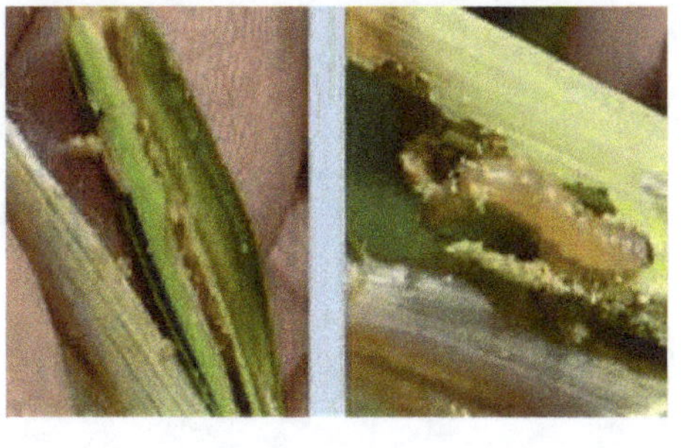

Larva feeding inside the central shoot

B. Root aphid, *Tetraneura nigriabdominalis* (Hemiptera: Aphididae)

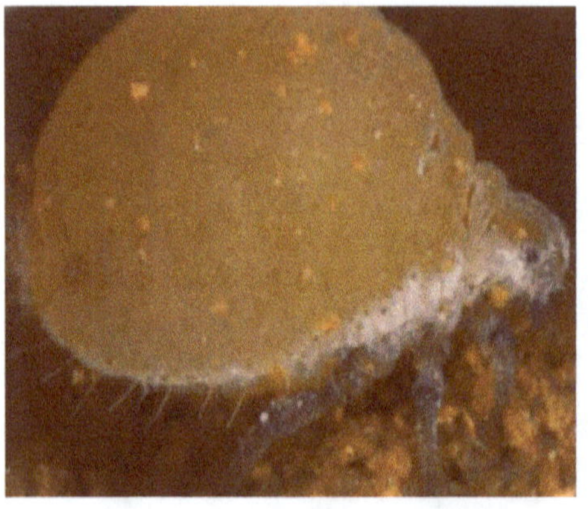

*Tetraneura nigriabdominalis*

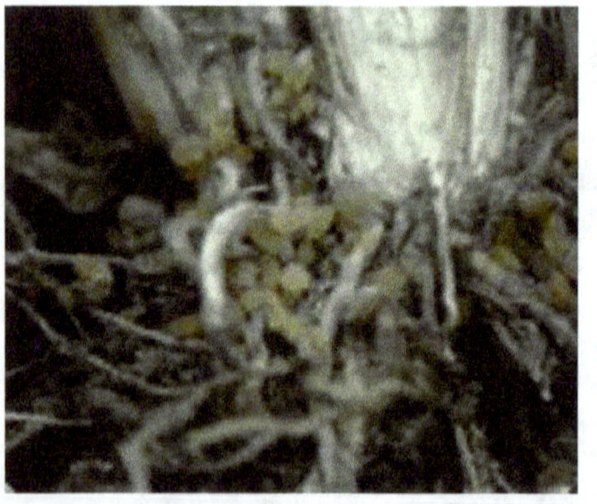

Adults and nymphs congregated at the base of roots

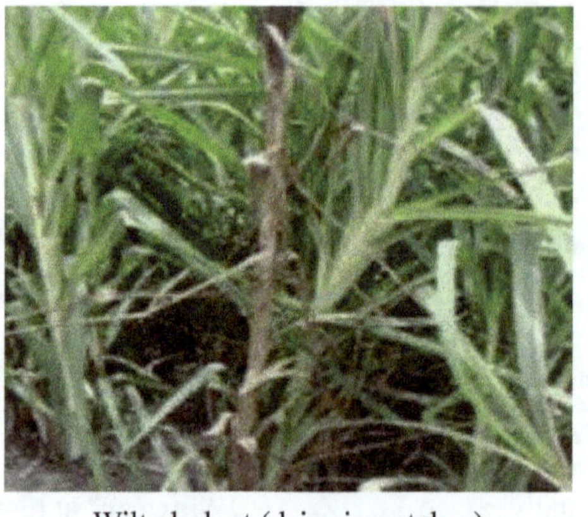

Wilted plant (dries in patches)

C. Earhead pests

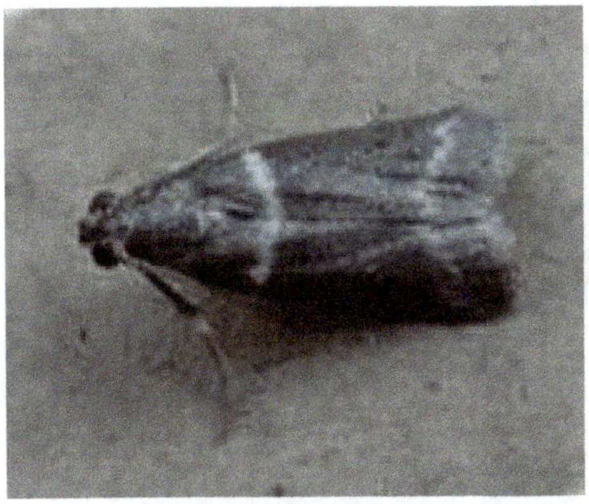

Earhead caterpillar *Cryptoblabes angustipennella* (Lepidoptera: Pyralidae)

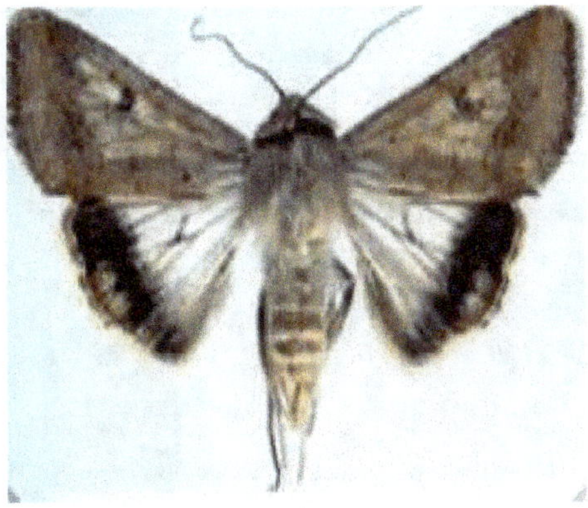

Gram caterpillar (*Helicoverpa armiger)* (Lepidoptera: Noctuidae)

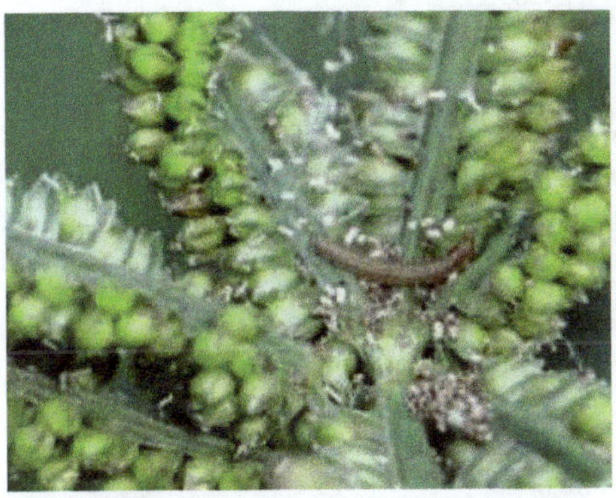

Larva feeds on 'developing grains' inside the 'earhead'

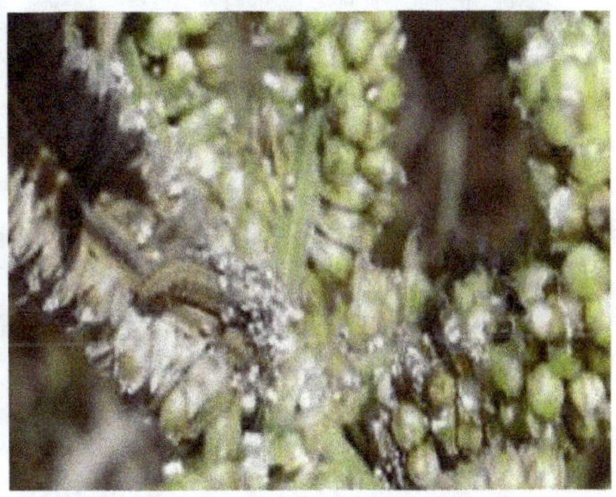

Damaged grains

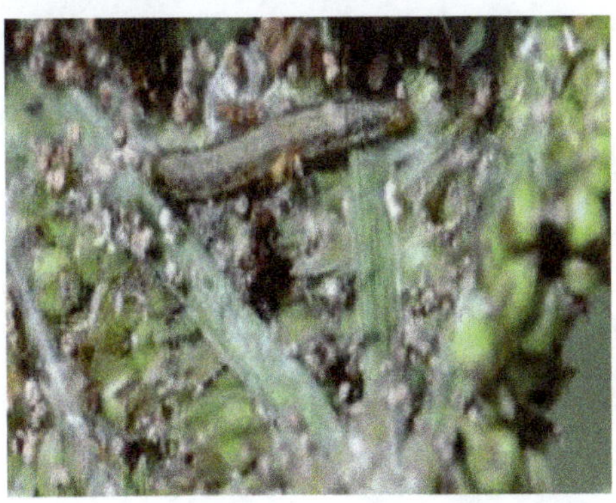

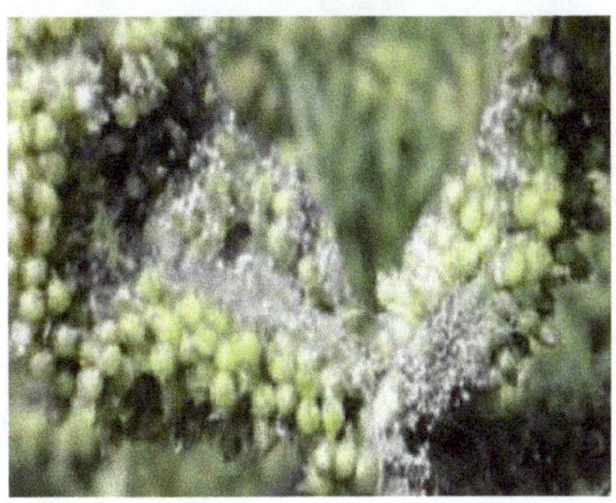

"**Webbing** and **fecal pellets** of the larva"

D. Ash weevil, *Myllocerus* spp., Curculionidae

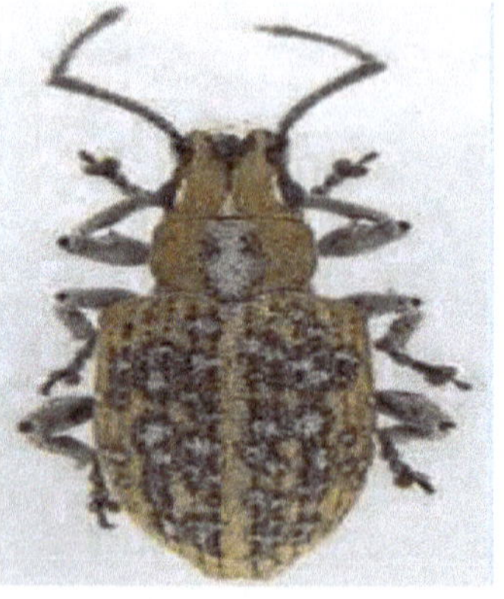

*Myllocerus discolor*

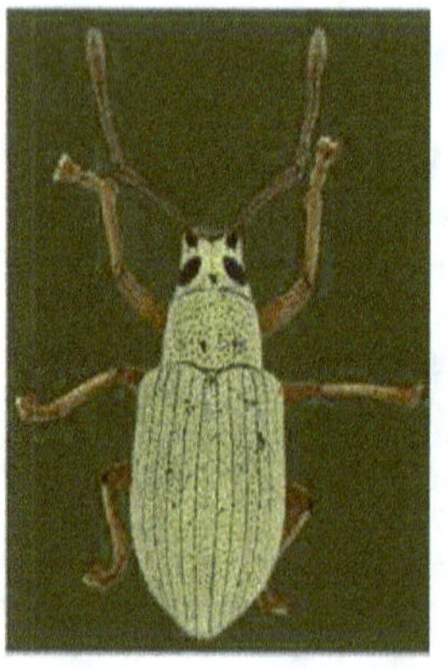

*Myllocerus viridanus*

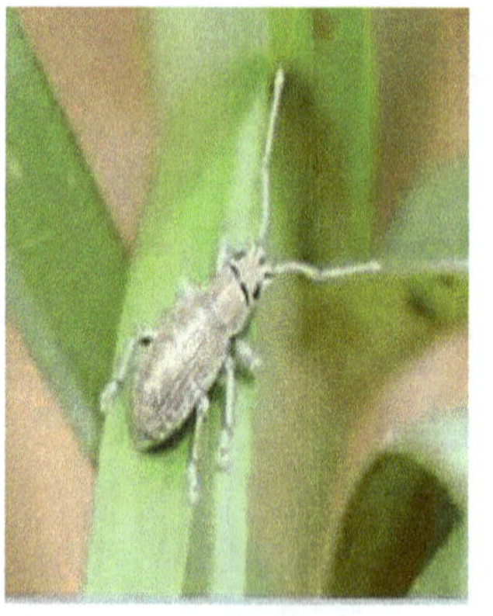

*Myllocerus subfasciatus*

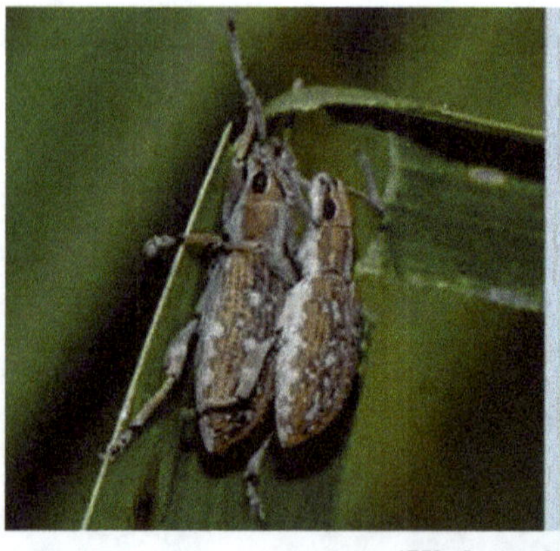

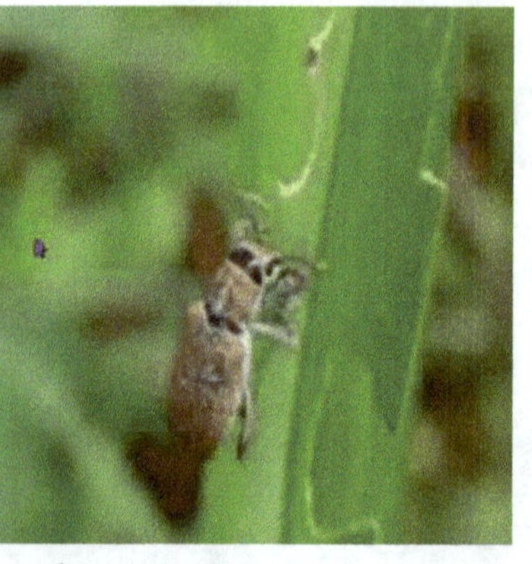

**'U' shaped** notches

E. Shoot fly, *Atherigona soccata* (Diptera: Muscidae)

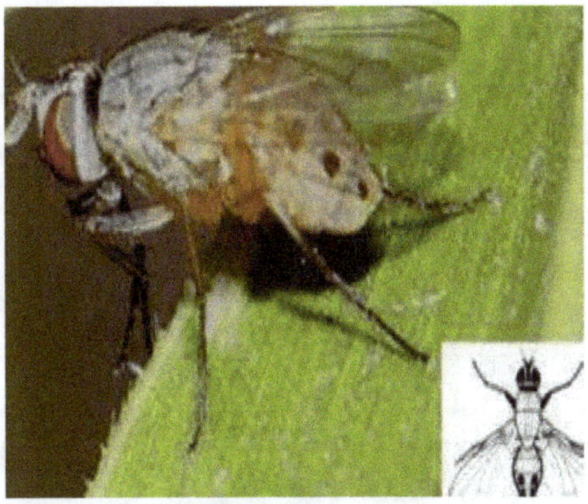

Adult

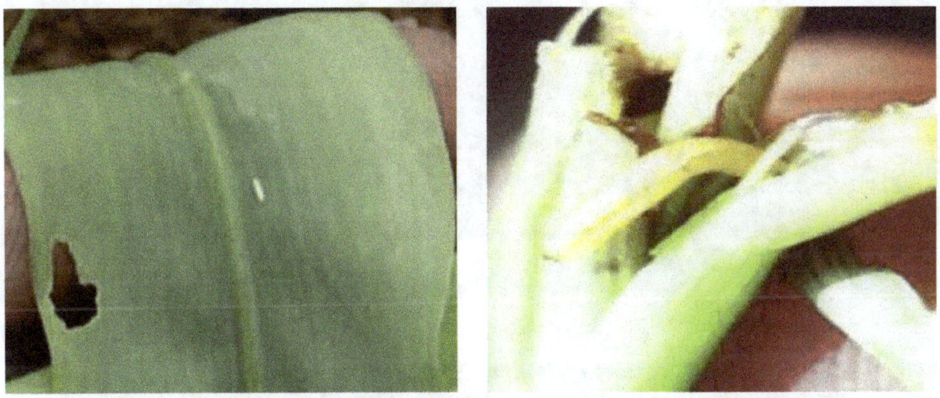

Maggot enters into the **'central shoot'** by making **'horizontal cut'**

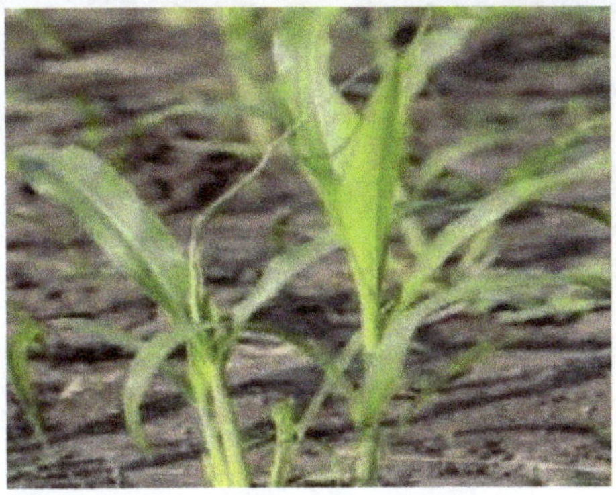

Dead heart

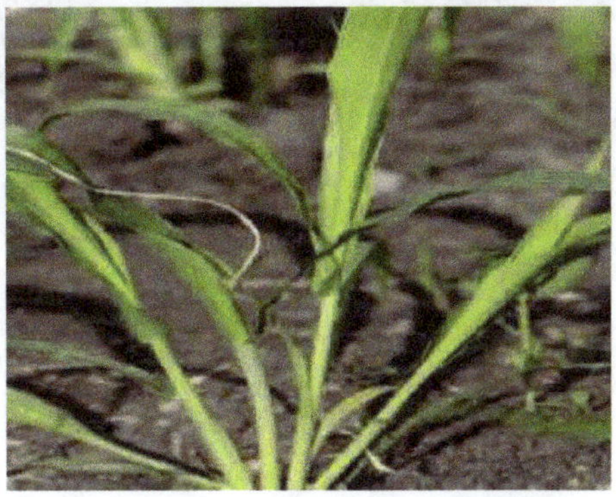

Production of '**side tillers / shoots'**

F. Stem borer, *Chilopartellus* (Lepidoptera: Crambidae)

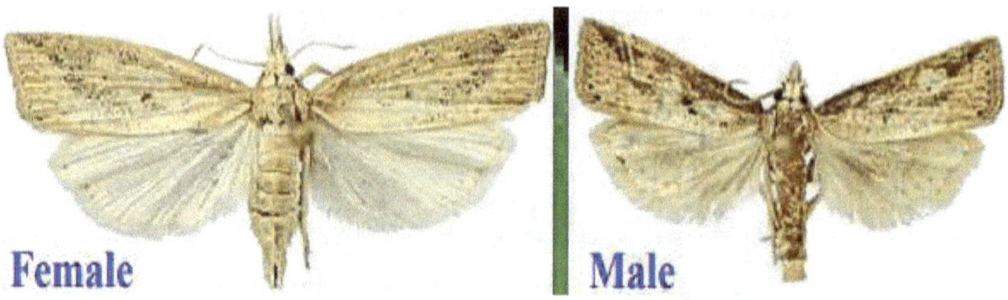


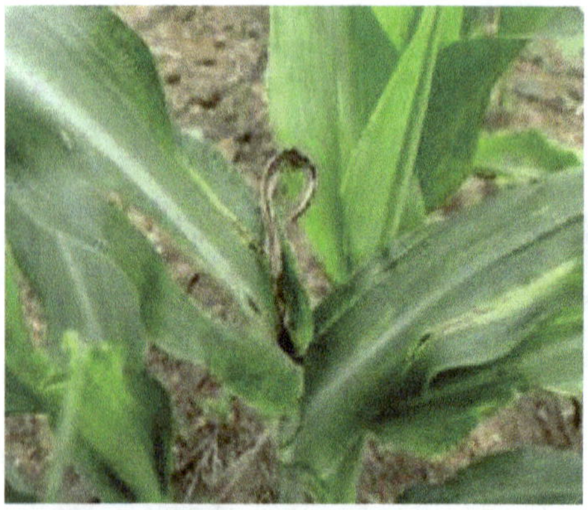

Dead heart

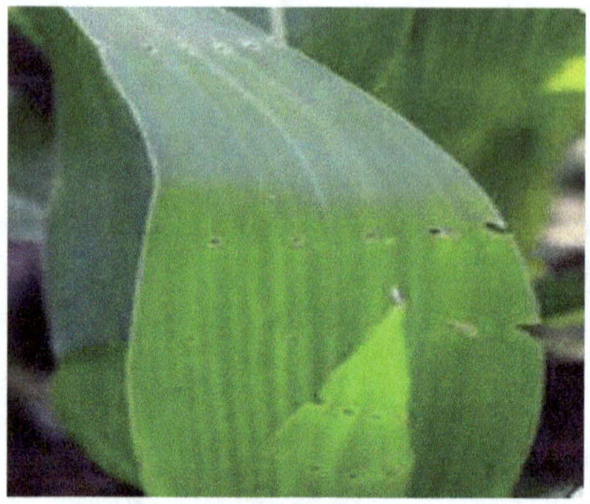

Series of pinholes

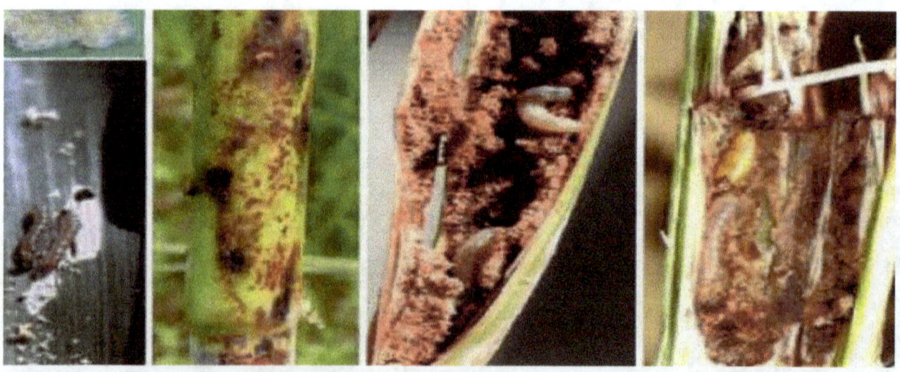

Larvae bores into the **stem** and feeds the **internal content**

G. Army worm *Mythimna separata* (Lepidoptera: Noctuidae)

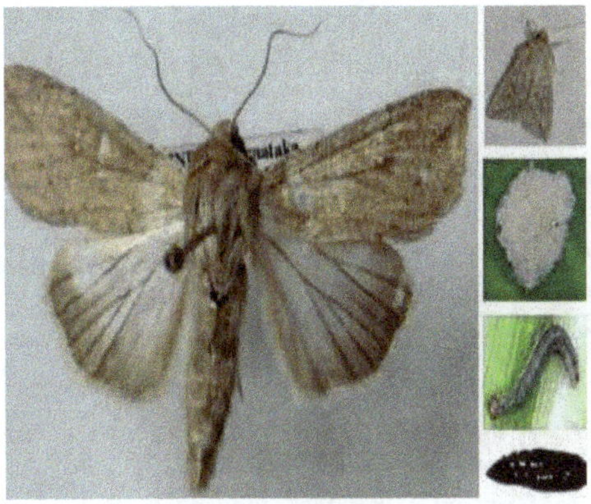

Adult

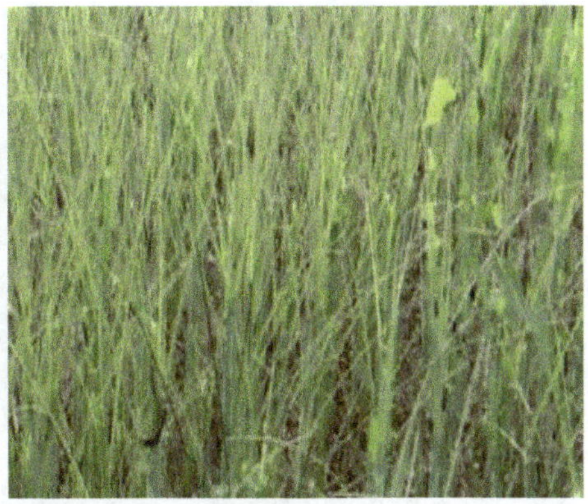

Defoliation

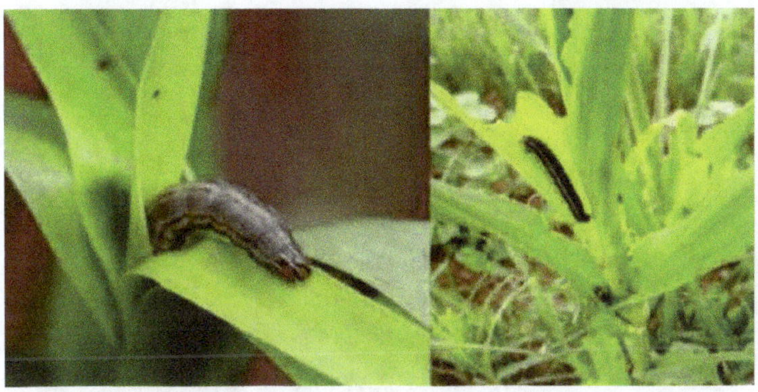

Larva feeds on 'developing grains' inside the 'earhead'

H. Shoot bug, *Perigrinus maidis* (Hemiptera: Delphacidae)

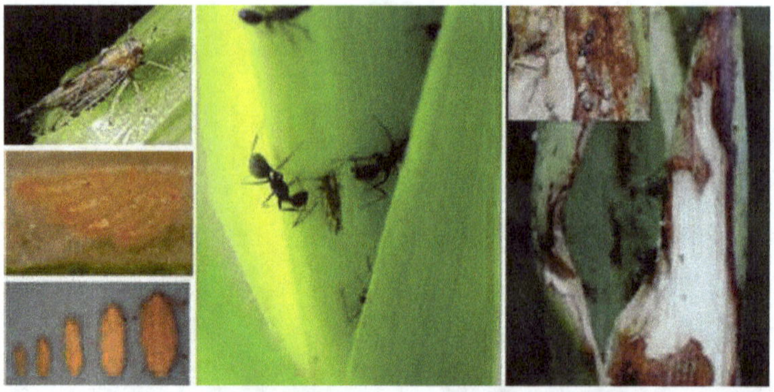

Nymphs & adults **'suck the sap'** from **'central leaf whorl'**& on leaf sheath of tender plants

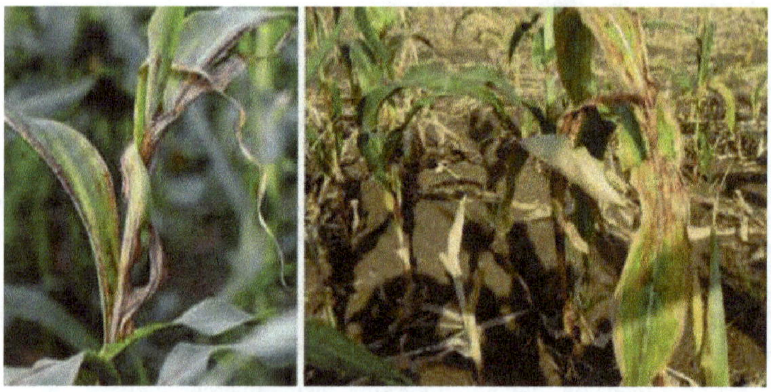

**Yellowing of leaves with stunted growth**; Under severe infestation, plants **'dry-up'**

I. Earhead midge, *Stenodiplosis sorghicola* (Diptera: Cecidomyiidae)

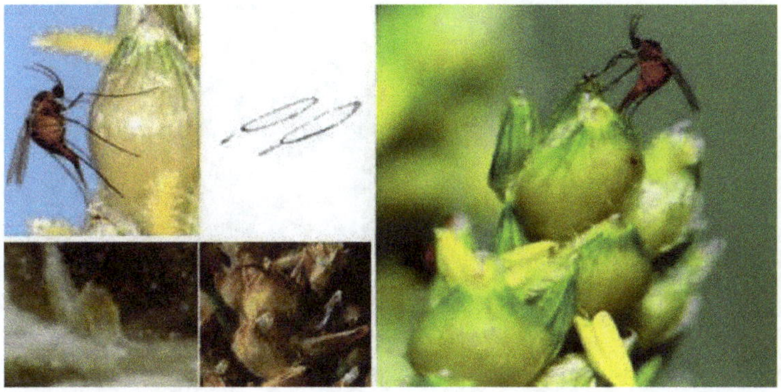

**'Maggot'** feeds on **'developing ovary'** inside the floret

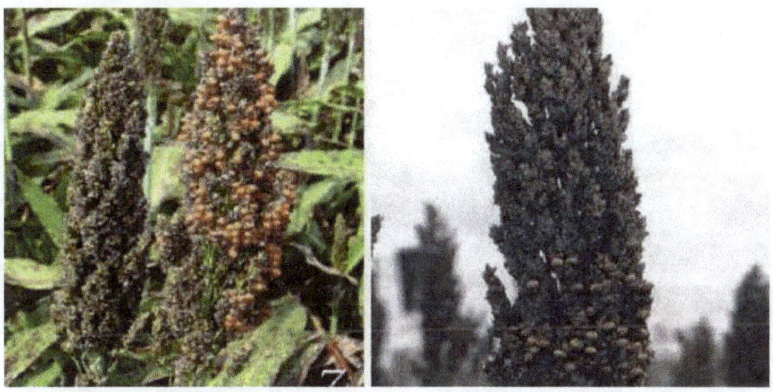

**'Chaffy ear-head'** or **'blighted grains'**

J. Earhead bug, *Calocoris angustatus* (Hemiptera: Miridae)

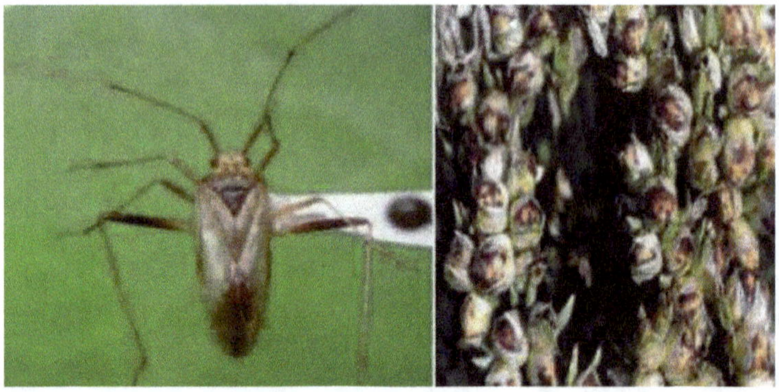

Nymphs & adults **suck the juice** from developing grainsat **milky stage** leading to **shrivelled or chaffy grains**& even ear-headappears uneven

K. Hairy caterpillar : *Euproctis subnotata*

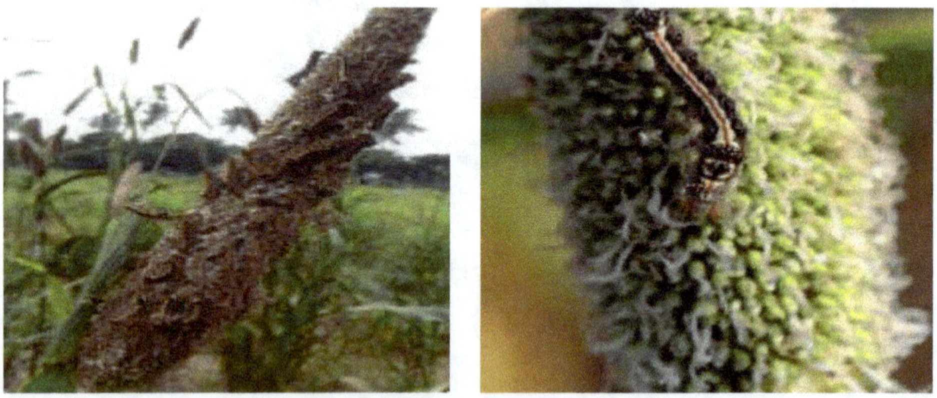

Larvae feeds on various parts of the plant

15

# Recent Approaches for Management of Insect Disease Problems in Pearl Millet

B C Anu[1]*, Rahul Singh Rajput[2] and Rishabh Raj[3]

[1] Krishi Vigyan Kendra, Turki, Muzaffarpur, Dr. Rajendra Prasad Central Agricultural University, Pusa, Samastipur, Bihar-848125

[2] Krishi Vigyan Kendra, Sukhet, Madhubani, Dr. Rajendra Prasad Central Agricultural University, Pusa, Samastipur, Bihar-848125

[3] Govind Ballabh Pant University of Agriculture and Technology, Uttarakhand-263153

**ABSTRACT**

Pearl Millet (*Pennisetum glaucum* L.) is one of the important crops that feed poor people living in semi-arid and arid tropics of Asia and Africa and provides nutritional security. It is generally cultivated in regions that are too hot, too dry or have soil constraints that prevent economic production of other staple food grain crops as a food, feed / fodder and fuel crop. It accounts for approximately 50% of the total world production of millets. One of the major factors, responsible for poor yield of pearl millet is the susceptibility to insect pest and diseases. During the growth and development, this crop is damaged by insect pests among which, shoot flies, white grubs, stem borers, leaf-sucking, and the panicle-attacking insects are considered economically important and downy mildew, blast, rust, ergot and smut are some of the major diseases attacking the crop. They individually or in combination lead to significant losses in yield and quality. Pest and disease outbreaks reduce millet yield and quality, leaving farmers with less income in comparison to cost of cultivation. With significant climatic changes, the introduction of high yielding hybrids, degradation of soil and water conservation measures, increasing cost of cultivation and fluctuating market rates for millet grains, current pest and disease management strategies need some changes. So, improvement in yield stability could be achieved through integration of different approaches like host plant resistance for pest and disease management along with further adoption of new crop cultivation technologies.

*Keywords*: Disease management strategies, Downy mildew, Host plant resistance, Nutritional security, Susceptibility, White grubs

## Introduction

The millet that is most frequently grown is pearl millet (*Pennisetum glaucum*). Unlike major cereal crops like maize or wheat, pearl millet can survive and tolerate

* Corresponding author.

challenging conditions like drought, low soil fertility, and high temperatures. Developing countries account for about 95% in production of pearl millet, which also account for the majority of the crop. Although, in the states like Gujarat, Rajasthan, and Haryana, the growing areas are getting smaller, still India stands as the largest producer of pearl millet in the world. It is generally grown as a dryland crop having a dual-purpose nature as grain and fodder and is irrigated occasionally in India, especially as a crop in summer. Even though pearl millet is used as primary food but recently there has been a shift in its use from primary food to feeds for animal, potable alcohol, different types of processed food, etc., it is now headed toward a more market-oriented crop.

Unlike most other cereals, this crop grows well in the driest and most marginal soils. It is grown in regions which are arid with frequent droughts, high temperatures, irregular and light rains, and infertile soils where water-holding capacity is low. In the north of India, during the rainy season pearl millet is grown; however, in the northwest and south, it may be grown during two or three seasons annually. Pearl millet can tolerate drought condition so it has a unique position among crops which are grown during thekharif season. Due to its unique property of quick growth and robust nature, in the arid as well as semi-arid tropical regions, it is used as fodder for cattle with high qualityas well as forage crop. The stalk of this crop is being used for thatching and as fuel. In India, asmajor source of dietary energy (360 kcal/kg) for the rural population, pearl millet is ranked fourth in position as significant cereal crop after major cereal crops like rice, wheat, and sorghum. It contains a lot of iron, calcium, phosphorus, and protein. Thiamine, riboflavin, and niacin are present in pearl millet grain in relatively high concentrations. Additionally, its grain is used for applications other than food like the production of ethanol and fodder for animals (Basavaraj *et al.,* 2010).

## Status of Pearl Millet distribution

Globally, it ranks as sixth highest producing crop after major cereal crops like maize, rice, wheat, rice, sorghum and barley (FAOSTAT, 2014). It is also regarded as one of the nutrition enriched and income generating crops for the smallholder farmers, contributing to their livelihoods and food availability (Patel *et al.,* 2015). Despite of the importance and values that pearl millet has it doesn't get the attention it deserves. It is grown globally on an area of 30 million hectares in the tropical regions of arid and semi-arid of Asia and is a main food for over 90 million poor people (Srivastava *et al.*, 2020).It is mostly cultivated under rainfed conditions in marginal lands and can produce grains with good quality even in drought. India is the top producer of pearl millet with a productivity of 1237 kg $ha^{-1}$over an area of 7.4 million ha.

Ninety percent of India's total production of pearl millet is produced in the major growing states of Rajasthan, Maharashtra, Uttar Pradesh, Gujarat, and Haryana. Rajasthan accounts for the largest share (about 4.283 million tonnes), followed by Uttar Pradesh, Haryana, Gujarat, Maharashtra and Tamil Nadu. It is mainly grown during the kharif season, but in some parts of Gujarat, Rajasthan, and U.P, it is also grown during the summer season (February-May) and, in the states of Maharashtra and Gujarat it is cultivated on a smaller scale, in the rabi season *i.e.*, November–February. Millets are correctly referred to as "nutricereals" because of their climate-smart nature with tremendous nutritional value. Additionally, Year 2018 was designated as the "Year of Millets" by Government of India and the Year 2023 is designated as the "International Year of Millets" by Food and Agriculture Organization (FAO) Committee on Agriculture (COAG) forum in an effort to mainstream millets, capitalize on their superior nutritional qualities, and promote their cultivation. In addition to grain, it is a crucial source of nutrition for livestock, particularly during the dry months when other feed sources are scarce. On the other hand, pearl millet is used as a chief food as well as feed for animal and poultry, as well as to make booze and health food (Yadav *et al.*, 2017).

## Nutritional value as health benefits

Pearl millet is climate resilient due to its low water requirement (200-600 mm), high temperature stability and drought tolerance. Millets' potential as "Nutri Cereals" can thus be used to increase food security in the future. Farmers began utilizing synthetic fertilizers, chemical pesticides, to meet this escalating demand. Over the past 50 years, this has upsurged the yield of pearl milletglobally (Savary *et al.*, 2017). In comparison to the main cereal crops like rice, wheat, maize, this crop is rich in nutritional supplements and cheaper as well, and has rich source of micronutrients like iron and zinc (Kumar *et al.*, 2016) amino corrosive composition sand protein for grazing animals. It is consider edan important energy source (Kanatti *et al.*, 2014). When compared to sorghum, it has high protein content,protein quality, and energy levels (Vadez *et al.*, 2012). As a result, lots of people depend on the yield of pearl millet for their personal as well as professional needs. Additionally, it has long been recognized as abiofuel crop of future (Lata, 2015). Therefore, it is a key component for the country's poor population's food security in dry regions. Dry stover of this millet is used as a basis of proportion for a large population of ox-like animals, which is thought to be the most essential source of supplying strength in the risky harvest domesticated animal farming system in water-restricted areas.

Pearl millet grains are primarily used for human consumption as different food. Compared to other major cereals, oats contain more micronutrients like iron and zinc, proteins (8–19%), antioxidants, soluble fat and insoluble fat, ash, dietary fibers (1.2 g per100 g), and fat (3–8%) with better digestibility of fat (Uppal *et al.*,

2015). Additionally, it contains a significant amount of minerals (2.3 mg per100 g), including phosphorous, potassium, iron,magnesium,copper,zinc, and manganese, as well as different vitamins like thiamine, riboflavin, and niacin (Weckwerth *et al.*, 2020).

## Major threat to Pearl Millet production

Insect pests and plant diseases like blast and rust negatively affect the quality and productivity of pearl millet (Jukanti *et al.,* 2016). These illnesses seriously jeopardize global food security and hurt farmers' livelihoods (Schütz *et al.,* 2011). Crop disease detection system must therefore be implemented. Due to feeding of various insect on plant parts at differentstages of growth, it causes huge economic losses like reduction inquality of grain, productivity, and yield of fodder (Bekoye and Dadie 2015, Kumar and Channaveer swami 2015). One of the main obstacles to millet production is the presence of disease and insect pests. Due to climate change, these issues are probably going to get worse in the future. Major diseases of millets include downy mildew, grain mould, smut, blast,rust, leaf spot, brown spot, and some viral infections (Table 1; Table 2).

**Table 1 :** Some common insect pests of Pearl Millet:

| S.No. | Common Name | Insect Species | Order | Family |
|---|---|---|---|---|
| **Borers** | | | | |
| 1. | Shoot fly | *Atherigona approximata* | Diptera | Muscidae |
| 2. | Stem borer | *Chil opartellus* Swinhoe | Lepidoptera | Pyralidae |
| 3. | Pink Stem borer | *Sesamia inferens* | Lepidoptera | Noctuidae |
| **Defoliators** | | | | |
| 4. | Grey weevil | *Myllocerus* spp. | Coleoptera | Curculionidae |
| 5. | White grub | *Holotrichia consanguinea* | Coleoptera | Scarabaeidae |
| 6. | Grasshopper | *Hieroglyphus* spp. | Orthoptera | Acrididae |
| 7. | Blister beetle | *Psalydolyttafusva* | Coleoptera | Meloidae |
| **Earhead feeders** | | | | |
| 8. | Earhead worm | *Cryptoblabes gnidiella* Milliere | Lepidoptera | Pyralidae |
| 9. | Earhead bug | *Calocoris angustatus* | Hemiptera | Miridae |
| 10. | Grain midge | *Geromyia penniseti* | Diptera | Cecidomyiidae |
| 11. | Semilooper | *Antoba silicula* | Lepidoptera | Noctudiae |
| 12. | Stink bug | *Nezara viridula* | Hemiptera | Pentatomidae |

## Economically important insect pests of Pearl Millet

### *1. Shoot fly*

**Scientific Name:** *Atherigona approximata* (Diptera: Muscidae)

**Distribution**: Throughout India

**Host range**: Pearl millet, sorghum, maize, finger millet etc.

**Damage symptoms**: This is a serious pest of pearl millet throughout India. During the cold weather season in TN (Tamil Nadu), the crop is attacked by this pest at seedling as well as boot leaf stages. The immature stage i.e., maggot after hatching from egg moves to ventral side of the leaf surface andcrawls between the leaf sheath and stem. Central leaf of the plant wilts and dries, it isknown as the "dead heart" due to the maggot which penetrates the soil and bores the inside of stem and cut the point which are growing. The infested plant makes side tillers that are susceptible to attack. In contrast to kharif season, the attack is more severe in the summer. In young plants, it results in dead hearts, and in mature crops, it results in chaffy grains.

**Bionomics**: Adult females lay white colour eggs which are like cigar in shape, on the lowersurface of leaf blades. The incubation period ranges from 2-3 days, and the oviposition period is between 37 and 48 hours long. The maggot is apodous and dirty white. Maggots are yellowcoloured and about 6 mm in length when mature. There are four larval instars and an 8–10 days larval period. Pupation takes place in the soil or at the base of stem for eight to ten days. The life cycle of shoot fly is about 17 to 21 days.

**Economic Threshold Level (ETL) of pest**: 1 egg / plant or 10% dead hearts

*2. Stem borer*

**Scientific Name**:*Chilo partellus* (Lepidoptera: Crambidae)

**Distribution:** Throughout India

**Host range**: Pearl millet, maize, sorghum, rice, sugarcane, finger milletetc.

**Damage symptoms**:The infestation starts 30 days after sowing up until the emergence of the earhead. The typical damage symptom is "dead heart" i.e., withering and deterioration of the central shoot. On the stem near to nodes, visible bore holes can be seen. Larvaefeed on tender leaves producing the "shot hole" symptom. Caterpillars sometimes internally tunnel in stem portions.

**Bionomics:** The adult is medium sized and straw-coloured. Female on an average lay 300 eggs which are flat and oval in shape and egg are laid in batches on the ventral surface of leaf. It takes about 2 to 5 days during incubation. The larval head is brown in colour and body is yellowish brown with 25 mm long prothoracic shield.Larval stage has seven instars and lasts for 28 to 50 days. Within the stem, it pupates before emerging as an adult within 7–10 days through the entry holes left by the larvae. The entire life cycle takes 30 to 40 days to complete.

**Economic Threshold Level (ETL) of pest**: 10% dead heart

### 3. *Pink stemborer*

**Scientific Name**: *Sesamia inferens* (Noctuidae: Lepidoptera)

**Distribution:**India, Malaysia,Pakistan, Burma, Taiwan,Bangladesh, South East Asia,Sri Lanka, Korea,China, Indonesia and Japan.

**Host range**: Sorghum, rice, maize, wheat, bajra, sugarcane, and barley, ragi, guinea grasses

**Damage symptoms**: Larva is the damaging stage and it bores the stem from inside causing damage to the central shoot resulting in its killing.

**Bionomics**:Wings of the adult moth arelight yellowish or straw-coloured and a white coloured body. The larva has a dark coloured head with pinkish-brown body. The entire life cycle takes 45 to 75 days to complete. 4-6 generations occur annually.

### 4. *White grub*

**Scientific Name**: *Holotrichia consanguinea* (Coleoptera: Scarabaeidae)

**Damage symptoms**: They are highly polyphagous pest which feeds on a variety of host plants. Plants' underground roots are harmed by grubs. Following feeding,plants exhibit varying degrees of yellowing and it further leads to wilting, which ultimately results in death of plants. White grubs attack young plants and it results in wilting of plant parts causing a characteristic purple colouration in the leavesintially, which further leads to the death of small plants, and a reduction in vigour. Dead heart is produced by the plants affected by white grub occasionally. Because they feed on apical buds and tender leaves, beetles are defoliating pests that cause significant damage to a variety of fruit trees, plantations, and forest trees.

**Economic Threshold Level (ETL) of pest**: 1 grub/m$^2$ area

### 5. *Earhead bug*

**Scientific Name**:*Calocoris angustatus* (Miridae: Hemiptera)

**Distribution:**Throughout India

**Host range**: Pearl millet, maize, sorghum etc.

**Damage symptoms**: The developing grains are suck by nymphs as well as adult when the grain is in the milky stage in the earheads. The affected grains contract, change color to black, and become chaffy or ill-filled. Older grains have noticeable feeding holes that leads to lower grain quality.

**Bionomics**:The colour of the adult bug- male is green, and the adult bug- femaleis green with brown coloured border. Female lays eggs which are blue in colour having shape of cigar eggs either in center of the florets or beneath the glumes. Each female produces 150–200 eggs. There is an egg period of 7-days. Nymphs are slim and have a green color. The color of the first instar is orange. Nymphal stage lasts 10 to 14 days. From egg to adult, the life cycle takes less than three weeks. When the paniclesripen at different time, at least 2 generations of the pest occurs which feed on the crop.

**Economic Threshold Level (ETL) of pest**: 10 nymphs or adults/earhead

**Table 2 :** Some of the common diseases of Pearl Millet:

| S.No. | Diseases | Causal Organism |
|---|---|---|
| | Downy mildew | *Sclerospora graminicola* |
| | Rust | *Puccinia penniseti* |
| | Smut | *Tolyposporium penicillariae* |
| | Ergot / Sugary disease | *Claviceps fusiformis* |
| | Pyricularia leaf spot or blast | *Puccinia substriata*var. *indica* |
| | Leaf spot by various fungi | *Bipolariss etariae* |
| | | *Cercospora penniseti* |
| | | *Curvularia penniseti* |
| | | *Dactuliophorae longata* |
| | | *Drechslera dematioidea* |
| | | *Myrothecium roridum* |
| | | *Phyllachora penniseti* |
| | | *Gloeocercospora sorghi* |
| | Leaf blight | *Exserohilum rostratum* |
| | | *Phyllosticta penicillariae* |
| | | *Rhizoctonia solani; Rhizoctonia zeae* |
| | | *Sclerotium rolfsii* |

## Important diseases of Pearl Millet

### *1. Downy mildew disease*

**Causal organism**: *Sclerospora graminicola*

InAsia and Africa, downy mildew is an extensive disease (Williams 1984) which causes approximately a grain yield lossof 20–40% annually (Hash *et al.,* 1999; Singh 1995).

**Symptoms:** Disease occurs in two stages (i) Downy mildew stage (ii) Green ear stage

**Downy mildew stage**: The affected leaf has white patches on the lower side of surface inform of white cottony growth. The entire lamina is covered by these patches, which eventually turn the lamina yellow. Sporangiophores and sporangia make up the down y growth.

**Green ear stage**: Earheads either partially or completely transform into green leafy structures. The main source of inoculum is the oospore.

**Epidemiology**: Development of disease is favoured by the higherrelative humidity *i.e.*, 85–90% RH) with a temperature range of 20–30°C. Under the favourable environmental and inoculum conditions, the development of disease only takes 7 days period from infection to spore production in susceptible host. The formation of sporangiophore and sporangia is favoured by low temperatures of 15–25°C.

### 2. *Rust*

**Causal organism**: *Puccinia penniseti*

**Symptoms:** On both leaf surfaces, infection appears as brownish yellow pustules. These stand in for the fungus' uredia. Black teliosori can be seen on leaves and leaf sheaths. Brinjal serves as a backup host.

**Epidemology:** Dew formation, clear, cool night temperature (approximately 20°C) and infection favour growth of disease. In India, post-rainy season crops tend to experience more severe rust than crops grown during the rainy or summer months. Closer spacing; the presence of numerous brinjal plants and other Solanum species, such as *S. xanthocarpum*, *S. pubescents*, and *S. torvum*.

### 3. *Smut Causal organism*

**Causal organism:** *Tolyposporium penicillariae*

**Symptoms:** When the grain sets, the disease is visible. On the earhead, green to black sori that are much larger than typical grains take the place of a few grains that are dispersed sporadically. The solid sorus wall is strong and encloses the powdery mass of smut spores which are present in balls.

**Epidemiology:** Smut infection starts with inocula that are contaminated by soil and seeds, not internally borne seeds. At threshing, teleutosporesremains in the soil from the florets which are previously infected and contaminate the fresh seeds. At the crop's flowering stage, a higher relative humidity of 80–95% and an ideal 25–35°C temperature is most conducive to smut infection and spread. Successive cropping with Pearl Millet is one of the cause of spread of this disease.

### 4. *Ergot / Sugary disease*

**Causal organism**: *Claviceps fusiformis*

**Symptoms**: From the spikelets, the tiny droplets of a pinkish, sticky fluid oozes out. The affected spikelets turn black, and the earhead develops a number of these dark, sticky patches. The growth of grains is prevented. Hyaline single-celled conidia are abundant in honey dew. Ovaries that have been infected later turn into sclerotia.

**Epidemology**: After inoculation, sclerotia become visible in 15-20 days under favourable conditions of relative humidity of 80-85% with a moderate 20-30°C Day temperature, and 15-20°C night temperature. Symptoms of honeydew appears in 4-6 days under these favorableconditions. The ergot sclerotia from the previously infected panicles are the primary inoculum source for the next crop, which fall on the soilduring harvesting or during threshing mixes with the uninfected seeds.

### 5. *Pyricularia leaf spot or blast: Causal organism: Puccinia substriata var. indica*

Blast disease, also known as pyricularia leaf spot, is particularly significant in cultivars of pearl millet used for forage. The disease was initially identified in India in Kanpur, Uttar Pradesh, and persisted for a considerable amount of time as a minor illness. Chronic losses in grain yield are caused by the disease and forage (Wilson and Gates 1993; Timper *et al.,* 2002).

**Symptoms**: The disease initially begins as large, necrotic spots that are grayish, water-soaked on the foliage. This causes chlorosis leading to premature drying and death of young leaves. A chlorotic halo that surrounds lesions frequently turns necrotic and resembles concentric rings. On the foliage, the lesions are typically limited to interveinal spaces. Large surface areas are covered by lesions as they spread and coalesce, resulting in tissue necrosis. When a cultivar is susceptible, the entire foliage appears burned. The only grain produced by severely infected plants is a small number of shriveled florets with no grains at all.

**Epidemology**: Cereal crops, including rice, foxtail millet, finger millet, pearl millet, and grasses are affected by *P. grisea*. The fungus has a wide range of hosts but is very specialized in those hosts. Higher relative humidity of >90% and moderate 25–30°C temperatures are more conducive to the development of infection and disease. When the weather is humid, the disease gets worse, especially when there are dense plant stands. The conidia are easily spread by the wind and spitting rain because the sporulation of pathogen starts on the lesions present on the foliage. These spores survive the winter in stubble and infect the following crop.

## Integrated pest management strategies

**Host plant resistance:** Although only few cultivated variety have shown ability of low to moderate levels of resistance to some of the most significant pests and diseases, HPR is a very effective management strategy. To reduce pest losses, higher levels of resistance are needed. Additionally, some sources of resistance exhibit poor agronomic traits. Resistant cultivars will offer a fair, sustainable, and eco-friendly pest management tool. In order to develop resistant or tolerant cultivar with desirable agronomic and grain characteristics, we must make an effort to transfer the pesttoleant and disease resistance traits into desirable genotypes.

It's important to understand the working mechanisms and inheritance pattern of resistance. Our ability to create cultivars with the desired levels of resistance has been hampered by knowledge gaps regarding the resistance mechanism, resistance inheritance, the sources of resistance and their diversity. To create genotypes with stable and long-lasting resistance, it is necessary to find out the genotypes which have different resistance mechanisms and then by using breeding programs can transfer to required geneotype .

## Development of genetically modified (GM) plants to combat insect pest problem

The use of biotechnological tools has the potential to ease some of these restrictions. In conventional genetic enhancement only possible within species and this barrier can be eliminated by using advance biotechnological tools. This allows the gene transfer from completely unrelated organisms to plant and make resistance GM plants to counter the insect pest problem. It would be most fruitful to combine genetic engineering with traditional plant breeding.

## Molecular marker-assisted selection

Selection of desired trait can do through molecular assisted markers which makes breeding programme more efficient and effective in comparison to convention method. The molecular markers can be identified at different stages ofplantbecause unlike the trait, they are not subject to environmental regulation and are therefore not affected by the plants' growing conditions. Expression of insect pest and disease resistance across seasons and or locations is associated with a number of challenges. To Find molecular markers for transfer of resistant traits into agronomically appealing and cultivars which are adaptive locally is necessary in such circumstances. This strategy is crucial for pyramiding resistance genes and ensuring material transfer across regions.

## Natural enemies (NE)

Major insect pests like *Helicoverpa* must be manage by this approach and natural enemies are crucial for this. The availability of glandular trichomes and exudates production in plantsare two factors limiting the efficacy and movement of NE. Our efforts to manage this pest can take on a new dimension if we search the genotypes with non-glandular traits to have a compatibility with NE. Armyworm and stem borers must be managed with the help of their natural enemies. Future pest management programs will be very concerned with quantifying how borer-tolerant germplasms and transgenics affect the efficiency and activity of NE.

## Biopesticides

The non-judicial use of synthetic pesticides has led concern about environmental pollution, human, pest resurgence as well as health risks. In comparison to synthetic insecticides, natural plant products and biopesticides are generally safe for use on humans, non-target organisms, and natural enemies. Recent advancements in the area of natural pest control products are very exciting. Environmentally friendly products like nuclear polyhedrosis virus (NPV), Bt toxins, and actinomycete-produced spinosads and avermectins are currently undergoing extensive testing. Numerous isolates of bacteria and fungi have been recognized as potential biocontrol agents.

Analysis of interactions at multiple trophic levels in relation to benefits vs crop damage and loss in yield is required for the efficientincorporation of different agronomic methods with HPR and biopesticides. Natural plant products have attracted a lot of attention from private to public institutions on domestic and international level. It is necessary to look into new approaches in cultural practices that can help to lower the pest incidence and damage. It has been demonstrated that many strains of *Trichoderma viride*, *T. harzianum*, and *Pseudomonas fluorescense* are effective against *A. flavus* in groundnut.

## Entomopathogenic microorganisms

Entomopathogenic microorganisms like *Beauveria bassiana*, *M. anisopliae* and commercial strains of *B. thuringiensis* that are commercially available are useful for control against insect pest.

## Botanicals

Most of the botanicals' hot water extracts demonstrated more activity than their corresponding compost washes. The growth of pearl millet is improved by a liquid extract of compost which made from *Datura metel, Azadirachta indica* and *Parthenium hysterophorus* leaves.

## Integrated diseases management strategies

**Cultural practices**: Deep summer ploughing, use of healthy and good quality seed for sowing purpose, timely sowing, proper seed rate and distance between plant to plant and also row to row, irrigation practice, weeding. These are the conventional approaches which have follow by farmers to manage diseases at early stage.

**Use of resistant varieties**: The utilization of different genotypes which have resistance traits varieties against diseases is least expensive and long-lasting approach in the disease management strategy. Growing of such genotypes also promote the environmental sustainability.

**Selection of seed and its treatment**: Make sure the seeds are properly examined by naked eyes and no admixture like ergot (Chepa), sclerotia are present in seeds. Farmers are also advised to use brine/salt solution treatment to identify the quality of seed if the seeds were not obtained or purchased from a certified/registered agency. Dipping of seed done in 10% slat solution for 10 minutes and then the floating materials are removed gently with the help of a perforated vessel and then thoroughly washed in normal water. The germination of the seed is hampered if any salt residue is left on the seed's surface. Finally, shade dry the seeds and treat them with any type of systemic fungicide such as carbendazim @ 2.0–2.5 per kg of seeds before sowing. Metalaxyl 35 % @ 6 g per kg of seed should be applied to treat downy mildew (green ear disease).

**Removal of diseased plants**: The millet crop should be uprooted and destroyed as early as possible if the signs of downy mildew disease started to show on the leaves and the diseased plants that were uprooted should not come into contact with healthy plants. Use mancozeb or zineb 0.25% solution for spray the crop with after removing the diseased plants from susceptible varieties of millet.

**Chemical methods**:Although this is the easy, quick and most efficient method ofmanagement of disease but using chemical fungicides excessively is not safe for crop as well as soil in integrated management of diseasesas they make pathogens more resistant to chemical treatments and also worsen soil quality. Crops and helpful microorganisms are also negatively impacted. For seed, soil treatment, and foliar spraying, always use the proper quantity of insecticides, fungicides, bactericides, insecticides, and weedicides. The reduction in use of chemical fungicidesneed to be reduced so that we can preserve thesoil microflora and fauna and environment by implementing use of biocontrol agents in Integrated Disease Management (IDM).

**Bio-control agents**: In this component, disease management is carried out using biological techniques such as soil treatment, seed treatment and foliar sprays by employing various microbes *i.e.,*fungus (*Trichoderma* spp.) and bacterium

(*Pseudomonas* spp.). For treatment of seed, a biofungicide (*Trichoderma*) should be used at a rate of 4-5 gram per kg seed while for treatment of soil 2.5 kg per ha of *Trichoderma* along with 100 kg of FYM is used.

## Conclusion

Pearl millet can be used to improve nutritional quality and combat malnutrition because it is multi-nutritional value and climatically resilient traits. The integration approach with various components can be helpful in reducing the losses by diseaseand pest as well as increase crop yields, it will be the focus of future management plans. These are the crops which now considered as the future crops to fight with arising climatic condition change. With significant climatic changes, anduse of high yielding varieties, degradation in soil conservation and water conservation methods, upsurge in cost of cultivation and variationin the rates for millet in market, present strategies in management of pest and diseaseneed some alteration. So, improvement in yield stability could be achieved through integration of different approaches like host plant resistance for pest and disease management.

## References

Basavaraj, G., Parthasarathy, Rao P., Bhagavatula, S. & Ahmed, W. (2010). Availability and utilization of pearl millet in India. Journal of SAT Agricultural Research, 8:1–6.

Bekoye, B.M. &Dadie, A. (2015). Evaluation des pertesen grains de mil dues aux insectes. European scientific journal, 11, 266–275.

FAOSTAT. (2014). FAO statistical yearbook. FAO, Rome. http://www.fao. org/3/a-i3590e. pdf. Accessed 12 Feb 2020.

Hash CT, Singh S.D., Thakur R.P. and Talukdar B.S. (1999). Breeding for disease resistance. In: Pearl Millet Breeding (pp. 337-379). Oxford & IBH.

Jukanti, A.K., Gowda, C.L.L., Rai, K.N., Manga, V.K. & Bhatt, R.K. (2016). Crops that feed the world 11. Pearl Millet (*Pennisetum glaucum* L.): An important source of food security, nutrition and health in the arid and semi-arid tropics. Food Security, 8(2), 307–329

Kanatti, A., Rai, K. N., Radhika, K., Govindaraj, M., Sahrawat, K. L., Srinivasu, K., *et al.* (2014). Relationship of grain iron and zinc content with grain yield in pearl millet hybrids. Crop Improv. 41, 91–96.

Kumar, S., Hash, C. T., Thirunavukkarasu, N., Singh, G., Rajaram, V. & Rathore, A., Senapathy, S., Mahendrakar, M.D., Yadav, R.S. & Srivastava, R.K. (2016). Mapping quantitative trait loci controlling high iron and zinc in self and open pollinated grains of pearl millet [*Pennisetum glaucum* (L) R. Br.]. Frontiers of plant science, 7:1636. doi: 10.3389/fpls.2016.01636

Kumar, A.D. & Channaveerswami, A.S. (2015). Pre and post emergence control measures for shoot fly incidence and its influence on seed yield of little millet (*Panicum sumatrense*). Journal of Experimental Zoology India, 18, 811–814

Lata, C., Muthamilarasan M. & Prasad M. (2015). Drought stress responses and signal transduction in plants. In: *The elucidation of abiotic stress signaling in plants* (pp: 195–225) Springer.

Patel, K., Gartaula, H., Johnson, D. & Karthikeyan, M. (2015). The interplay between household food security and wellbeing among small-scale farmers in the context of rapid agrarian change in India. Agriculture and Food Security, 4, 16. https://doi.org/10.1186/s40066-015-0036-2)

Savary, S., Bregaglio, S., Willocquet, L., Gustafson, D., Mason-D'Croz, D., Sparks, A.H., Castilla, N., Djurle, A., Allinne, C. & Sharma, M. *et al.* (2017). Crop health and its global impacts on the components of food security. Food Security, 9, 311–327.

Schütz, H., Jansen, M. &Verhoff, M.A. (2011). How to feed the world in 2050. Archiv für Kriminologie, 228, 151–159.

Singh S.D. (1995). Downy mildew of pearl millet. Plant Disease, 79, 545-550.

Srivastava, R.K., Singh, R.B., Lakshmi, V., Srikanth P., Pusuluri B., Satyavathi M., *et al.* (2020). Genome wide association studies and genomic selection in Pearl millet: Advances and Prospects. Frontiers in Genetics,10, 1389. doi: 10.3389/fgene. 2019. 01389

Timper, P., Wilson, J.P., Johnson, A.W. & Hanna, W.W. (2002). Evaluation of pearl millet grain hybrids for resistance to *Meloidogyne* spp. and leaf blight caused by *Pyricularia grisea*. Plant Disease, 86, 909-914.

Uppal, R.K., Wani, S.P., Garg, K.K. &Alagarswamy, G. (2015). Balanced nutrition increases yield of pearl millet under drought. Field Crops Research, 177, 86–97. doi: 10.1016/j.fcr.2015.03.006

Vadez, V., Hash, T., Bidinger, F.R. &Kholova, J. (2012). Phenotyping pearl millet for adaptation to drought. Frontiers in physiology, 3, 1-12.

Weckwerth, W., Ghatak, A., Bellaire, A., Chaturvedi, P. & Varshney, R.K. (2020). PANOMICS meets germplasm. Journal of plant biotechnology, 18, 1507–1525. doi: 10.1111/pbi.13372

Williams, R.J. (1984). Downy mildews of tropical cereals. Advances in Plant Pathology, 2, 1-103.

Wilson, J.P. & Gates, R.N. (1993). Forage yield losses in hybrid pearl millet due to leaf blight caused primarily by *Pyricularia grisea*. Phytopathology, 83, 739-743.

Yadav, O.P., Singh D.V., Vadez, V., Gupta, S.K., Rajpurohit, B.S. & Shekhawat, P.S. (2017). Improving pearl millet for drought tolerance – Retrospect and prospects. Indian journal of human genetics, 77(4), 464- 474.

# 16

# Exotic Fruits in India: Production, Nutritional Benefits and Medicinal Properties

Bijayalaxmi Sahoo[1,2*], Itishree Nayak[1], Parameswaran C[1], Khirodkumar sahoo[2]

[1] Crop Improvement Division, ICAR-National Rice Research Institute, Cuttack-753006, Odisha, India

[2] Department of Biotechnology, Ravenshaw University, Cuttack-753003 , Odisha, India

**ABSTRACT**

Exotic fruits are varieties that are not native to the area and are managed to grow beyond their natural habitat. The term "exotic fruits" is mostly used in advanced countries to refer tropical fruits that are unfamiliar to developed-country consumers. Exotic fruit are low in calorie, high in fiber, minerals, and vitamins. Furthermore,They also have antioxidant, anti-inflammatory, antimicrobial and anticancer properties. Their sweet tastes and colors make them more appealing to customers. Exotic fruits that grown around the world such as durian, akebi, rambutan, salak, pandanus, Lutqua, Elephant apple, carambola, buddha's hand, kiwi and many others. In recent years, a variety of exotic fruits such as star fruit, finger citron, jackfruit, kiwi, dragon fruit, persimmon, Indian hog plum, avocado, langsat, passion fruit mangosteen, and others have been grown in India. Many fruits contain vitamin C and iron, which help with immunity and the production of haemoglobin and myoglobin. In recent years, the exotic fruits business has been heavily influenced by customer demand and the health benefits they provide. The exotic fruit market is expected to expand further as they are becoming more popular among consumers due to their high nutritional value and delicious flavour. So, the focus of this chapter was on the cultivation, nutritional benefits, and medicinal properties of exotic fruits.

*Keywords*: Exotic fruits, low in calorie, high in fiber, Mangosteen, star fruit, finger citron, immunity, nutritional value and delicious flavor

## Introduction

The second-largest producer of exotic fruits in the world is India. That's because a country with a diverse climate and cultural background can produce a wide range of fruits and is not limited to mango, banana, and citrus fruit production (Agrifarming, 2022). The term exotic refers towards something non - resident in an unusual way (Wakchaure *et al.,* 2021). However many exotic fruits are tropical

* Corresponding author.

in nature. Fruits and vegetables are the primary sources of bioactive compounds such as vitamins, secondary metabolites and have a high antioxidant potential. Vitamins are necessary for the growth of both plant and animal bodies. Most exotic fruits are rich in vitamin C, one of the most crucial vitamins. Exotic fruits are high in antioxidants, so efforts to promote fruit consumption should be maintained for public health benefits. There are different categories of fruits like, berry, capsule, nuts, drupe, pome, multiple fruit, legumes and aggregate fruit.Fruits are significant food items in our daily diets because they contain a variety of bioactive nutritional supplements that improve our bodies' ability to fight off various diseases (Devalaraja *et al.,* 2011). Vitamins are necessary building blocks for the development of both plant and animal bodies.Among the vitamins, vitamin C is essential because it functions as a significant antioxidant and boosts the activity of white blood cells, strengthening a variety of immune systems. Expert on vitamin C and Nobel Prize winner "Linus Pauling" advised taking 2000–5000 mg daily to avoid getting sick (Ariharan *et al.,* 2012). Since more specialty and conventional grocery stores have increased and diversified their selection of these "unusual" fruits over the past few years, they have gained popularity. Mangosteen is one of the sweetest exotic fruits that tastes like candy. In recent years, a variety of exotic fruits such as star fruit, finger citron, jackfruit, kiwi, dragon fruit, Indian hog plum, avocado, langsat, mangosteen, and others have been grown in India (Wakchaure *et al.,* 2021).

**Table 1:** List of exotic fruits, their scientific name and origin

| Common name | Scientific name | Country of Origin |
|---|---|---|
| Passion fruit | *Passiflora edulis* | South America (Brazil) |
| Dragon fruit (Pitaya) | *Selenicereus undatus* | Mexico and Central America |
| Soursop | *Annona muricata* | South America or caribbean |
| Cherimoya (Aka custard apple) | *Annona cherimola* | Ecuador and Peru |
| Acai | *Euterpe oleracea* | South ABD Central America (Brazil) |
| Jackfruit | *Artocarpus heterophyllus* | Rainforests near India and Malaysia |
| Pineapple Guava (Feijoa) | *Accasel lowiana* | South America |
| Quince | *Cydonia oblonga* | Turkey |
| Lychee | *Litchi chinensis* | South China |
| Rambutan | *Nephelium lappaceum* | Malaysia and Indonesia |
| Mangosteen | *Garcinia mangostana* | Southeast Asia and Thailand |
| Star Fruit | *Averrhoa carambola* | Southeast Asia |
| Horned Melon (Kiwano) | *Cucumis metuliferus* | Africa |
| Persimmon | *Diospyros kaki* | China |
| Buddha's Hand | *Citrus medica* | India |

## Dragon fruit

The botanical name of Dragon fruit is *Selenicereus undatus,* belongs to the family Cactaceae and genus Hylocereus. According to Fournet (2002), this genus is primarily distinguished by climbing vine cacti with aerial roots that produce attractive berries with large scales. Dragon fruit has a very appealing color, mellow pulp that melts in your mouth, and edible seeds that are embedded in the pulp that are black in color. This fruit also has a tremendous amount of nutritional value, which draws growers from all over India to cultivate it. It is a lovely flower that blooms at night and is known by the names "Noble Woman" or "Queen of the Night".The fruit is also known as pitaya, that makes it likely "the scaly fruit" due to its bracts or scales on its skin. There are many different varieties of dragon fruit grown worldwide such as,

*Hylocereus undatus*: -Pitahaya is another name for it, and it has pink skin and white flesh. It is well-known among dragon fruit varieties.

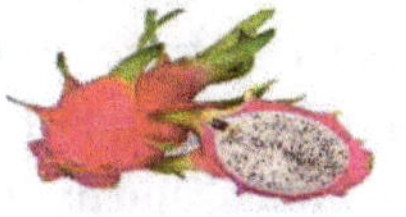

*Hylocereus costaricencis*: -This variety is also known as Costa Rican Pitaya. Its fruits are magenta in color and have skin that is pink with violet-red flesh. This type of dragon fruit is simple to grow in India.

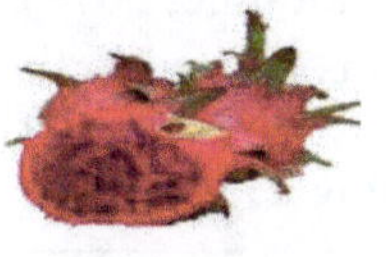

*Hylocereus polyrhizus*: - This variety is also known as Red Pitaya, and it has pink skin and red flesh.Among the various dragon fruit varieties, this one is the most lucrative.

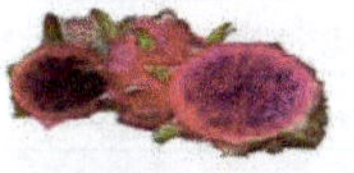

*Hylocereus megalanthus*: - its skin is known for being yellow with white flesh. When compared to other dragon fruit varieties, it is gorgeous (Tractor junction, 2021).

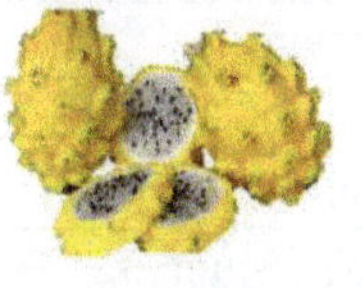

### *Origin and production*

Dragon fruit is originated in Mexico, Central America, and South America. Due to strong consumer demand, dragon fruit is currently being grown as a super fruit in India. The tropical climate is ideal for growing dragon fruit. From clay loam to loamy sand, a variety of soils can be used to grow this fruit. However, the best soil for its cultivation is sandy soil with sufficient organic matter and an ideal drainage system; for protected cultivation, the annual rainfall requirement is 50 cm, and the required temperature range is 20°C to 30°C. The ideal pH range for growing dragon fruit is 5.5 to 7. Cuttings are the most typical way to propagate dragon fruits. For field planting, cuttings of about 20 cm in length should be used. Two days prior to potting, pile up these cuttings.

However, seeds can also be used to spread it but, the seeds take a very long time and do not retain the traits of the mother plant. Comparatively speaking, this plant uses less water than others. As a result, you can frequently water it during the planting, flowering, and fruit-development stages and in hot and dry weather. As the plant matures, it develops aerial roots from the branches; therefore, it is advised to have a round or circular metal frame to maintain the balanced dragon shrub with a spacing of 8x8 ft. This will ensure the proper upright growth and development of the plant. When the skin turns from bright green to red or pink, it is ready for harvest. Three to four days after the fruit's skin color changes is the better time to harvest dragon fruit (Hossain *et al.,* 2021).

### *Nutritional benefits*

Dragon fruit has few calories, is high in fiber, high water content (80%) and contains significant amounts of a number of vitamins and minerals. Several nutrients are present in trace amounts in dragon fruit. Additionally, it contains a lot of fiber, magnesium, and iron. Itcontains plenty of antioxidants like betalains, carotenoids, flavonoids, and hydroxycinnamates, which shield cells from damaging free radicals (Healthline, 2019). Omega-3 and 6 fatty acids are among the polyunsaturated fatty acids located in the seeds of dragon fruit (Table 2).

**Table 2 :** Nutritional facts for a serving of 100grams

| **Calories** | **60 Kcal** |
|---|---|
| Fat | 0 grams |
| Carbohydrates | 13 grams |
| Fibre | 3 grams |
| Protein | 1.2 grams |
| Vitamin C | 3% of the RDI |
| Iron | 4% of the RDI |
| Magnesium | 10% of the RDI |

*RDI (Recommended Dietary Intake)

### *Medicinal properties*

- Due to its high fiber content, dragon fruit helps with digestion.
- It is helpful for controlling type 2 diabetes, lowering the risk of colon cancer, and maintaining a healthy body weight.
- Since it contains vitamin C and carotenoids, it boosts the immune system response against diseases and infections.
- Prebiotic fiber found in dragon fruit helps the growth of good bacteria in your gut.
- Aids in lowering cholesterol level, preventing arthritis, fight against aging etc.

## KIWI

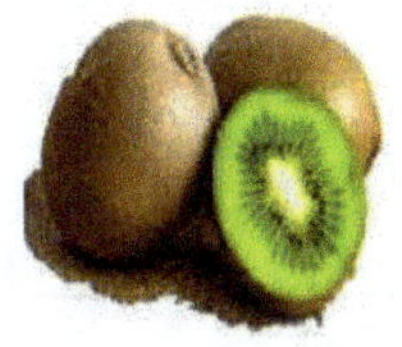

Kiwi (*Actinidiadeliciosa*), a woody vine with edible fruit from the family Actinidiaceae and genus Actinidia and is also referred to as kiwifruit or Chinese gooseberry.As a true berry, kiwi fruit is globular or elliptic in shape and has furry brownish green skin. There are innumerable eatable purple-black seeds are engrained throughout the firm, transparent green flesh, which also has a white center (Petruzzello, 2023). Kiwis come in two main varieties *Actinidia deliciosa* and *Actinidia arguta*, or hardy and fuzzy kiwis, respectively. One of the more recent vines created for growing in cooler climates is hardy kiwi. They lack hair, are green, and are small, but they are incredibly flavorful and can withstand conditions that the fuzzy kiwi cannot.

### *Origin and production*

The plant is native to Taiwan and mainland China, as well as being commercially produced in California and New Zealand. The fruit can be consumed raw or cooked and has a mildly acidic flavor. In India, mid hills of Himachal Pradesh, Uttar Pradesh, J&K, Sikkim, Meghalaya, Arunachal Pradesh, and Kerala are where kiwis are primarily grown. Kiwis grow best in sandy loam soils that are deep, rich, and well-drained. Around 16ºC to 19ºC is the ideal temperature for normal growth, flowering, and fruiting. High temperatures are unfavorable for the development and growth of kiwis (Lee, 1990). The majority of plant reproduction occurs vegetatively through cuttings and grafting. Typically, planting takes place in January. To promote brisk growth, the plants are severely pruned to a height of about 30 cm. In September and October, when the fruit is still in its early stages of development irrigation is provided. It has been noticed that irrigation at intervals of 10-15 days is beneficial. While commercial production of kiwi begins at the age of 7-8 years, the kiwi vine begins to bear fruit at the age of 4-5 years. After harvest, the fruits are rubbed with a rough cloth to get rid of any stiff hairs that might have grown on their surface. To get to the market, hard fruits are transported. Then, two weeks later, they become softer and edible (Portland nursery, 2023).

### *Nutritional benefits*

Kiwi fruit (Table 3) is rich in nutrients and have advantages for the digestive, immune, and metabolic systems in addition to bettering nutritional status (Patel hiral, 2022). Although kiwi fruit isn't frequently referred to as a "super food," it contains many essential vitamins and minerals and can improve your health. A wide variety of nutrients, including fiber, vitamin C, folate, copper, potassium, antioxidants, vitamin E, and vitamin K, are present in kiwis. Although the skin and seeds are edible, several people actually prefer to scrape the skin off because of its fuzzified texture (WebMD, 2022; Richardson *et al.,* 2018)

**Table 3 :** Nutritional facts for a serving of 100grams

| Calories | 61 Kcal |
|---|---|
| Fat | 0.5 grams |
| Carbohydrates | 15 grams |
| Fibre | 3 grams |
| Protein | 1.1 grams |
| Sugar | 9 grams |
| Sodium | 3mg |

*Medicinal properties*

- Kiwis have a lot of health benefits and are high in dietary fiber and vitamin C. This sour fruit can boost immunity, digestive and heart health.
- Vitamin C promotes the routine formation of collagen, which is necessary for the proper activity of blood vessels, bones, cartilage, as well as skin.
- When compared to other commonly consumed fruits, kiwifruit has relatively high levels of vitamin E. Vitamin E aids in the protection of cells against oxidative stress.
- Kiwifruit is frequently mentioned as a good source of dietary folate. During pregnancy, folate aids in the growth of maternal tissue (Crane, 2001).

## Star fruit

The woody plant species known as *Averrhoa carambola*, which bears the common name "star-fruit" is a member of the Oxalidaceae family.The showy fruits have an oblong shape, are longitudinally 5 to 6 angled, and have an orange-yellow-colored thin, waxy skin. The juicy fruits have a crisp texture, a yellow interior when ripe, and a star-shaped cross-section when cut.The smell of oxalic acid, which is present in the fruits, ranged between plants from strong to mild. The flavor varies as well, varying from immensely sour to lightly sweetish. Star fruit comes in two flavors: sweet and sour. Typically pale green in color, sweet star fruit trees produce relatively small-sized fruits. Darker leaves and a dark yellow color when ripe characterize sour star fruit.

*Origin and production*

The star fruit is thought to have originated in either Sri Lanka or the Indonesian islands of the Moluccas.It distributed across the whole of Asia and has been grown for centuries. Star fruit is widely cultivated in southern China, India, and the Philippines. Carambola trees grow well in a variety of well-drained soils. Trees thrive in soils that are moderately acidic to neutral in pH (Frey melia, 2021).

*Nutritional benefits*

Star fruits (Table 4) are fat free cholesterol free and rich in antioxidants, vitamin C and fibre content. Star fruit is high in polyphenolic flavonoids, an antioxidant phytonutrient. Quercetin, epicatechin, and gallic acid are some of the important flavonoids found.These compounds protect the body from the harmful effects of oxygen-derived free. It is high in B-complex vitamins like folates, riboflavin, and pyridoxine (vitamin B-6).These vitamins work together as cofactors for enzymatic reactions in metabolic activities and also in different synthetic functions within the body. Minerals and electrolytes like potassium, phosphorus, zinc, and iron are also found in trace quantities. As a crucial component of body and cell fluids, potassium helps to control blood pressure and heart rate, thereby offsetting the deleterious effects of sodium (Nutrition and you, 2023).

**Table 4 :** Nutritional facts for a serving of 132grams

| Calories | 41 Kcal |
|---|---|
| Fat | 0.4 grams |
| Carbohydrates | 8.9 grams |
| Fibre | 3.7 grams |
| Protein | 1.4 grams |
| Sugar | 5.3 grams |
| Sodium | 2.6 mg |

*Medicinal properties*

- Nutrient-rich starfruit is particularly high in fiber and vitamin C. To help with digestion, nutritionists advise consuming fiber-rich foods like star fruit.
- Additionally, it has a lot of beneficial nutrients and very few calories. As a result, starfruit is a great option for people trying to lose weight.
- This tropical fruit contains a lot of potassium, which is crucial for maintaining cardiovascular health and controlling the body's blood pressure. However, eating star fruit will supplement your body's intake of vitamin A and will support and improve your vision.

## Finger citron

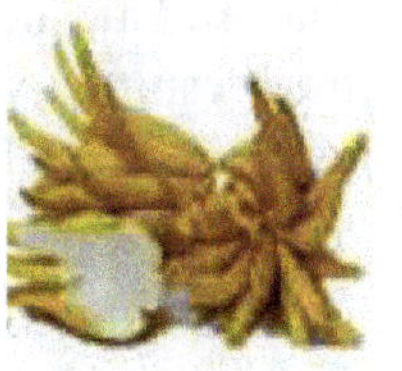

The finger citron (*Citrus medica*), also known as Buddha's hand and a member of the rutaceae family, is a small, shrubby tree that can reach a height of 2.4 meters. The golden fruit of the Fingered Citron, which is between 15 and 30 cm long, has projections that resemble fingers on a hand. Purplish to dark brown are the colors of immature fruits. It's interesting to note that the fruit has no pulp or seeds and is primarily composed of super thick and rough peels (rind). Rather, it is packed with albedo, a white, spongy tissue that bears a sweet taste (National parks, 2021). The bitter-sweet, bright, and floral flavor of Buddha's Hand citron is mainly utilized as a zest for flavouring savory and sweet applications (Specialty produce, 2023).

### *Origin and production*

This particular variety of citron is believed to have come from northeastern India and was brought to China by Buddhist monks sometime just after fourth century A.D.In China, the "Fo-shou" or Buddha's hand citron is used as an offering at Buddhist temple altars and is regarded as an icon of pleasure and long life (Michele Warmund, 2013). Most citrus and citron trees grow well in well-drained, well-tilled soil. Sandy soils are preferred over loams or rocky soils, and the soil pH should be 5.5-7.The optimum temperature for growing Buddha's Hand Citron is around 65 degrees Fahrenheit (18 °C).They thrive in temperatures ranging from 50 to 100 degrees Fahrenheit (10-38 °C) (Michele Warmund, 2013). Seed, stem cuttings, and leaf cuttings can all be used to propagate this species. It should be grown in full sun in moist, well-draining soil. When grown in a large container, it can reach a height of 0.3 to 0.9 m.Fruits can be picked while still green to make succade for confectionery and baking, or while still yellow to make essential oils used to flavouring candy and specialty alcoholic drinks (Klein, 2014).

## Nutritional benefits

The Buddha's hand may not contain many nutrients, but it is rich in calcium, dietary fiber, and vitamin C. It contains no sugars, proteins, carbohydrates, or fats. Buddha's hand is loaded with aromatic organic substances like coumarin, limonin, and diosmin as well as volatile oils. The Buddha's hand's chemical makeup is crucial in the treatment of numerous illnesses.

### *Medicinal properties*

- Aromatic organic molecules identified in the Buddha's hand, such as coumarin, limonin, diosmin, and bergapten, are painkillers. They are also anti-inflammatory, which aids in the reduction of swelling and pain.
- The mild alcoholic compound in Buddha's hand acts as a cough suppressant to treat respiratory diseases. It aids in the removal of phlegm and cough from the pharynx, as well as the relief of pain and the facilitation of breathing.
- This boosts the body's immunity and protects against common infections such as the common cold and flu. Vitamin C defends the body from pathogen attack and fights infections.

- This fruit's anti-inflammatory properties aid in the reduction of inflammation in the gastrointestinal system and intestine. It treats diarrhea and reduces pain and cramps.
- Buddha's hand is an old remedy for menstrual cramps, mood swings, and bleeding. Its antioxidant and anti-inflammatory properties aid in the relaxation of lower abdominal muscles and the reduction of pain (Kriti Jain, 2018).

## Jackfruit

*Artocarpus heterophyllus*, also known as jackfruit, is a tropical climacteric fruit in the mulberry family Moraceae. It is referred to as "the rice tree" in Sri Lanka. The jackfruit, which can grow up to 60 cm (about 2 feet) long and weigh up to 18 kg, is the biggest tree-borne fruit in the world (about 40 pounds). It is ellipsoidal and aggregate, made up of numerous "bulbs" of flesh that contains seeds encircling a stringy core, all of which are covered by a bumpy rind.

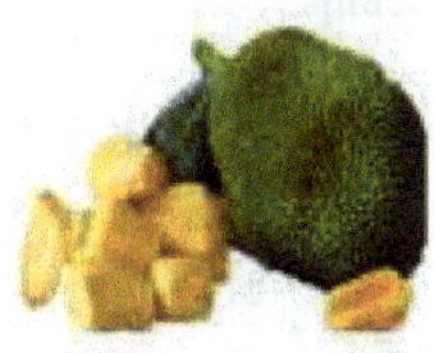

### *Origin and production*

In countries like India, Malaysia, Central and Eastern Africa, the Caribbean, Florida, Brazil, Australia, Puerto Rico, and many Pacific Islands, jackfruit grows in tropical and subtropical climates. India is the biggest jackfruit producer. These trees are frequently grown outside of orchards, in contrast to other fruit-bearing trees. They are roadside vegetation in their home countries, meant to block the sun or the wind. They can also be planted in woodlots and grow in forests (Madhura, 2020). Jackfruit tolerates a wide range of soil types, including shal-low limestone, sand, and rocky substrates, but does best in deep, well-drained soils of moderate fertility. The tree can survive in soils with a pH range of 5.0 to 7.5 and the optimum temperature is between 32 and 35 °C (90 and 95 °F) (Elevitch and Manner, 2006).

### *Nutritional benefits*

The seeds of the jackfruit (Table 5) are a good source of protein, potassium, calcium, and iron, while the flesh is a good source of vitamin C. In addition, jackfruit contains B vitamins, such as vitamin B6, niacin, riboflavin, and folic acid, which are particularly crucial for a healthy nervous system. This makes it different from other fruits (Ranasinghe *et al.,* 2019).

**Table 5 :** Nutritional facts for a serving of 100grams

| Calories | 95 Kcal |
|---|---|
| Fat | 0.64 grams |
| Carbohydrates | 23.2 grams |
| Fibre | 1.5 grams |
| Protein | 1.72 grams |
| Sugar | 19.1 grams |
| Vitamin C | 13.7 mg |
| Calcium | 24 mg |

### *Medicinal properties*

- Jackfruit is high in potassium, and foods that are high in potassium can help lower blood pressure.
- The seeds of the jackfruit, in particular, are a reliable source of both soluble and insoluble fiber .
- Jackfruit contains nutrients that could aid in preventing the development of stomach ulcers or sores.
- With intermediate level of Glycemic Index, jackfruit may aid in the treatment of type 2 diabetes.

## Mangosteen

Mangosteen (*Garcinia mangostana*), also known as purple mangosteen, is a beautiful tropical tree belongs to family Clusiaceae. Mangosteen is also known as Kaattampi, Kokam, Hannu, and Kao in India. Mangusta is the name for mangosteen in Hindi. It is an evergreen tree that reaches almost 20 meters in height. The primary region of production is Southeast Asia. Due to its flavor and the advantages of mangosteen fruit, mangosteen trees are also referred to as the "Queen of Fruit." Its fruit is roughly the size of a golf ball and is spherical in shape. Its pericarp is thick and woody, but not particularly hard. You are easily peelable off by hand. The interior flesh is tender like lychee. The four sections that make up the flesh are both sweet and acidic (Kaur *et al.*, 2020).

### *Origin and production*

Most botanists believe that the mangosteen (*Garcinia mangostana*) originated in Malaysia or the Indonesian SundaIslands.The fruits are cultivated in India's southwest region. Kerala and Tamil Nadu typically experience tropical weather with high humidity and consistent rainfall. These regions have extensive cultivation of this rare fruit because the environmental conditions are favorable for its growth. Mangosteens thrive in sandy loam soil that seems to be high in organic matter. A pH of slightly acidic, well-draining soil will benefit the plants even more. The fruit is tropical and necessitates a temperate climate. It requires high humidity and an average annual temperature of 5-35 °C (Patil and Appaiah, 2015).Themangosteen season lasts from April to June and again from July to October during the monsoon season.

## Nutritional benefits

Vitamins B1, B2, C, E, folic acid, copper, manganese, carbohydrates, and fiber are all abundant in mangosteen. Mangosteen is primarily composed of vitamin B1, manganese, and vitamin E.It has numerous antioxidants in addition to an abundance of minerals. Mangosteen contains a substance known as Xanthones, one of the best and most potent antioxidants.

**Table 6 :** Nutritional facts for a serving of 100grams

| Calories | 73 Kcal |
|---|---|
| Fat | 0.58 grams |
| Carbohydrates | 17.91 grams |
| Fibre | 1.8 grams |
| Protein | 0.41 grams |
| Magnesium | 13 mg |
| Vitamin C | 2.9 mg |
| Calcium | 12 mg |

### *Medicinal properties*

- The fruit has anti-inflammatory, anti-aging, and anti-diabetic properties that are also attributed to the presence of Xanthones, Folate, and Vitamin C.
- Mangosteen fruit and roots have been used for women's menstrual problems since ancient times. Mangosteen or its extract can treat symptoms like pre/post menstrual cramps and pain, mood swings, etc.
- The high potassium, copper, magnesium, and manganese content of mangosteens contribute to the body's ability to keep its blood pressure at a healthy level.
- Mangosteen is beneficial for skin care because it has anti-inflammatory, antibacterial, antifungal, anti-allergic, and antioxidant properties. It restores damaged cells, guards against UV rays and many skin issues like eczema, allergies, skin aging, and bacterial infections.
- Mangosteen has no saturated fat, no cholesterol, and few calories. So, it has a good reputation for weight management (Yaacob and Tindall, 1995).

## Avocado

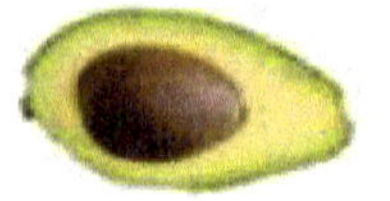

The edible fruit of the avocado tree, *Persea americana,* also known as the alligator pear, belongs to the Lauraceaefamily. Fruits from avocado trees have bumpy skin and green or yellowish creamy smooth flesh that is buttery in texture and flavor.The fruit can range in size from being no bigger than an egg in some Mexican races to occasionally weighing 1-2 kg in others. Green to dark purple is the color range, and the shape can be either circular pear-shaped with such a long, slender neck. The fruit's outer skin can vary in texture from being rough and woody to being no thicker than an apple's.

### *Origin and production*

Avocados are widely grown in warm climates and are indigenous to the Western Hemisphere from Mexico south to the Andean regions. Tamil Nadu, Skking Karnataka, and Maharashtra produce the majority of the avocados consumed in India. Although they can be cultivated in a variety of soil types, avocados are delicate to inadequate drainage. They thrives in humid, warm weather that is typical of tropical and semitropical regions and require a PH of 5-7. Avocados cannot grow in salty environments. They cannot withstand flooding. It is intolerant of frost, dry cold wind, and both. Thus, the climate of North India is not suitable (Tripathi *et al.,* 2014). Avocado plants grown from seeds start producing fruit after five to six years of plantation, fruits mature and become greenish-yellow. The fruit is ready to be picked when the color of the seed coat inside the fruit changes from yellowish-white to dark brown. Six to ten days after harvesting, mature fruits ripen. The fruits remain hard for the duration of their life on the tree, only softening after harvest (Binitakumari, 2022).

## Nutritional benefits

Avocados (Table 7) are high in fiber and possess more good fat than carbohydrate, making them popular on low-carbohydrate diets, such as those used to treat diabetes. Because it is one of the highest-fat plant foods, it is popular in both vegetarian and vegan diets. Avocado is one of the best fruits in terms of antioxidant content. They are high in vitamin B, C, E and K. (Hurtado-Fernández *et al.,* 2018).

**Table 7 :** Nutritional facts for a serving of 100grams

| Calories | 160 Kcal |
|---|---|
| Fat | 14.66 grams |
| Carbohydrates | 8.53 grams |
| Fibre | 6.70 grams |
| Protein | 2 grams |
| Magnesium | 29 grams |
| Vitamin C | 10 mg |
| Calcium | 12 mg |

### *Medicinal properties*

- Eating an avocado-rich diet appears to reduce low-density lipoprotein (LDL) "bad" cholesterol while increasing high-density lipoprotein (HDL) "good" cholesterol.
- It contains the highest concentration of omega-3 fatty acids, plant hormones such as beta-sitosterol and stigmasterol, and phytosterols.Avocados are high in anti-inflammatory compounds, which help to reduce internal inflammation in the body.
- High in fiber content and low in carbs, avocado serves as weightloss diet.
- Avocado contains beta-sitosterol, a natural plant sterol.Regular intake of beta-sitosterol and other plant sterols aids in the maintenance of healthy cholesterol levels. They also keep your heart arteries and veins in good condition.
- Avocado is an excellent source of minerals, vitamins, antioxidants, and fatty acids. As a result, it is necessary for healthy skin. They are high in vitamin C and E, which give your skin a natural glow (Duarte *et al.,* 2016).

## Indian hog plum

Indian Hog plum (Spondia spinnata) commonly known as 'Ambate' or 'Ambadekaai' belongs to Anacardiaceae family. It is an ovoid, 4–5 cm long, yellow, fleshy drupe with a finely textured edible pulp. Unripe fruits are very sour, while ripe fruits have a hard stone and are sweet-sour (Cherdthong *et al.,* 2019).

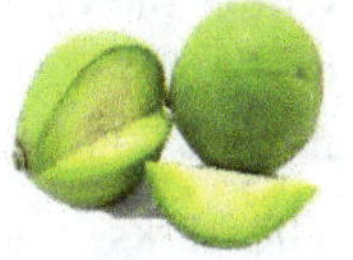

### *Origin and production*

Indian Hog Plum (Table 8) can be found growing wild or cultivated all across the tropical Indian subcontinent, Andaman Islands, Sri Lanka, Myanmar, Thailand, Malaysia, China, and the Philippines.This plant can be found growing very well in India's tropical and Himalayan regions, but it is rarely seen in the country's western regions. It can survive in a variety of climates, including dry, tropical, and subtropical ones. It prefers soils with good drainage and can withstand drought, but it cannot withstand frost. It frequently grows in open woodlands, scrublands, along rivers and streams, and it can grow in either full sun or full shade.

### *Nutritional benefits*

The nutrient-rich Indian hog plum is a small, round fruit. In addition to other antioxidants, it is a source of vitamins C and A. It also has trace amounts of calcium, iron, and vitamin B. Moreover to its nutritional value, Indian hog plum is known for its distinct flavor and is frequently used in traditional recipes.

**Table 8 :** Nutritional facts for a serving of 100grams

| | |
|---|---|
| Calories | 48 Kcal |
| Fat | 3 grams |
| Carbohydrates | 4.6 grams |
| Fibre | 1 grams |
| Protein | 0.7 grams |
| Phosphorous | 11 mg |
| Vitamin C | 21 mg |
| Calcium | 36 mg |

### *Medicinal properties*

- It is an excellent source of minerals like iron, which aids in the synthesis of hemoglobin and myoglobin, two proteins that transport oxygen throughout the body's systems.
- Hog plums are high in dietary fiber and thus beneficial to digestive health (Rymbai *et al.,* 2016).
- It is a fruit free of fat, sodium, cholesterol, and other unhealthy fats, as well as a good source of vitamin K, which supports healthy bones.
- One of the vitamins that can be found in hog plums is thiamine, which has many different jobs to do in the body, including assisting with nerve conduction and muscle contraction.
- The barks, juice, and fruit in general have medicinal properties that render them beneficial to traditional herbalists for natural remedies. The leaves serve as antiseptics and are used to make antiseptic soaps, treat sore throats, coughs, malaria, and other related illnesses.

## Langsat

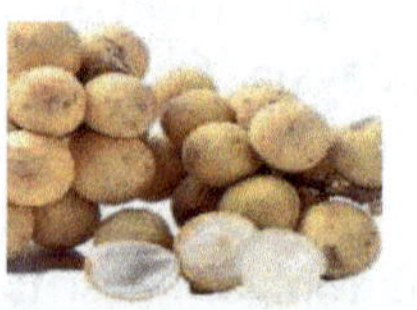

The evergreen *Lansium domesticum*, also known as langsat or lanzones, is a member of the Meliaceae family and typically reaches heights of 5 to 10 meters in cultivation but 10 to 30 meters in the wild.The fruits have a diameter of about 37mm and are produced in clusters of 2 to 30. Each fruit has 5 or 6 segments of fragrant, white, opalescent, juicy flesh as well as 1 to 3 fairly substantial and bitter seeds. These seeds occasionally have a tendency to stick to the flesh very firmly, which can cause the fruit to become bitter.

### *Origin and production*

The edible fruit of the langsat (*Lansium domesticum*), which is native to western Southeast Asia, is grown there. It also grows well in the Nilgiris and other humid regions of South India, as well as in southern Thailand and Vietnam.langsat plants grows best in fertile, well-drained, slightly acidic, humus-rich soil and prefers a pH between 6 and 6.5, tolerating between 5.5 and 7.5 The recommended temperature range for growth is 12 to 40 °C, with the ideal temperature falling between 20 and 35 °C. It cannot withstand prolonged dry seasons and requires a humid environment with plenty of moisture.

According to reports, the ideal annual rainfall range for growth is between 1,400 and 2,200 mm, with the range being 1,000 to 3,000 mm. The seeds used to grow langsats typically have a limited viability and must be planted within 1-2 days of being removed from the fruit. In a nursery seedbed, sow in a shaded area. After 10 days, germination can begin, and 90% of seeds will germinate within a month. Multiple seedlings from polyembryony are quite typical.

*Nutritional benefits*

Langsat (Table 9) fruit is high in vitamins C, A, and B, and also contains minerals like calcium, potassium, and iron. It is also high in carbohydrates and dietary fiber. The fruit is commonly consumed raw, but it also has the potential to make jams, jellies, and other preserves.

**Table 9 :** Nutritional facts for a serving of 100grams

| Calories | 41 Kcal |
|---|---|
| Protein | 0.8 grams |
| Carbohydrates | 9.5 grams |
| Fibre | 2.3 grams |
| Potassium | 275 mg |
| Phosphorous | 30 mg |
| Vitamin C | 2 mg |
| Thiamine | 89 mcg |

*Medicinal properties*

- The leaf extract is utilized to treat inflammation in the eyes as eyedrops.
- The resin is administered to stop diarrhea and intestinal spasms and is non-toxic.
- Fever, intestinal spasms, diarrhea, and malaria are all treated with dried pericarp. The active ingredient of the pericarp seems to be a resin.
- The ground-up seed is used as a vermifuge and febrifuge.

## Conclusion

Exotic fruits have several health advantages because they are organic and natural. Including these fruits into your daily diet, will help in improving your health.

Exotic fruits are packed with the vitamins, minerals, and antioxidants that we need on a daily basis, just like other seasonal fruits. Exotic whole fruits, peels, leaves, and waste materials do have natural ability to be the effective antioxidant properties sources for food or pharmaceutical products. Because exotic fruits and vegetables require less technology to develop, developing countries are capable of handling them. Primary and secondary industries are typically important in developing countries. Exotic fruit farming in Indian agriculture will result in new production methods and be able to satisfy consumer demand.

## References

Agrifarming (2022). How to start exotic fruit farming in India: A production and growing guide for beginners. Retrieved September 20, 2022. https://www.agrifarming.in/how-to-start-exotic-fruit-farming-in-india-a-production-and-growing-guide-for-beginners

Ariharan, V. N., Kalirajan, K., Devi, V. N., & Prasad, P. (2012). An exotic fruit which forms the new natural source for vitamin-C. *Rasayan J Chem*, *5*(3), 356-359.Dragon fruit: An exotic super future fruit of India

Binitakumari (2022). Avocado Farming in India: Cultivation Practices, Varieties, Yield, Profitability and much more. In: Krishijagran

Cherdthong, A., Unnawong, N., Khonkhaeng, B., &Prachumchai, R. (2019). Dietary Hog Plum (*Spondiaspinnata* (Lf) Kurz) Could Modulate Fermentation Process, and Feed Digestibility, As Well As and Reduce Protozoal Population. *Adv. Anim. Vet. Sci*, *7*(12), 1054-1059.

Crane, J. H. (2001). The carambola (star fruit). University of Florida Cooperative Extension Service, Institute of Food and Agriculture Sciences, EDIS.

Devalaraja, S., Jain, S., & Yadav, H. (2011). Exotic fruits as therapeutic complements for diabetes, obesity and metabolic syndrome. *Food research international*, *44*(7), 1856-1865.

Duarte, P. F., Chaves, M. A., Borges, C. D., & Mendonça, C. R. B. (2016). Avocado: characteristics, health benefits and uses. *Ciência rural*, *46*, 747-754.

Elevitch, C. R., & Manner, H. I. (2006). *Artocarpus Heterophyllus* (jackfruit), Moaceae *(mulberry Family)*. Permanent Agricultural Resources Publishers.

Frey melia., (2021). Retrieved December 23, 2021 Star Fruit Nutrition Facts and Health Benefits. https://www.verywellfit.com/star-fruit-calories-carbs-nutrition-facts- 417-4575

Healthline. What Is Dragon Fruit and Does It Have Health Benefits? Retrieved January 25, 2019. https://www.healthline.com/nutrition/dragon-fruit#nutrition

Hossain, F. M., Numan, S. M., & Akhtar, S. (2021). Cultivation, nutritional value, and health benefits of Dragon Fruit (*Hylocereus* spp.): A Review. *International Journal of Horticultural Science and Technology*, *8*(3), 259-269.

Hurtado-Fernández, E., Fernández-Gutiérrez, A., & Carrasco-Pancorbo, A. (2018). Avocado fruit—*Perseaamericana*. In *Exotic fruits* (pp. 37-48). Academic Press.

Kaur, G., Singh, A., & Dar, B. N. (2020). Mangosteen (*Garcinia mangostana* L.). *Anti-oxidants in Fruits: Properties and Health Benefits*, 83-101.

Klein, J. D. (2014). Citron cultivation, production and uses in the Mediterranean region. *Medicinal and Aromatic Plants of the Middle-East*, 199-214.

Kriti Jain. (2018, July 19). *Health Benefits of Buddha's Hand / Fingered Citron*. Medindia. Retrieved on Feb 09, 2023 from https://www.medindia.net/patients/lifestyleandwellness/health-benefits-of-buddhas-hand.htm.

Lee, S. H. (1990). Kiwifruit resources and production in China. *Acta Horticulturae*, (282), 57-63.

Madhura, (2020): Where Does Jackfruit Come From and How Is It Grown?. In: The Food Unfolded Magazine

Michele Warmund (2013). Buddhas hand citron- A truly extraordinary fruit. In: University of Missouri Plant Science & Technology.

National parks. (2021). Fingered Citron. https://www.nparks.gov.sg/nparksbuzz/oct-issue-2021/facts/fingered-citron

Nutrition and you, 2023. Star fruit (Carambola) Nutrition facts. https://www.nutrition-and-you.com/star-fruit.html

Patel hiral., (2022). Kiwi Fruit – Benefits, Nutrition & Kiwi for Weight Loss. Retrieved September 19, 2022.https://www.healthifyme.com/blog/kiwi-fruit-benefits/

Patil, M. M., &Appaiah, K. A. (2015). Garcinia: Bioactive compounds and health benefits. *Introduction to Functional Food Science*, *1*, 110-125.

Petruzzello, M. (2023). Kiwi. *Encyclopedia Britannica*. Retrieved January 13, 2023. https://www.britannica.com/plant/kiwi-fruit

Portland nursery, 2023. Kiwi vines. https://www.portlandnursery.com/fruits/kiwi

Ranasinghe, R. A. S. N., Maduwanthi, S. D. T., & Marapana, R. A. U. J. (2019). Nutritional and health benefits of jackfruit (*Artocarpusheterophyllus* Lam.): a review. *International journal of food science, 2019*.

Richardson, D. P., Ansell, J., & Drummond, L. N. (2018). The nutritional and health attributes of kiwifruit: a review. *European journal of nutrition*, *57*, 2659-2676.

Rymbai, H., Deshmukh, N. A., Jha, V. A., Verma, V. K., War, F. G., Paul, D., ... & Roy, A. R. (2016). Indian Hog Plum. *Breed. Underutilized Fruit Crop*, *13*, 183-190.

Specialty produce, 2023. Buddhas Hand Citron. https://specialtyproduce.com/produce/Buddhas_Hand_Citron_2036.php

Tractor junction (2021). Dragon Fruit Cultivation: Complete Information About Dragon Fruit. Retrieved December 16, 2021. https://www.tractorjunction.com/blog/dragon-fruit-cultivation-complete-information/

Tripathi, P. C., Karunakaran, G., Sakthivel, T., Sankar, V., Senthilkumar, R., Muralidhara, S. R., ... &Begane, N. (2014). Avocado cultivation in India. *Bulletin, Central Horticultural Experiment Station Indian Institute of Horticultural Research Chettalli, Kodagu, Karnataka, 14.*

Wakchaure, G. C., Kumar, S., Meena, K. K., Rane, J., & Pathak, H. (2021). Dragon Fruit Cultivation in India: Scope, Constraints and Policy Issues. *Technical Bulletin*, (27), 47.

WebMD (2022).Health Benefits of Kiwi. RetrievedSeptember 09, 2022 https://www.webmd.com/diet/health-benefits-kiwi

Wild 'n' free(2019). Lanzones Fruit – Health Benefits and Nutrition Facts. https://wnfdiary.com/lanzones-fruit-health-benefits/

Yaacob, O., & Tindall, H. D. (1995). *Mangosteen cultivation* (No. 129). Food & Agriculture Org..

# 17

# Flourishing the Climate Resilient Fruit Crops to Ensure Global Food and Nutritional Security

Amit Layek[1*], Kaushik Pramanik[1] and Debarati Seal[2]

[1] Department of Agricultural Entomology, Bidhan Chandra Krishi Vishwavidayalaya, Mohanpur, Nadia, West Bengal, India. Pin-741252.

[2] Department of Agronomy, Bidhan Chandra Krishi Vishwavidayalaya, Mohanpur, Nadia, West Bengal, India. Pin-741252.

**ABSTRACT**

We are in a grave danger as a result of numerous disruptive anthropogenic activities and the abasement of nature. Nowadays unpredictable climatic change is occurring across the entire planet. Due to this dramatic climate change, fruit crops were mostly impacted. Humans depend on plants for food and nutritional security, both of which are necessary for maintaining a healthier livelihood. We need to concentrate on sustainable production of fruit crops as a potential solution to guarantee that nutritional security and their availability even under changeable climate circumstances. Despite changing climatic conditions, it is possible to grow fruit crops such as fig, phalsa, wood apple, aonla, karonda, barbados cherry, and dragon fruit. In addition to being nutrient-dense in the changing climate, these fruit crops are also likely a substitute for reducing the damage. In this chapter we discussed the production strategy of these fruits and highlighting their role in the betterment of humanity.

*Keywords*: Production; Ecology; Climate change; Nutritional security; Fruit crops.

## Introduction

A major global threat to food security, agriculture, and public health is climate change (Schnitter and Berry 2019; Gregory *et al.*, 2005). India is extremely concerned about climate change. The prospect of climate change is concerning because of the country's varied topography, natural resource-based livelihoods, related climatic changes, and resource limitations to adapt to the rising frequency of extreme climatic events, catastrophes, and disasters (Rasul *et al.*, 2020). Changes in climate has a direct and indirect impact on many areas of food security, particularly in the agricultural and animal sectors. The major source ofemployment

* Corresponding author.

and income for more than 70% of the world's poor people is agriculture, which they practise on a daily basis. The majority of cereal and pulse crops that we consume for food are annual crops that aren't as affected as fruit crops, which are generally perennial. Climate change has considered to be most impacted by fruit crops. This is due to the fact that fruit crops have distinct and intricate flowering and fruit set patterns. Climate is a crucial environmental component that has an impact on the production of fruit crops.Changes in plant physical traits like canopy improvement, vitality, biological traits such as fruit set ability and reduced fruit weight, in addition to quality parameters such as less colour development, reduction shelf-life, poor juice material, and increased pest attack, were the major contributors to poor fruit quality as well as decreased fruit production (Jangra *et al.*, 2013). The effects of changes the climate must be handled as soon as possible because they are mostly caused by manmade activities that are not sustainable.

The most likely solution is to choose fruit cultivars that are climate sensitive in order to maintain nutritional security through the availability of fruits. It is thought that these fruit crops are substantially more resistant to moisture stress and heat stress. They are the fruit crop of the future that is climate-smart. Fruit crops like wood apples, figs, Barbados cherries, phalsa, pumello, dragon fruit, bael, pumello and aonla, are said to require less moisture and transpire at a slower pace.These fruit crops may also be able to withstand severe drought and moisture stress.In the climate change context and rising demand for fruits, there are possibilities to pursue as well as obstacles to face. Existing fruit producers want to know how they may change to impending changes and keep producing. New business owners want to discover which fruits are currently suitable for production in their nations. Not all fruit crops can be cultivated in every region of the world. The consequences of climate change on fruits, including dangers, potential adaptations, and opportunities in new locales, have only received a very scant amount of study until date. This chapter seeks to summarise the present state of information on these topics, focusing on tropical and subtropical fruit trees. Additionally, climate change is altering the habitat ranges of both plants and animals (Pereira *et. al.,* 2010). For instance, if average global temperatures rise, plant and animal populations may migrate to other latitudes with more hospitable climates. So, it is possible that crops that were formerly fruitful in one location are no longer so, or vice versa. Climate change has always been a dynamic factor, influencing everything from the origin of life on Earth through ongoing evolutionary processes.

Although change is a part of nature, the rate of climate change has considerablyrisen over the past 10 years as a result of the abusive exploitation of the environment and natural resources. Because of how quickly the climate is changing and how much human interference is causing it, we have reason to be concerned about it.The changing climatic pattern has caused a shift in the growing season in many regions of the world, transforming the lifecycles of pollinators such as bees. This causes the bees to be out of rhythm with the blossoming times of plants and trees. This inconsistency can impair both pollinators and plants' ability to live and reproduce, reducing availability of food throughout the food chain. Not just is the food chain impacted, but so is nutritional security. Pollinators are necessary for the growth of fruit production in all climates, tropical to temperate regions. Most temperate crop pollinators are introduced into orchards from outside to ensure proper pollination and, as a result, crop productivity. Pollinator populations are also impacted by fluctuating climatic conditions. Another factor that affects dramatically with climate change is the rainfall pattern, which leads to a lack of soil water required for crop life. Bore well clogging is a common occurrence connected with regular drought caused by climate change.

Temperatures are also rising noticeably, and uncertainty in climatic forecasting has a significant impact on vegetation (Olesen and Bindi, 2002). The majority of fruit crops, including guava, papaya, mango and others, typically experience flower drop when extremely low temperatures predominate during flowering, which reduces fruit yield (Dinesh and Reddy, 2012). Mango flowers in the present season have a poor sex ratio as a result of high temperatures during floral bud differentiation. Increasing temperatures prohibit coloured guavas from developing their desired fruit colours and limit quality grape production, which ultimately reduces the area available for cultivation and market demand (Zemni *et. al.*, 2005; Rajan, 2008). The abundance and sex ratio of flowers are similarly influenced by temperature. The crop's season-long fruiting potential is directly impacted by this. Low nighttime temperatures are necessary for the development of attractive fruit peel colour in fruit crops including grapes, colored guava, and mandarins. Fruits from warm climates are sweeter as the difference in day and night temperatures rises, which is undoubtedly impacted by bad weather. These are just a few examples; the true scenario is considerably larger, and if necessary, precautions are not followed, the problem may escalate. Another terrible effect that changes of climate is pest and disease transit, which can become severe under hot and humid circumstances that favour pathogenesis and epidemiology of both major and minor pests such as fruit fly, which is gradually becoming a severity of the risk to guava. Another banana disease, black leaf streak, may become more damaging as global temperatures rise.

Given the shifting climate scenario, previously inert diseases or pests may become a big danger. In adverse conditions, crop planting dates may be shifted or varieties with short life cycles introduced to rescue the farmer from severe crop failure, which isn't possible in fruit production. Breeding of fruit trees to create varieties with abiotic tolerance is a complicated and time-consuming process. Fruit crops, despite being resistant in nature, particularly tropical and subtropical fruits, can migrate to higher elevations when temperatures rise. The sluggish way makes it difficult for crops to modify at the same rate as weather changes, their biological cycle as well as ecological niche. By doing this, several important species could go extinct. As a result, we need to start a trend of growing climate-hardy fruitcultivars that can endure physiologically and delivera sufficient quantity of fruit under a scenario with climate change.

## Climate Change Impact on Horticultural Fruit Crops

The replacement of high-cooling required apple producers like Royal Delicious with less cooling required producers as well as other fruit crops including plum, peach, kiwi, pear, and vegetables has been demonstrated. In the middle hills of the Shimla district, there is a movement away from full-scale potato and apple production. This has been confirmed by the Himachal Pradesh apple production and snowfall patterns. Apple production per acre decreased from 10.8 to 5.8 tonnes. A simple illustration of climate change is this (Awasthi *et al.*, 2001). Many abiotic components that have emerged as a result of climate change have an impact on the metabolic, anatomic, morphological, and biochemical properties of the different horticulture fruit crops. One of most important environmental variables that impact the yield of fruit are temperature, droughts, acidity, precipitation, changes in concentration of CO2, and insect-pest outbreaks (Gora *et al.,* 2019).

## Impact on temperature

Extreme temperature changes the plant's structure, anatomy, and physiology, which impacts fruit set, fruit quality, weight and size of fruit, as well as germination of seeds, flower shedding, gametophyte fertilisation, enhanced plant, and pollen viability. (Gora *et al.,* 2019). Cold and hot waves have badly harmed several fruit orchards (Malhotra, 2017). Temperature influences flowering in annual fruit crops such as mango. It has a tendency towards plant development, and when the temperature goes up, it produces more leaves, which influences the phenology of flowersIt must be noted that late developing inflorescences had higher percentages of hermaphrodite flowers, which was associated with high temperature changes (Singh *et al.,* 1966; Balogoun *et al.,* 2016). The principal indications of heat stroke in mango trees, whether bearing or not, are burned leaves and dead twigs. The main effects of climate change on mango were increased reproductive flushes, early or delayed flowering, reduce fruit development, reproductive buds transforming into vegetative ones, changes in fruit maturity, and so on (Rajan *et al.*, 2011). Higher temperatures of 31$^{o}$C to 32$^{o}$C usually accelerate the maturity rate of banana plants, which reduces the time needed for formation of bunch (Turner *et al.*, 2007). Banana bunches become choked when temperatures exceed 38$^{o}$C.

In contrast, in case of low temperatures for cross-pollinated crops like pistachios and walnuts, where inadequate cold can reduce pollination, which have lowers crop yields. The ideal temperature for fruit development of temperate fruits like plum, apple, cherry, pears, etc. is between 20ºC and 25 °C. Conditions like fog, rain, or cold temperatures were discovered to have a detrimental effect on sour cherry pollination in the USA (Haokip *et al.,* 2020). Horticultural crops suffer losses from the unusually cold waves that range from 10% to 100% of their return, depending on the crops and varieties (Hazarika, 2013). Cold or dry circumstances during the immature fruit stage have been associated to extreme fruit breaking (Yang *et al.,* 2010).

The low temperature has two impacts on mandarins: it initiates blossoming and ends bud dormancy. Developing inflorescences are in a greater sensitivity of dormancy than vegetative buds, and the early stages of bloom initiation seem to occur even before winter rest period (Reddy *et al.,* 2017). Low temperatures had an impact on the acidity level in core oranges, which led to low TSS (Peng *et al.,* 2000). Hence, only crops that are climate-appropriate should be planted. Since papaya is extremely susceptible to frost, it is not ideal for the climate in Punjab. Physiological issues and their accompanying issues are caused by horticultural crops being exposed to more heat stress (Gora *et al.,* 2019). The following are a list of key physiological problems and their related causes in fruit crops (Table 1).

**Table 1:** Table of crucial physiological dysfunction and their relative effect in fruit crops are as follows:

| Fruit crop | Disorders | Caused due to |
|---|---|---|
| *Emblica officinalis* | Unfruitfulness | Temperature |
| *Mangifera indica* | Spongy tissue | High Temperature |
| *Aegle marmelos* | Fruit cracking | Deficiency of nutrients |
| *Eriobotrya japonica* | Purple spot | Temperature |
| *Mangifera indica* | Black tip | Harmful Gases like CO and SO2 |
| *Citrus* sp. | Granulation | Water moisture |
| *Mangifera indica* | Jhumka | Lack of pollination |
| *Mangifera indica* | Fruit drop | Lack of pollination |
| *Vitis vinifera* | Flower and berry drop | High temp, Lack of pollination |
| *Punica granatum* | Fruit cracking | Variation in day & night temperature |

*Source*: (Mishra *et al*., 2016)

## The risks of CO2 consumption

The atmosphere of the Earth is mostly composed of N (78.1%), $O_2$ (20.9%), Ar (0.93%), and $CO_2$ (0.031%) (Lide, 2009). Because nitrogen and oxygen are practically transparent to ground radiation, they play no significant influence in global warming. The greenhouse gas effect is principally caused by water vapour,

$CO_2$, and trace amounts of other gases such as methane, nitrous oxide, and ozone, which absorb radiation leaving the Earth's surface (IPCC, 2001). Photosynthesis and Growth rise as a consequence of high-water usage efficiency because of the decreased stomatal conductance, stomatal aperture, and transpiration caused by the air around the leaf blade had more carbon dioxide than usual (Stöckle *et al.*, 2009). As shown in Table 2**.** The substantial use of fuel for soil treatment results in very large emissions of $CH_4$, $CO_2$, and $N_2O$.

**Table 2 :** Emissions of $CO_2$, $CH_4$, and $N_2O$ from Fruit Production to Consumption

| Fruits | Emissions | | | |
|---|---|---|---|---|
| | $CO_2$ | $N_2O$ | $CH_4$ | Total |
| | $CO_2$ Equivalents/kg Product over a 100-years of Time Period | | | |
| *Malus domestica* | 0.80 | 0.02 | 0 | 0.82 |
| *Citrus* sp. | 1.1 | 0.10 | 0 | 1.2 |
| Tropical fruit | 11 | 0.23 | 0 | 11 |

Adapted from Carlsson-Kanyama and Gonza´ lez, 2009.

## Drought

Drought is a territorial phenomenon and its features depend on its frequency, duration, and climatic location. Although there is no single definition of what constitutes a drought, it is a natural disaster that has significant economic, social, and environmental effects on a large section of the population (WMO, 2006). Plants that are currently suffering severe water shortages are more vulnerable to water stress caused by a lack of rainfall, just like during heat waves. Dry soil prevents the decomposition of organic matter and root growth, further reducing soil fertility. Droughts do, however, have additional effects since they enhance soil erosion because plant cover is diminished; this is especially problematic on steep slopes. A consequence of changes of climate will be an increase in the frequency and length of droughts that are more severe, as was the case in late 2011 in the Horn of Africa, where 13 million people experienced starvationAccording to predictions, 10% of the earth's crust will be completely dry by 2050, up from the current 2%. Thirty percent of the earth's surface will be completely dry by the finish of the twenty-first century.

## Solar radiation

In addition to playing a crucial role in the creation of biomass and, ultimately, the yield of fruit crops, solar radiation that is noticeable a vital energy source for plants to engage in photosynthetic activity (Koyama *et al.*, 2012). If soil moisture is sufficient, more carbohydrates will be created and accessible for filling and enhancing the sweetness of fruits if climate change results in high light intensity for extended periods of time (Sherman and Beckman, 2003). In this situation, plants must have a smaller leaf area to yield the same quantity of fruit as they did before to climate change due to higher radiation and heat (Fischer *et al.*, 2012a). When photoinhibition occurs as a result of changes in radiation levels or temperature, the plants' ability to efficiently perform photosynthetically would be severely hampered. The canopy heats up due to increased radiation absorption and decreased transpiration (stomatal closure), which impacts the meristem heat while affecting the ambient air temperature. Depending on the ambient temperature range, this can increase or slow down plant growth (Pritchard and Amthor, 2005). Due to a lack of carbohydrates, prolonged low radiation with diffused or decreased light stimulates the longitudinal expansion of delicate vegetative structures (Dwivedi and Dwivedi, 2012). For this reason, proper and moderate plant and branch densities, tree height and crown shape, which are controlled by pruning and espalier, as well as the direction of the lines from the north toward the south, are crucial elements to maximise light absorption in plantations (Fischer and Orduz-Rodriguez, 2012).Since floral onset, flower bud distinction, fruit development, size, colour, and organoleptic quality are all directly impacted by the reduction of light intensity, the reproductive phase is more negatively impacted than the vegetative phase (Fischer *et al.*, 2012b). High levels of solar heat result in apples with excellent colouring (due to enhanced anthocyanin production) as well as thicker cuticles and epidermis, which are resistant to infections and insect pests.

## Rainfall

Rainfall is yet another noticeable impact brought on by climate change. Crop productivity is decreased by uneven or nonexistent rainfall, particularly in rainfed regionsInsect-pests, diseases, and floods caused by high rains in areas with insufficient drainage can affect crop yield, as will the proliferation of beneficial microbes. The look and flavour of ripe mango fruits may be negatively impacted by changes in precipitation patterns. Rainfall has a negative impact on fruit set, growth, and production at the time of flowering. Due to prolonged and severe precipitation, excessive fruit production and flower drop happen in some locations. Poor fruit output is a result of pests influenced by untimely precipitation (Makhmale*et al.,* 2016). Fruits in high-rainfall areas are susceptible to a number of diseases throughout their development stage, including anthracnose in mango fruit (Ploetz, 2003). Pollen from the flower's stigma washed away by rain during blossoming, which led to poor or nonexistent fruit development. Due to unseasonal rain that was followed by a severe dew attack, which slowed fruit setting, increased fruit drop, and also enhanced the heavy incidence of sooty mould and powdery mildew in mango, there was a reported 80–90% loss in mango production in Gujarat (Rajatiya *et al.,* 2018).

## Crop Enhancement Techniques

### *Diversification*

Diversity is a useful strategy for minimising the impact of changing climate. In suitable climatic situation, a single crop can produce a lot, but variety can stabilise the production system and reduce insect pest and disease attack. Farmers throughout the world use a diverse crop system to combat uncertainty and variance in growth, and fruit trees offer beneficial chances to diversify crops. using fruit crops like kiwis, olives, peaches apricots and walnuts to diversify (Subedi, 2019). creation of genotypes that are disease, insect, salinity, moisture stress, and drought resistant.

## Use of Mulching

Mulching enhances the soil's microclimate, nutrient uptake, and health. It also helps to conserve soil moisture. Another important tactic is the adoption of mulches. Thin translucent mulch or black film should be used to solarize the soil, while silver mulch is recommended for insect repellant purposes. In comparison to the control, it should be highlighted that the plastic mulch improved yield percentages in the following crops: papaya (64.24%), mango (45.23%), banana (33.95%), ber (27.06%), guava (25.93%), pineapple (14.63%), and litchi (12.61%) (Patil *et al.*, 2013) and highest runner plant output was seen in strawberries when treated with white-on-black plastic mulch at a warmer region (Cook, 2002).

## Policy for Climate Change Adaptation in Agriculture

In order to ensure food security in the face of climate change, policies must work towards a climate - resilient and reliable agricultural sector that recognizes the requirements of those who are most at risk, such as women and children, while also enhancing nutritional quality. This is important because good nutrition makes people more resilient to the effects of climate change, such as disease outbreaks and poor hygiene. In order to prevent nutrient loss during food processing and storage, as well as during crop production (where ironically, increasing crop yields does not always result in greater nutrition for the population). As was previously mentioned, the adaptation must be extremely local and concentrated on the demographics and geographic features of the area, regardless of how small. The basic premise is that there is no one solution, and that neither more output nor technical advancement would necessarily result in greater food security in the face of climate change. Technical improvement must be considered in adaptation strategies, but they must also take into account the traditional agricultural methods used by small farmers and indigenous groups.

## Climate-resilient fruit crops

Fruit crops like pomegranates, wood apples, aonla, karonda, barbados cherries, and dragon fruit are thought to have lower moisture requirements and lower transpiration rates. Moreover, temperature variations have little impact on their flowering and fruiting. These plants could therefore be the next-generation climate-smart fruit crop.

### *1. Dragon fruit (Hylocereus undatus)*

This is a new tropical and subtropical fruit that is primarily found in urban and peri-urban regions. This fruit is a cactaceae family and has a great tolerance for drought. As a result, the fruit crop has a great tolerance for drought. When it reaches a specific height, the fruit is born in the intersection of the cladode. Temperature and light levels may have an impact on the flowering of dragon fruit. The flower may bloom at around 4 p.m. on warm, cloudy days while the withering may not begin until 1 a.m. on cool days. Flowers stay open overnight if pollination does not occur during that time. The maximum temperature at which dragon fruit may be grown is 45ºC. Moreover, it can thrive in rainfed environments. It may grow in rainfall ranging from 100 to 2000 mm, with periods of alternately dry and rainy weather (Swamy *et. al.*, 2004).

### *2. Phalsa (Grewia asiatica)*

Phalsa is a subtropical fruit plant that may be grown anywhere, with the exception of high altitude. Up to an elevation of 1,000 m, the plant grows successfully. In regions with distinct summer and winter seasons, the plant thrives. Due to their perennial nature, the plants usually lose their leaves as winter draws near before going dormant. In warmer climates, however, there is no dormancy and no leaf shedding. It can grow in a range of temperatures, from 3 °C to 45 °C. Plants can withstand brief frost. however, needs to be protected from the extremely low temperatures. Fruit must be allowed to ripen, develop the proper fruit colour, and develop acceptable eating qualities in warm or hot temperatures. The plant is well-known for its fruit, which is packed with nutrients and is frequently consumed as a beverage. Moreover, it can endure drought for longer days. This is one of the tropics, subtropics, and desert regions' upcoming crops.

### *3. Pumello (C. grandis / C. maxima)*

The pummelo is a tropical or almost tropical fruit that grows natively at sea level at low elevations. Pummelo may flourish in both semi-arid and warm sub-tropical climates. This can be explained by the fact that it requires the least amount of water of any citrus species. In addition, there are no strict or precise temperature requirements for flowering. It requires a lot of heat yet can withstand heat waves and drought. Even at 45ºC, pummelo is reported to produce a considerable amount of fruit. This citrus species' excellent disease and pest tolerance is its best quality. Mani *et al.* (2017) examined the variety of flowering, fruiting, and physic - chemical characteristics of various pummelo procurements cultivated throughout North Bengal and noted a wide range in fruit quality. This study came to the conclusion that pummelo fruit can be produced effectively in high temperature regions with little rainfall.

### *4. Wood apple: Feronia limonia*

The plant grows naturally in dry plains of India and Ceylon and is rather common. The plants can withstand tough soil conditions and environmental conditions because they have robust, deeply penetrating roots. Before processing methods were established in the middle of the 1950s, the fruit was considered a "poor man's food" in India. While unripe, the fruit is widely used in India as a cardiac and liver tonic, a way to stop persistent diarrhoea and illness, and a potent remedy for coughs, sore throats, and gum disorders. Wood apple having the fundamental capacity to tolerate extreme drought stress and can even survive in dry soil. Wood apples are known to withstand temperatures as high as 45ºC. Even in conditions with little water, it may produce a lot of fruit and flowers.

### *5. Ber (Ziziphus mauritiana)*

In the plains of northern India, the ber fruit tree, which belongs to the Rhamnaceae family, is one of the oldest cultivars. Whereas the majority of other fruit trees either fail to grow or perform extremely poorly, it can even thrive on marginal grounds or subpar soils. It is known as both the poor man's apple and the king of fruits from arid regions. The nation is home to three primary species. The primary species of commercial significance, with its numerous variations, is *Z. mauritiana.* It is highly valued for its leaves, which are protein-rich and used as animal fodder (Pala). The third one *Z. rotundifolia*, also produces edible fruits, albeit ones that are smaller. It serves as the rootstock for the commercial ber crops. Jujubogenin, obelin lactone, and saponins are all found in the seeds. In addition to vitamins A, B, protein, calcium, and phosphorus, jujube fruits also contain a fair quantity of vitamin C. (Jawanda and Bal, 1978). It is a resistant, annual fruit tree that provides farmers with little access to capital with a variety of products like fruits, fodder, and fuel wood. It's the only fruit crop that can be cultivated in a wide range of soils and climates, from sub-tropical to tropical, and still produce adequately. The physiological makeup of the branches helps to reduce moisture loss. Furthermore hairy, the leaves are ideal for reducing water loss through stomata. As a result, it can resist severe drought conditions and protracted dry spells.

### 6. *Aonla (Emblica officinalis)*

India has been growing aonla, a member of the Euphorbiaceae family, since the Vedic period. It has achieved commercial status as a consequence of extensive research and development, and it has also demonstrated that it has the potential to be a fruit crop for dry ecosystems. It may be cultivated in a variety of agro-climatic and soil conditions and is resilient, prolific in bearing fruit, and highly lucrative even with minimal maintenance.The fruits are valued for their nutritional, medical, and therapeutic properties and are a good source of pectin, iron, calcium, phosphorus, and vitamin C (4–9 mg/g). The fruit serves as the primary component of the Ayurveda medicines Chayvanprash and triphala. The tree can tolerate prolonged dry spells as a result of its pure deciduous nature and robust physiology. Because the leaves have a little surface area, less moisture is lost by transpiration. Aonla can grow healthily at temperatures close to 50ºC and can withstand frost. (Chaube, 2000).

### 7. *Pomegranate (Punica granatum)*

A commercially important fruit crop in dry and semi-arid environments is the pomegranate, which belongs to the family Lythraceae. Due to its propensity for an arid climate, commercial pomegranate orchards can be found in Maharashtra, Gujarat, Rajasthan, Andhra Pradesh, and Karnataka. Its xerophytic traits and hardiness make it a great crop for dry, rain-fed pastures and uneven ground, where other fruits cannot thrive. In addition to being a favourite table fruit, it is also used to make squash and juice. An important condiment known as anardana is made from dried seeds. Moreover, the peel is used to colour clothing and has therapeutic benefits. Pomegranates can withstand temperatures of up to 50°C in the regular season and 42°–45°C in the prime fruiting season. Moreover, it requires little water and can endure prolonged dry spells.

### 8. *Kair (Capparis decidua)*

Rajasthan's western Thar Desert, a perennial woody shrub or small tree known as kair, which serves a variety of purposes, grows extensively and carelessly. It has many branches, is leafless, bushy, and flourishes in even the most unfavourable climatic circumstances and on infertile soils. It is ideal for preventing soil erosion caused by wind and water as well as stabilising sand dunes. The plant thrives in extreme climatic circumstances as a result of its xerophytic adaptation. It's unripe berry-shaped fruits are filled with proteins, minerals and carbohydrates which are used both as fresh vegetables and to make pickles. Fruits that have been dehydrated are utilised as vegetables during the off-season, either on their own or in combination with other dried vegetables. In general, residents in hot, arid locations place a great value on it. Natural reproduction happens by seeds and root suckers, while vegetative reproduction via hard wood cuttings has been attempted. Kair has a good adaptation to semi-arid and desert environments. It can also endure a dry, hot summer.

### *9. Karonda (Carissa carandas)*

Karonda is a subtropical and dry tropical evergreen spiky shrub or small tree that can grow to a height of 3 metres. Wastelands and marginal areas both support its successful growth. Moreover, the plant can be used to create a beautiful, densely thorned hedge around in any fruit orchard. It produces a large number of beautiful, berry-like fruits that are abundant in vitamin C, minerals including iron, calcium, magnesium, and phosphorus, as well as edible. In addition to being appropriate for preserving, mature fruit contains a large level of pectin, which may be used to produce jelly, jam, squash, syrup, and pickles that are highly sought after on the global market. The plants are able to take full use of monsoon rain because their primary flowering season is from March to April, and the fruits mature from August to September. While others flower from October to November, some varieties and plant types do both. Karonda can tolerate temperatures as high as 45$^{0}$C. It is amazing how well-adapted the plant is to tolerate dry seasons. The tree can withstand dry conditions and high temperatures without losing its ability to bear fruit in the coming season.

### *10. Bael (Aegle marmelos)*

The hardy fruit crop bael, which belongs to the Rutaceae family, is indigenous and may be produced effectively in dry environments. It is renowned for both its medicinal and nutritional benefits. Unripe fruits are used to treat diarrhoea and dysentery and are in high demand in traditional medical systems like Ayurveda and ripe fruits are laxatives. Many researchers have isolated and identified a variety of chemical components, including alkaloids, coumarins, and steroids, from the leaves, wood, root, and bark of the bael tree. Fruit's marmelosin content is regarded as a cure-all for stomach problems. The tree can endure even in the most hostile environments because of its innate thorniness. In dry places with temperatures well above 400C, it can be observed flourishing ferociously.

## Conclusion

One of the most pressing concerns confronting the world is feeding a population of 9 billion people by 2050 without increasing greenhouse gas emissions. Climate change will have a stronger impact on food security in developing countries, which are already the most vulnerable to its consequences. Malnourished people are less able to tolerate the adverse impacts of climate change, also including disease outbreaks, resulting in a destructive cycle. To achieve food security in the face of climate change, the agricultural sector in developing countries must undergo a considerable transformation. Sustainable or climate-smart farming, which includes traditional practises, nature, and the vital role of rural women in developing countries, must take into account the synergy between both the potential for adaptation and the prospects for reduction given. This agriculture system change requires funding.This is now insufficient, and there is a noticeable "financial gap" as a result. In addition to funds from aid programmes for development, agriculture needs access to resources to fight climate change. The main problem is that, up until now, the agriculture industry really hasn't played a significant role in international treaties aiming at decreasing greenhouse gas emissions, therefore there are no methods in place to evaluate its contribution. This could change. One of the decisions reached at the Durban Conference was to have the Subsidiary Group for Technical and Scientific Advice investigate issues pertaining to agriculture. As the agricultural industry participates in carbon pricing, emerging countries' adaptation and mitigation efforts must take food security into account to prevent them from becoming dominated by vast territories being taken over for bioenergy or monoculture. Prevention must never jeopardise the safety of the food supply.

## References

Abd El-Rhman, I.E. (2010). Physiological studies on cracking phenomena of pomegranates. J. Appl. Sci. Res, *6*(6), 696-703.

Awasthi, R.P., Verma, H.S., Sharma, R.D., Bhardwaj, S.P. & Bhardwaj, S.V. (2001). Causes of low productivity in apple orchards and suggested remedial measures. *Productivity of Temperate Fruits. Solan: Dr. YS Parmar University of Horticulture and Forestry, 18.*

Balogoun, I., Ahoton, L.E., Saïdou, A., Bello, D.O., Ezin, V., Amadji, G.L., Ahohuendo, B.C., Babatounde, S., Chougourou, D.C. and Ahanchede, A. (2016). Effect of climatic factors on cashew (*Anacardium occidentale* L.) productivity in Benin (West Africa). Journal of Earth Science & Climatic Change, *7*(1).

Bhargava, R., Singh, R. S., Pal, G. & Sharma, S. K. (2011). Physiological disorders in fruits in arid region: A review. Indian J. Arid Hort, *6*(1-2), 1-10.

Carlsson-Kanyama, A. & González, A. D. (2009). Potential contributions of food consumption patterns to climate change. The American journal of clinical nutrition, 89(5), 1704S-1709S.

Chaube, R.P. (2000). Aonla cultivation in sub tropics and semi-arid, Ecology and Ecosystem, 13(3): 12-17

Cook, S.M. (2002). Runner plant production and the effect of light intensity on flower and fruit development in day-neutral strawberries.

Dinesh, M.R.andReddy, B.M.C. (2012). Physiological basis of growth and fruit yield characteristics of tropical and Sub-tropical fruits to temperature. Tropical Fruit Tree Species and Climate Change. 45.

Dwivedi, P. & Dwivedi, R. S. (Eds.). (2010). *Physiology of abiotic stress in plants.* Agrobios (India).

Fischer, G. &Orduz-Rogríguez, J.O. (2012). Ecofisiologíaenfrutales (No. Doc. 26022) CO-BAC, Bogotá).

Fischer, G., Parra-Coronado, A. and Miranda. D.(2016). La calidadposcosecha de losfruto-senrespuesta a losfactoresclimaticosenelcultivo. Agron. Colomb. Supl. 1.

Friend, D.J.C. (1981). Effect of night temperature on flowering and fruit size in pineapple (*Ananas comosus* [L.] Merrill). Botanical Gazette, 142(2), 188-190.

Gariglio, N., Castillo, A., Juan, M., Almela, V. &Agustí, M. (2003). Effects of fruit thinning on fruit growth, sugars and purple spot in loquat fruit (*Eriobotrya japonica* L. indl.). The Journal of Horticultural Science and Biotechnology, 78(1), 32-34.

Gora, J.S., Verma, A.K, Singh, J., Choudhary, D.R. (2019). Climate Change and Production of Horticultural Crops. In Agricultural Impacts of Climate Change; 1:45-61.

Gregory, P.J., Ingram, J.S. &Brklacich, M. (2005). Climate change and food security. Philosophical Transactions of the Royal Society B: Biological Sciences, 360(1463), 2139-2148.

Haokip, S.W., Shankar, K. &Lalrinngheta, J. (2020). Climate change and its impact on fruit crops. Journal of Pharmacognosy and Phytochemistry;9(1):435-438.

Hazarika, T.K. (2013). Climate change and Indian horticulture: opportunities, challenges and mitigation strategies. International Journal of Environmental Engineering and Management;4(6):629-630.

IPCC, 2001. Climate change, 2001: Impacts, adaptations and vulnerability. In: McCarthy, J.J., Canziani, O.F., Leary, N.A., Dokken, D.J., White, K.S. (Eds.), Contribution of Working Group II to the Third Assesment Report of the Intergovernmental Panel on Climate Change. Cambridge University Press, Cambridge.

Jangra, M.S.& Sharma, J.P. (2013) Climate resilient apple production in Kullu valley of Himachal Pradesh. International Journal of Farm Sciences.3(1):91-98.

Jawanda, J.S., Singh, R. & Pal, R.N. (1974). Effect of growth regulators on floral bud drop, fruit character and quality of ''Thompson Seedless" grape (*Vitis viifera* L.). Vitis. 13(3):215-221.

Katrodia, J.S., Rane, D.A. &Salunkhe, D.K. (1985). Biochemical nature of spongy tissue in Alphonso fruits. In II International Symposium on Mango. 231:835-839.

Koyama, K., Ikeda, H. Poudel, P.R.&Goto-Yamamoto, N. (2012). Light quality affects flavonoid biosynthesis in young berries of Cabernet Sauvignon grape. Phytochem. 78, 54-64.

Lide, D.R., (2009). CRC Handbook of Chemistry and Physics. 90th ed. CRC Press, Boca Raton, pp. 2804.

Makhmale, S., Bhutada, P., Yadav, L. & Yadav, B.K. (2016). Impact of climate change on phenology of Mango–The case study. Ecology, Environment and Conservation Paper. 22:119-124.

Malhotra, S.K. (2017). Horticultural crops and climate change: A review. Indian Journal of Agricultural Sciences. 87(1):12-22.

Mani, A., Yadav, V.K.,Dey K. & Ghosh, A.(2017). Flowering, fruiting and physiochemical properties of pummelo. Bulletin of Environment, pharmacology and life sciences, 6(4): 432-437.

Mishra, D.S., Tripathi, A. &Nimbolkar, P.K. (2016). Review on physiological disorders of tropical and subtropical fruits: Causes and management approach. International Journal of Agriculture, Environment and Biotechnology. 9(6):925-935.

Negi, S.S. (1999) Mango production in India. In VI International Symposium on Mango. 509:69-78.

Olesen, J.E. & Bindi, M. (2002), Consequences of climate change for European agricultural productivity, land use and policy. European Journal of Agronomy.16(1):239-262.

Pandey, S.N. (1998). Mango cultivars. Mango Cultivation, International Book Distributing Company, Lucknow, India. 39:99.

Patil, S.S., Kelkar, T.S. &Bhalerao S.A. (2013). Mulching: A soil and water conservation practice. Research Journal of Agriculture and Forestry Sciences ISSN, 2320, 6063.

Peng, L., Wang, C., He, S., Guo, C. & Yan, C. (2000) Effects of elevation and climatic factors on the fruit quaity of Navel orange. South China Fruits. 29(4):3-4.

Pereira, J.M., Goncalves, B., Bacelar, E., Cunha, J.B., Coutinho, J.&Correia, C.M. (2009) Effects of elevated $CO_2$ on grapevine (*Vitisv inifera* L.): Physiological and yield attributes. Vitis, 2009; 48(4): 159-165.

Ploetz, R.C. (2003). Diseases of tropical fruit crops. CABI.

Pritchard, S.G. &Amthor, J.S.(2005). Crops and environmental change. Food Products Press, The Haworth Press, New York, NY.

Rajan, S. (2008). Implications of climate change in mango. Impact Assessment of Climate Change for Research Priority Planning in Horticultural Crops. Central Potato Research Institute, Shimla. 36-42.

Rajan, S., Tiwari, D., Singh, V.K., Saxena, P., Singh, S. & Reddy, Y.T.N. (2011). Application of extended BBCH scale for phenological studies in mango (*Mangifera indica* L.). Journal of Applied Horticulture. 13(2):108-114.

Rajatiya, J., Varu, D.K., Gohil, P., Solanki, M., Halepotara, F. & Gohil, M.(2018). Climate Change: Impact, Mitigation and Adaptation in Fruit Crops. Int. J Pure App. Biosci. 6(1):1161-1169.

Rasul, G., Pasakhala, B., Mishra, A., & Pant, S. (2020). Adaptation to mountain cryosphere change: issues and challenges. Clim. Dev.12, 297–309.

Saini, R.S., Singh, S. &Deswal, R.P.S. (2004). Effect of micro-nutrients plant growth regulators and soil amendments on fruit drop, cracking, yield and quality of bael (*Aegle marmelos* Correa) under rainfed conditions. Indian Journal of Horticulture. 61(2):175-176.

Schnitter, R., & Berry, P. (2019). The climate change, food security and human health nexus in Canada: a framework to protect population health. Int. J. Environ. Res. Public Health. 16, 2531.

Sherman, W.B. & Beckman, T.G. (2003). Climate adaptions in fruit crops. Acta Hortic. 622, 411-428.

Singh, R.N. (1966). Sex expression in mango with reference to prevailing temperature. In Proc. Amer. Soc. Hort. Sci. 89:228-230.

Stöckle, C.O., Marsal, J. & Villar, J.M. (2009). Impact of climate change on irrigated tree fruit production. In VI International Symposium on Irrigation of Horticultural Crops. 889:41-52.

Sun, P., Mantri, N., Lou, H., Hu, Y., Sun, D., Zhu, Y.*et al*. (2012). Effects of elevated CO2 and temperature on yield and fruit quality of strawberry (*Fragaria ananassa* Duch.) at two levels of nitrogen application. PloS one.7(7).

Swamy,P.R. Ramanujan, S.E.&Venkata, P. (2004), Dragon fruit- Botany and physiology, Intern. Journal of Ecosystem and sustainance, 11(2): 196-203.

Turner, D.W. & Fortescue, J.A. Thomas, D.S.(2007). Environmental physiology of the bananas (*Musa* spp.). Brazilian Journal of Plant Physiology.19(4):463-484.

WMO, (2006). Drought monitoring and early warning: concepts, progress and future challenges. Message from Ban Ki-Moon.

Yang, W.H., Zhu, X.C., Deng, S.C., Wang, H.C., Hu, G.B., Wu, H. *et al*. (2010). Developmental problems in over-winter off-season longan fruit. I: Effect of temperatures. Scientia horticulturae. 126 (3):351-358.

Zemni, H., Souid, I., Ben Salem, A., Fathalli, N., Mliki, A., Ghorbel, A., Hammami, M. & Hellali, R. (2005). Aromatic potential of grapevines cultivated in Northern and Southern Tunisia. Acta horticulturae.

Zong, R.F., Shao, P.F., Hu, X.Q. & Dai, L.Y. (1979). Preliminary studies on fluctuations in the components of the juice sac and rind in citrus fruit granulation. Scientia. Agri. Sincia. 3:60-64.

# 18

# Vegetables: A Food to Ensure Economic and Dietary Security

Debarati Seal[1*], Amit Layek[2] and Kaushik Pramanik[2]

[1] Department of Agronomy, Bidhan Chandra Krishi Viswavidayalaya, Mohanpur, Nadia, West Bengal, India, Pin-741252

[2] Department of Agricultural Entomology, Bidhan Chandra Krishi Viswavidayalaya, Mohanpur, Nadia, West Bengal, India, Pin-741252.

**ABSTRACT**

Vegetables are becoming increasingly significant for providing a steady supply of food and nutrients. Producing vegetables is a crucial component of agricultural diversification plans and offers a sizable economic prospect for decreasing rural unemployment and poverty in emerging nations.Despite being the most commonly accessible supplier of vitamins and minerals for human wellbeing, vegetables still have untapped monetary and nutritive potentiality.To fully realise the economic viability of vegetables, governments will be required to increase their involvement in agricultural production (inclusive of high yielding cultivars, avoiding synthetic pesticides, and controlled farming), good post-harvest management, nutrition security, and market accessibility.To properly utilise the nutritional content of vegetables, consumers must be aware of how they improve health and be able to purchase them at fair prices or grow these themselves.As a result, it's important to encourage the consumption and production of vegetables through a combination of supply-side measures and behaviour modification messaging that highlights their importance for a balanced diet.Vegetables have enormous economic and nutritional potential, but to fully realise it, governments and donors must give them far more consideration than they already do. Making investments in vegetables a top priority today would increase the economic potential of smallholder farmers and guarantee that everyone has accessibility to a diet rich in nutrients.

*Keywords*: Vegetable, Food, Nutrition security, Economic viability, Balanced diet.

## Introduction

The idea of availability of cereals, tubers, and roots —the basic crops which offer reasonably priced resources of nutritional energy—has long been linked to food and nutritional security. But as the idea of food security has ingrained nutrition

* Corresponding author.

security into it and the need of dietary variability for optimum health has risen to the forefront, this picture is shifting. Consuming a variety of food groups in the proper amounts is necessary for a healthy, high-quality diet. Worldwide, the number of people who experienced hunger decreased by 795 million in 2015 (FAO *et al.,* 2015), demonstrating improvement in assuring appropriate accessibility of suitable basic meals as assessed by calorie intake. However, according to WHO data from 2016, an estimated 2 billion individuals suffer from inadequate micronutrient requirements, and an additional billion people around the world are obese or overweight (Ng *et al.,* 2014).

Micronutrients required for healthier diets can be found in large amount in vegetables and fruits. Vegetables contain potassium, which aids in maintaining healthy blood pressure, dietary fibre, which lowers cholesterol level in blood and may reduce the chances of heart problems, folate (folic acid), which lowers the risk of birth deformities, vitamin A, which supports healthy eyes and skin, and vitamin C, which not only supports good oral health but also enables the body to absorb iron. In order to avoid chronic diseases (particularly heart diseases, malignancies, and diabetes) and provide essential micronutrients (notablyiron, calcium, zinc, vitamin A, and iodine), the World Health Organization (WHO) advises a minimal consumption of 400 g of fruits and vegetables each day (WHO, 2015; WHO/FAO, 2003). Today's consumers, including those with greater earnings, are thought to be falling short of this goal. It is necessary to devote more resources to addressing this nutritional gap and facilitating customers to access the nutritive value of vegetables.

Vegetable cultivation, processing, and commercialization present possible prospects which may be particularly alluring to young people since they require little land, are technologically advanced, and yield big profits quickly. A unique need for female labour is also frequently created by the lower degrees of mechanisation in vegetable cultivation and the requirement for attentive produce handling. Such employment might be advanced by public expenditures in training, infrastructure and subsidies to promote vegetable supply chains.

Yet, the relatively low levels of support that national and international funders provide to government-sector vegetable research and development have constrained vegetables' potential to have advantageous financial and nutritional consequences. In contrast to products high in micronutrients, public and corporate investment in agriculture are still mostly concentrated on staple crops and oil crops (Haddad *et al.,* 2016; Pingali, 2015).When the private sector invests in vegetables in low-earning nations, it typically concentrates on a small number of key vegetables including, onions, tomatoes, peppers, green beans, cucumbers and lettuce. In accordance with the Sustainable Development Goals, this chapter examines how vegetables may, firstly, open up new doors for small-holder farmers in low-earning tropical and subtropical nations and, secondly, improve nutrition and food security as well as the health of billions of consumers.

## The role of vegetables in the world food economy

Cucurbits (pumpkins, squashes, cucumbers, and gherkins), alliums (onions, shallots, and garlic), chilies and tomatoes are the four vegetables that dominate the world's food industry. These vegetables are appropriately referred to as "global" because they are eaten in almost every country, despite having a wide range of shapes, sizes, colours, and flavours. While the sale of imported veggies generates substantial streams of revenue, traditional vegetables frequently have better nutritive qualities (Yang and Keding, 2009). Such as, 100 g of the green leaves of amaranths, vegetable cowpea, African nightshade or jute mallow, can meet above 100% of a pregnant woman's vitamin A requirements (World Vegetable Center, 2017).

Increasing affluence and population expansion are the main factors driving the increase in vegetable demands. Vegetable accessibility per person increases by 0.5% for every 1% rise of per capita income in emerging parts of the country.Thus, middle-income nations with a large population produces the major portion of the world's fruit and vegetable production (77% of the total value). China produces 24% of the world's fruit and contributes 45% of the value of the world's vegetable crop (FAO, 2017). India stands in second place, contributing 8% and 7% of the world's overall supply of vegetables and fruits, respectively.

According to FAO statistics on foodstuff balance sheets, vegetable availability per person in upper-middle earning nations has risen to proportion seen in high-earning nations, and supply in middle-earningnation is improving at a similar trend. Today, on average, middle-income nations produce enough vegetables and fruit to satisfy the FAO/WHO recommendations of 200g of fruit and 200g of vegetables daily (WHO/FAO, 2003). Contrarily, low-earning nations have experienced little expansion in their mean vegetable production, and the amount available is far below the level advised for consumption. However, this situation may be partially offset by the utilisation and manufacture of more conventional vegetables, which are not included in the FAO information.

It's also possible that vegetable agricultural productivity is not increasing as quickly as it could. The creation of novel crop management strategies, new varieties, and advancements in postharvest processing and handling are all dependent on systematic research activities. There is information that government financing for vegetable innovation (as a subset of the "specialty crops" industry) is lower than anticipated, despite the financial importance and benefit to human health of vegetables. This is true even in high income nations like the United

States (Alston and Pardey, 2008). Rarely is public research funding in less and mediumearningnations sufficiently broken down to evaluate expenditures in vegetable research individually (Pray *et al.,* 2011).

Investment in private sector research is crucial, especially for vegetables. It is challenging to gather information on private-sector investment in vegetable R&D. Nevertheless, the enormous industrial consolidation that has occurred globally and the fierce competition for market dominance within the sector are evidence of its significant economic worth (Howard, 2009).However in China and India, which are regarded as principals in this field, only approximately 5% of all research funding comes from the private sector (Hu *et al.,* 2011; Pray and Nagarajan, 2012). A small number of "global" vegetables with great economic value, such as tomatoes, chillies, onions, and cucumbers, are the focus of most private sector investment in vegetable research.

## Enhancing the accessibility of a varied range of safe vegetables

Production must rise to keep up with the market's rising requirement for vegetables at fair rates. This can be accomplished by intensifying already-existing specialist vegetable systems and diversifying dietary staple crop systems to incorporate vegetables, especially in peri-urban settings (Beed *et al.,* 2015). Yet, increasing the availability of vegetables depends critically on ensuring their safety in the supply. This section begins by discussing the significance of taking steps to guarantee that vegetables are safe to consume before examining three major obstacles to growing the supply of vegetables: enhancing on-farm productivity, lowering post-harvest loss, and enhancing market access.

## Making sure that vegetables are healthful to consume

At the growing stage, plant diseases and insect pests can seriously harm the majority of crops. Some insects and pathogens can decrease productivity and result in flaws or strange shapes. Farm managers frequently apply inappropriate amounts of pesticides to prevent these financial risks since consumer put a greaterprice on the quality of fresh product presented in markets. High-value crops receive far more pesticide application than low-value crops, and farmers typically use preventative spraying to safeguard their capital (Riwthong *et al.,* 2015 for Thailand).This approach exposed farm workers and their families to pesticide leftovers that may have a negative impact on their own wellbeing, in addition to raising customer worries about potential health risks and food safety (Praneetvatakul *et al.,* 2013). Moreover, the utilization of organic waste in vegetable cultivation, the utilizations of dirty water to irrigate crops or direct pollution by cattle, birdsor wild animals, are all examples of ways that vegetable sources might get contaminated with foodborne diseases (Heaton and Jones, 2008; Ha *et al.,* 2008; Park *et al.,* 2012).

Hence, customers are consequently becoming more cautious regarding the safety of vegetables. If pathogens or maximum pesticide residue limits are consistently found in vegetables, customers would link fresh vegetables with health hazards rather than advantages and lower intake. Modernizing supply chains (such as using supermarkets' refrigerators and quality control systems) only offers a temporary solution. According to studies (e.g. Duedu *et al.*, 2014), vegetables available in supermarkets had lower levels of microbial contamination than vegetables sold at wet markets, but both may still contain contamination (e.g. Wanwimolruk *et al.*, 2016).

Innovative market channels have emerged in several middle-income nations with the goal of providing consumers with a more reliable source of freshly harvested vegetables, some of which are recognised as meeting safety and quality criteria. Similar or less expensive programmes are growing in other nations, for instance, organic farmers directly distributing weekly baskets of different veggies to consumers.Vegetable growers and producer organisations are finding new ways to engage with customers and provide them with a source of healthy, high-quality vegetables using conventional phone-based methods or online applications. To achieve their goals of ensuring food safety, policymakers must establish appropriate standards for the cultivation and handling of vegetables as well as systems for ensuring compliance, such as routine pathogen and pesticide testing at key markets and the release of test results to the general public.

## Enhancing on-farm production

Vegetable farming yields might vary greatly. For example, Nigerian growers barely produce 4 t/ha of tomatoes on average (FAO, 2017; average 2012–2014). On the contrary, farmers in Cameroon produce 13 t/ha of crops, those in India produce 21 t/ha, and those in China produce as much as 51 t/ha (FAO, 2017). These variations are the result of the wide variation in growing environments and input usage. This variation suggests that there is room for innovation to raise on-farm production. Here, we concentrate on three crucial innovation areas: varietal enhancement, disease and pest control, and protective farming.

## Improved vegetable varieties

A key component of raising farm production is the accessibility of high-quality vegetable seeds. Investments in hybrid variety research and development as well as the marketing of seeds that are properly conform with particular production restrictions have been connected to the increased supply of vegetables around the world. The creation and production of high-quality vegetable seeds has benefited from public policies that have encouraged private investment. It's interesting to learn about the history of vegetable seeds in India. The Indian government imposed strong regulations on the seed industry up to 1988, barring entry of major domestic and international corporations and limiting the importation of seed for use in commercial or research endeavours (Pray *et al.,* 2001). Few private seed firms existed, there was little demand for hybrid types, and the majority of farmers either recycled their own seed or received their supplies from the unofficial seed industry (Kolady *et al.,* 2012; Pray *et al.,* 2001).

Private seed sector development, and the vegetable seed business in particular, received a huge boost from later seed sector liberalisation and better breeders' rights protection. Today, high-quality vegetable seeds are accessible almost everywhere in India. There is a fiercely competitive seed market, and there are hundreds of hybrids with various fruit and plant features that are high yielding and widely resistant to common pests and diseases (Schreinemachers *et al.,* 2016b). According to estimates, the Indian vegetable seed business is currently worth $580 million annually and expanding at a rate of 5% (Kapur, 2017). The accessibility of a wide variety of seeds will be crucial for coping with climate change. Pest control that is both secure and long-lasting.

New types of both imported and domestic vegetables must be produced while balancing the challenges of nutritional properties and commercial demand. Despite the fact that many of these traditional vegetables seem to be far more nutrient-dense than worldwide vegetables, information on their nutritional profiles in raw and prepared forms is still limited. More knowledge is required regarding how nutrient profiles change depending on growing conditions, varietal choice, processing, and cooking techniques, and conclusively how much of these nutrients are absorbed by the human body, which depends on a number of additional factors, including people's health status (Sriwichai *et al.,* 2016). Increased research demonstrating the health advantages of traditional vegetable consumption, along with increased access to better or modified indigenous seed cultivers, may open up new business options for growers, processors, and distributors of vegetables.

## Effective and safe pest prevention

Pests and diseases of crop plants are frequently cited by farmers as these are the primary cause of risk since they lower productivity and adversely impact the commercialization of the commodity. It appears that climate change may increase the severity of pest and disease stresses (Bebber *et al.,* 2013), hence techniques of reduction may become even more crucial in the future. Experiences at the World Vegetable Centre suggests three main groups of actions that could be helpful: using bio control techniques, grafting high-yield seedlings onto highly resistant rootstocks, and investing in protected growing environment. Bio-control techniques, which involve the utilization of living creatures like parasites or predator insects to manage pests, have a great deal of promise to replace conventional pesticides, enhancing food safety and reducing productivity risks.

The rapid growth of the global commerce in synthetic pesticides, farmers' higher confidence with the efficacy of agrochemicals, and a lack of risk consciousness and biological control method knowledge, however, prevent the spread of such technologies in so many places (Schreinemachers *et al.,* 2015). The execution of safer procedures are hampered by the fact that regulatory frameworks frequently regard bio pesticides (pesticides made from natural ingredients like those of the neem plant) in the same way as synthetic insecticides (Srinivasan, 2012). Another method that shows promise for preventing diseases and pests is vegetable grafting. Grafting is a standard technique for growing fruits and vegetables in high-income nations, although it was less frequent in Southeast Asia or Africa. For example, compared to non-grafted plants, the grafted tomato plants produced a yield advantage of roughly 37% (Genova *et al.,* 2013). Moreover, grafting provided new business options for smaller companies, allowing them to trade and process the increased tomato supply in addition to producing their own grafted plants.

## Protected cultivation

The adoption of protected agricultural systems can help reduce the prevalence of pests and illnesses. These systems provide producers greater control over the surroundings in which they create. They might also enable producers to grow vegetables apart from the "normal" growing season (often determined by temperature and rainfall). Outside of this season, production brought to market may fetch much higher prices. Technology range from basic bamboo and plastic sheet rain shelters to fully functional greenhouses that enable year-round production. In Asia, the utilization of protected farming techniques is expanding quickly (Kang *et al.,* 2013; Nair and Barche 2014). According to a research conducted in Bangladesh, seasonal revenue of farmers improved by 48% after getting training on how to cultivate tomatoes during the hot, rainy season utilising inexpensive rain shelters, heat-resistant cultivars, and phytohormones that cause flowering (Schreinemachers *et al,* 2016c).

Although protected farming is still mostly underutilised in Africa, there is immense possibility in the vicinity of medium- to large-sized cities where there is a market demand for vegetables. Yet, the necessary inputs are frequently just not accessible, necessitating both private and public expenditure to import or generate the necessary resources. The adoption (or promotion) of protected farming would profit from more public policy backing. Farmers might need to look for finance, improve their book-keeping abilities to monitor financial flows, and utilize market data to better idea of production.

## Reduce post-harvest losses

Vegetable production chains generally experience substantial postharvest losses, which are in the amount of 30 to 50% of agricultural output volumes in so many poor nations (FAO, 2011). With the right variety selection and the application of sound agricultural methods, these losses can be reduced on-farm. Financial losses can be decreased by using straightforward farm innovations like picking produce at the proper time of day, separating and grading it, and using the right packaging close to the farm gate.

To enhance market performance for high-value perishable vegetables, post-farmgate expenditures are required in logistics, cold storage systems, and market intelligence systems. The "hidden middle" of vegetable value chains, as Reardon (2015) referred to it, is a crucial area that is changing quickly in many middle-income nations. Interventions after harvest are difficult because they need for coordinated modifications throughout the entire vegetable production chain, starting from from farmers' input suppliers to retailers. Documenting whatever works and what doesn't in vegetable supply chain interference is urgently needed.

## Expanding market accessibility

Improved accession to national, regional, and global vegetable markets can offer farmers significant financial incentives to start growing vegetables, as Muriithi and Matz (2015) shown for Kenya. Produced to stringent market criteria, packed to maintain freshness, and sent by air or sea directly to stores in Europe, producers there have successfully entered the vegetable export industry. Examples include fresh Asian vegetables and French beans. These exports to Kenya are estimated to be worth $1 billion USD annually (Fernandez-Stark *et al.,* 2011).

Due to the expansion of contemporary retail, including supermarkets, many emerging countries have also witnessed a change in conventional value chains (Reardon *et al.,* 2003). If properly handled, this might be advantageous for both customers and farmers. To satisfy the requirements for quality, consistency, and amount of contemporary shop, it is necessary for farmers to upgrade their abilities to use technological advances, engage in contracts, and invest in infrastructure and equipment. Reardon and Gulati (2008) reported that in Indonesia, tomato producers who supplied supermarket channels made a net profit that was 33–39% greater than those who supplied traditional markets. Chege *et al.* (2015) shown that in Kenya, providing supermarkets improved household intake of micronutrients as well as household revenues.

## Raising the consumption of vegetables to boost nutrition

Dietary priorities for low-income populations frequently centre on consuming enough calorie-dense foodstuffs to satisfy daily requirements. In comparison to food staples, vegetables are somewhat costly per calories of energy, therefore it makes sense that people don't prioritise buying vegetables. To reach the dietary recommendation levels of 400 g per day, greater accessibility of vegetables is essential yet insufficient. Also, it's unlikely that increased wealth will lead to enough fruit and vegetable consumption. Despite increases in average salaries, vegetable intake has dropped significantly in several countries (Global Panel, 2016).

The pattern of foodstuff intake can change over time, reflecting more than just obtainability and cost (Kearney, 2010; Traill *et al.,* 2014). Vegetables aren't always a part of family meals for a variety of compelling reasons, including tastes, evolving lives, convenience, eating habits, poor nutritional awareness, and worries about food safety. Little children come to mind as a population section that simply doesn't "like" vegetables. In certain cultures, eating vegetables is associated with being poor or of low social standing.In some cultures, eating animal products like dairy and meat is seen as a sign of greater social standing or as being more nutrient-dense than eating plants. However, there are societal taboos in some communities. For instance, Cameroonian study participants believed that eating amaranth promotes male impotence (Kamga *et al.,* 2013).

Furthermore, there is a movement towards the consumption of highly processed foodstuffs, which contain rising amounts of salts, sugars and edible oils, in both high- and low-earning nations (Popkin *et al.,* 2012). As a result, even when vegetables are easily accessible and reasonably priced, there is still a discrepancy between the prescribed and real consumption of vegetables. Consumer habits must change in order to reap the health and nutritional benefits linked to the recommended intakes of vegetables.

## Behaviour change communication on vegetable utilization

Several countries have government efforts that encourage the intake of vegetables and nutritional knowledge, such as the UK's "Five a Day" initiative. Moreover, dietary variety and healthy eating habits are encouraged by educational initiatives in hospitals, schools, and marketplaces. Nongovernmental organisations routinely carry out these campaigns and programmes in Africa and Asia, but there has also been an increase in the dissemination of data about nutritional quality as a consequence of national and regional organisations' increased emphasis on nutrition (e.g., Scaling Up Nutrition movement participants). Although there is still a dearth of impact data, some of them are encouraging. In northern Tanzania, for instance, Ochieng *et al.* (2017) assessed the effects of campaigns encouraging the consumption of traditional vegetables of Africa on dietary patterns among rural and urban households and discovered substantial growth in the dietary patterns of kids below 5 years old as well as of women in reproductive age. Research in high-earning nations demonstrate that straightforward informative strategies, such as linking vegetables with superhuman abilities or providing vegetable dishes catchy names, can encourage kids to choose healthier eating choices. Additional "nudges" to alter food choices include simply chopping up vegetables or putting them on the plate before meat and other staples (Appleton *et al.,* 2016; Wansink *et al.,* 2012).

For the sake of increasing the "nutrition awareness" of social security and food safety net programmes and promote better diets, it has been frequently suggested to utilise monetary incentives (either vouchers or cash) to persuade low-earning customers to buy a wider variety of foodstuffs, including vegetables. The Healthy Incentives Pilot in the United States revealed that offering financial incentives connected exclusively to the purchase of vegetables and fruits produced favourable outcomes in terms of both behaviour and prospective nutritional benefit (Bartlett *et al.,* 2014). Aninvestigationabout the food preferences of low-earning populations in Ecuador indicated that vouchers were the most successful at promoting the intake of vegetables (Hidrobo *et al.,* 2014).

## Kitchen gardens and vegetable consumption in remote areas

Home garden initiatives that focus on dietary quality connect practical instruction in vegetable cultivation with behaviour change communications for health and nutrition (World Vegetable Center, 2016). These interference deal with vegetable accessibility, requirement, and use all at once. According to several studies (DFID, 2014; Galhena *et al.,* 2013; Olney *et al.,* 2009; Schreinemachers *et al.,* 2016a), this multifaceted strategy is particularly successful at improving vegetable usage in low-income rural families who are susceptible to micronutrient deficiencies.

While women primarily choose and prepare meals, home garden treatments frequently target them, but it's also sometimes crucial to include grandfathers and men in behavioural modification communication. Home gardens appear to support empowerment of women in Bangladesh (Bushamuka *et al.,* 2005; Patalagsa *et al.,* 2015), however research is still needed to confirm that in rest of the nations.

## School lunches or meals

School lunches or meals are a satisfactory starting point for changing kids' nutriment, and currentresearches have shown that they have a positive nutritional effects (Global Panel, 2015; Kristjansson *et al.,* 2006). When fresh fruit and vegetables are included in school meal programmes together with staple food grains,vegetable oil, pulses,dairy, and meat, nutritional advantages can be maximized.However, there is currently no proof whetherit can successfully supplement school meals with fresh seasonal vegetables and fruits. Recently there has been a lot of interest in locally produced school meals that combine the purchase of ingredients from nearby farms with the provision of school lunches (Gelli *et al.,* 2010). The potential for the fields of agriculture, health, and education to effectively collaborate for the well-being of kids and neighbouring farmers both is starting to become apparent.

One such integrated strategy to change kids' eating habits towards nutritious food selection, such as vegetables and fruits, is school garden programmes, which combine health and nutrition teaching with practical gardening practise. The goal of school garden interventions is to introduce kids to fresh produce at an early age and help them form lifelong dietary habits and attitudes about food. In Bhutan and Nepal, schoolchildren aged 10 to 15 participated in a recent evaluation of the integrated effects of school gardens associated to complementing lessons along with informational activities regarding farming and nutriment (Schreinemachers *et al.,* 2017a, 2017b). These programs indicated a considerable rise in youngster's knowledge and awareness of fruits and vegetables as well as their expressed predispositions for consuming them, but no appreciable changes in children's consumption of these foods or nutritional status. This shows that only school garden efforts are insufficient to improve food standard and that, in low-earning regions, substantial links to school meals or home gardening initiatives may be necessary.

## Enhancing nutrition by altering food systems

There is rising awareness that the modern food systems do not provide diets that are getting healthier and better (Global Panel, 2016). In particular for low-income customers, agricultural strategies are heavily biased in favour of boosting the yield of the agricultural crops (grains, fruits and tubers), which are the main supplier of energy. Yet, when incomes rise, more foodstuffs with additional sugars, salt, and fats are consumed, lowering the nutritious value of the diet. Additionally, even in rural areas, food and beverage consumption that is highly processed or even ultra-processed is rising rapidly (Tschirley *et al.,* 2015). These foods do not promote the kinds of varied, nutritionally balanced foods that are required for health, despite being more practical and frequently more affordable than those of fresh meals that are richer in nutrients.

## Conclusion

The best supplies of micronutrients for optimal health can be found in vegetables, which are nutritional powerhouses. Vegetables enrich diets with variety, flavour, and nutritional value. The most obvious and cost-effective strategy to improve everyone's nutrition may be to place a stronger emphasis on vegetables. Vegetables are also the backbone of prosperous agricultural economies. Vegetables are a crucial component of any agricultural growth strategy since increased vegetable productivity has the potential to produce more money and jobs than other areas of the agricultural sector. Nonetheless, today's population is still underestimating the value of vegetables in both the economic and dietary senses. It is necessary to broaden the perspective and shift the long-standing emphasis away from staple food crops. Governments and donors should give increasing postharvest losses, improving affordability, and expanding market access higher priority than they already do. It is essential to take precautions to ensure the safety of vegetables. As knowledge of the relationships among nutritional health and quality advances, policymakers need to be prepared to back further efforts to improve the consumption of vegetables. The persistent discrepancy between prescribed and actual vegetable consumption must be overcome if the Sustainable Development Goals pertaining to enhancing nutritional and food security and good health are to be accomplished. The moment has come to focus more on the vegetable sector, giving new and smallholder farmers in particular greater opportunity to generate money and employment while also encouraging more varied, nutritious, and high-quality diets for everyone.

## References

Alston, J.M. &Pardey, P.G.(2008). Public funding for research into specialty crops. *HortScience*, 43 (5), 1461–1470.

Appleton, K.M., Hemingway, A., Saulais, L., Dinnella, C. & Monteleone, E. (2016). Increasing vegetable intakes: rationale and systematic review of published interventions. *European Journal of Nutrition*, 55, 869–896.

Bartlett, S., Klerman, J., Olsho, L., Logan, C., Blocklin, M., Beauregard, M., Enver, A., Wilde, P., Owens, C. & Melhem, M.(2014). Evaluation of the Healthy Incentives Pilot (HIP): Final Report. Prepared by Abt Associates for the U.S. Department of Agriculture. Food and Nutrition Service, Washington, D.C.

Bebber, D.P.,Ramotowski, M.A.T. & Gurr, S.J.(2013). Crop pests and pathogens move polewards in a warming world. *Nature Climate Change*, 3 (11), 985–988. http://dx.doi. org/10.1038/nclimate1990.

Beed, F., Dubois, T. & Yang, R.Y. (2015). Nutrition implications of urban and peri-urban agriculture. *Agricultural Development*, 26, 7–11.

Bushamuka, V.N., Pee, S., Talukder, A., Kiess, L., Panagides, D. & Taher, A.(2005). Impact of a homestead gardening program on household food security and empowerment of women in Bangladesh. *Food Nutrition Bulletin*, 26. http://dx.doi.org/10.1177/156482650502600102.

Chege, C.G.K., Andersson, C.I.M. & Qaim, M.(2015). Impacts of supermarkets on farm household nutrition in Kenya. *World Development*, 72, 394–407.

DFID. (2014). Can Agriculture Interventions Promote Nutrition: Agriculture and Nutrition Evidence Paper. Department for International Development, London.

Duedu, K.O., Yarnie, E.A., Tetteh-Quarcoo, P.B., Attah, S.K.,Donkor, E.S. & Ayeh-Kumi, P.F. (2014). A comparative survey of the prevalence of human parasites found in fresh vegetables sold in supermarkets and open-aired markets in Accra, Ghana. *BMC Research Notes*, 7, 836.

FAO. (2011). Global Food Losses and Food Waste – Extent, Causes and Prevention. Food and Agriculture Organization of the United Nations, Rome.

FAO.(2017). FAOSTAT. FAO Statistics Division. Food and Agriculture Organization of the United Nations, Rome(Available online at) http://www.fao.org/faostat/en/#data (Accessed 2 February 2017).

FAO, IFAD, WFP.(2015). The State of Food Insecurity in the World 2015. In: Proceedings of Meeting the 2015 International Hunger Targets: Taking Stock of Uneven Progress. Food and Agriculture Organization of the United Nations (FAO), Rome.

Fernandez-Stark, K., Bamber, P. & Gereffi, G.(2011). The Fruit and Vegetables Global Value Chain: Economic Upgrading and Workforce Development. Center on Globalization, Governance and Competitiveness, Duke University, Durham, NC.

Galhena, D., Freed, R. & Maredia, K.(2013). Home gardens: a promising approach to enhance household food security and wellbeing. *Agriculture & Food Security*, 2, 8.

Gelli, A., Neeser, K. & Drake, L.(2010). Home Grown School Feeding: Linking Small Holder Agriculture to School Food Provision HGSF Working Paper Series #1, HGSF and Partnership for Child Development, Imperial College London

Genova, C., Schreinemachers, P.&Afari-Sefa, V.(2013). An Impact Assessment of AVRDC's Tomato Grafting in Vietnam. AVRDC – The World Vegetable Center, Shanhua, Taiwan.

Global Panel.(2015). Healthy Meals in Schools: Policy Innovations Linking Agriculture, Food Systems and Nutrition. Policy Brief. Global Panel on Agriculture and Food Systems for Nutrition, London, UK.

Global Panel.(2016). Food Systems and Diets: Facing the Challenges of the 21st Century. Global Panel on Agriculture and Food Systems for Nutrition, London, UK.

Ha, N.T., Kitajima, M., Hang, N.V., Matsubara, K., Takizawa, S., Katayama, H., Oguma, K. &Ohgaki, S.(2008). Bacterial contamination of raw vegetables, vegetable-related water and river water in Ho Chi Minh City, Vietnam. Water Science & Technology, 58 (12), 2403–2411. http://dx.doi.org/10.2166/wst.2008.435.

Haddad, L., Hawkes, C., Webb, P., Thomas, S., Beddington, J., Waage, J. & Flynn, D.(2016). *A new global research agenda for food*, 540, 30–32.

Heaton, J.C. & Jones, K.(2008). Microbial contamination of fruit and vegetables and the behaviour of enteropathogens in the phyllosphere: a review. *Journal of Applied Microbiology*, 104 (3), 613–626. http://dx.doi.org/10.1111/j.1365-2672.2007.03587.x.

Hidrobo, M., Hoddinott, J., Peterman, A., Margolies, A. & Moreira, V.(2014). Cash, food, or vouchers? Evidence from a randomized experiment in northern Ecuador. *Journal of Development Economics*, 107, 144–156. http://dx.doi.org/10.1016/j.jdeveco.2013.11.009.

Howard, P.(2009). Visualizing Consolidation in the Global Seed Industry: 1996–2008. Sustainability, 1 (4), 1266.

Hu, R., Liang, Q., Pray, C., Huang, J. & Jin, Y.(2011). Privatization, Public R & D policy, and Private R & D investment in China's agriculture. *Journal of Agricultural and Resource Economocs*, 36 (2), 416–432.

Kamga, R., Kouamé, C. & Akyeampong, E.(2013). Vegetable consumption patterns in Yaounde, Cameroon. *African Journal of Food Agriculture, Nutrition andDevelopment*, 13.

Kang, Y., Chang, Y.C.A., Choi, H.S. & Gu, M., (2013). Current and future status of protected cultivation techniques in Asia. *ActaHorticulturae*, 33–40.

Kapur, A. (2017). 10 vegetable seed companies fuelling growth of agriculture. Rural Mark:Integr. *Urban Rural Mark*, 46–49.

Kearney, J.(2010). Food consumption trends and drivers. *Philosophical Transaction ofthe Royal Society B: Biological Sciences*, 365, 2793–2807.

Kolady, D.E., Spielman, D.J. & Cavalieri, A.(2012). The impact of seed policy reforms and intellectual property rights on crop productivity in India. *Journal of Agricultural Economics*, 63, 361–384.

Kristjansson, B., Robinson, V., Petticrew, M., MacDonald, B. & Krasevec, J. (2006). School Feeding for Improving the Physical and Psychosocial Health of Disadvantaged Students Campbell Systematic Reviews, 14.

Muriithi, B.W. & Matz, J.A.(2015). Welfare effects of vegetable commercialization: evidence from smallholder producers in Kenya. *Food Policy*, 50, 80–91. http://dx.doi.org/10.1016/j.foodpol.2014.11.001.

Nair, R.& Barche, S. (2014). Protected cultivation of vegetables – present status and future prospects in India. *Indian Journal of Applied Research*, 4, 245–247.

Ng, M., Fleming, T., Robinson, M., Thomson, B. & Graetz, N. (2014). Global, regional, and national prevalence of overweight and obesity in children and adults during 1980–2013: a systematic analysis for the Global Burden of Disease Study 2013. Lancet 384, 766–781.

Ochieng, J., Afari-Sefa, V., Karanja, D., Kessy, R., Rajendran, S. & Samali, S. (2017). How promoting consumption of traditional African vegetables affects household nutrition security in Tanzania. *Renewable Agriculture and Food Systems*, 1–11.

Olney, D.K., Talukder, A., Iannotti, L.L., Ruel, M.T. & Quinn, V. (2009). Assessing impact and impact pathways of a homestead food production program on household and child nutrition in Cambodia. *Food and Nutrition Bulletin*, 30, 355–369.

Park, S., szonyi, B., Gautam, R., Nightingale, K., Anciso, J. & Ivanek, R. (2012). Risk factors for microbial contamination in fruits and vegetables at the preharvest level: a systematic review. *Journal of Food Protection*, 75 (11), 2055–2081. http://dx.doi.org/10.4315/0362- 028x.jfp-12-160.

Patalagsa, M.A., Schreinemachers, P., Begum, S. & Begum, S.(2015). Sowing seeds of empowerment: effect of women's home garden training in Bangladesh. *Agriculture and Food Security*, 4, 24. http://dx.doi.org/10.1186/s40066-015-0044-2.

Pingali, P.(2015). Agricultural policy and nutrition outcomes – getting beyond the preoccupation with staple grains. *Food Security*, 7, 583–591.

Popkin, B.M., Adair, L.S. & Ng, S.W.(2012). Global nutrition transition and the pandemic of obesity in developing countries. *NutritionReviews*, 70 (1), 3–21. http://dx.doi.org/10.1111/ j.1753-4887.2011.00456.x.

Praneetvatakul, S., Schreinemachers, P., Pananurak, P. & Tipraqsa, P.(2013). Pesticides, external costs and policy options for Thai agriculture. *Environmental Science and Policy*, 27, 103–113. http://dx.doi.org/10.1016/j.envsci.2012.10.019.

Pray, C. & Nagarajan, L.(2012). Innovation and Research by Private Agribusiness in India (IFPRI Discussion Paper 1181). International Food Policy Research Institute, Washington, D.C.

Pray, C.E., Gisselquist, D. & Nagarajan, L. (2011). Private investment in agricultural research and technology transfer in Africa. In: Proceedings of Conference Working Paper 13, prepared for the ASTI/IFPRI-FARA Conference Agricultural R & D: Investing in Africa's Future. Analyzing Trends, Challenges, and Opportunities, Accra, Ghana 5–7 December 2011. International Food Policy Research Institute (IFPRI), Washington, D.C.

Pray, C.E., Ramaswami, B. & Kelley, T.(2001). The impact of economic reforms on R & D by the Indian seed industry. *Food Policy*, 26, 587–598.

Reardon, T.& Gulati, A. (2008). The Supermarket Revolution in Developing Countries. Policies for "Competitiveness with Inclusiveness" (IFPRI Policy Brief2). International Food Policy Research Institute, Washington, D.C.

Reardon, T., Timmer, C.P., Barrett, C.B., Berdegu, X.E.& Julio.(2003). The rise of Supermarkets in Africa, Asia, and Latin America. *American Journal of Agricultural Economics*, 85 (5), 1140–1146.

Riwthong, S., Schreinemachers, P., Grovermann, C. & Berger, T.(2015). Land use intensification, commercialization and changes in pest management of smallholder upland agriculture in Thailand. *Environmental Science and Policy*, 45, 11–19. http://dx.doi.org/10. 1016/j.envsci.2014.09.003.

Schreinemachers, P., Afari-Sefa, V., Heng, C.H., Dung, P.T.M., Praneetvatakul, S. & Srinivasan, R.(2015). Safe and sustainable crop protection in Southeast Asia: status, challenges and policy options. *Environmental Science and Policy,* 54, 357–366.

Schreinemachers, P., Bhattarai, D.R., Subedi, G.D., Acharaya, T.P. & Chen, H.P.(2017a). Impact of school gardens in Nepal: a cluster randomized controlled trial. *Journal of Development Effectiveness*, 9 (3), 329–343. http://dx.doi.org/10.1080/19439342.2017 .1311356.

Schreinemachers, P., Patalagsa, M.A. & Uddin, N. (2016a). Impact and cost-effectiveness of women's training in home gardening and nutrition in Bangladesh. *Journal of Development Effectiveness*, 8 (4), 473–488. http://dx.doi.org/10.1080/19439342.201 6.1231704.

Schreinemachers, P., Rai, B.B., Dorji, D., Chen, H.-p., Dukpa, T., Thinley, N., Sherpa, P.L. & Yang, R.-Y. (2017b). School gardening in Bhutan: evaluating outcomes and impact. *Food Security*, 9 (3), 635–648. http://dx.doi.org/10.1007/s12571-017-0673-3.

Schreinemachers, P., Rao, K.P.C., Easdown, W., Hanson, P. & Kumar, S. (2016b). The contribution of international vegetable breeding to private seed companies in India. *Genetic Resources and Crop Evolution*, 64 (5), 1037–1049. http://dx.doi.org/10.1007/s10722- 016-0423-y.

Schreinemachers, P., Wu, M.-h., Uddin, M.N., Ahmad, S., Hanson, P. (2016c). Farmer training in off-season vegetables: effects on income and pesticide use in Bangladesh. *Food Policy*, 61, 132–140. http://dx.doi.org/10.1016/j.foodpol.2016.03.002.

Srinivasan, R. (2012). Integrating biopesticides in pest management strategies for tropical vegetable production. *Journal of Biopesticides*, 5, 36–45.

Sriwichai, W., Berger, J., Picq, C. & Avallone, S. (2016). Determining Factors of Lipophilic Micronutrient Bioaccessibility in Several Leafy Vegetables. *Journal of Agricultural and Food Chemistry*, 64, 1695–1701.

Traill, W.B., Mazzocchi, M., Shankar, B. & Hallam, D. (2014). Importance of government policies and other influences in transforming global diets. *Nutrition Reviews*, 72, 591–604.

Tschirley, D., Reardon, T., Dolislager, M. & Snyder, J. (2015). The Rise of a Middle Class in East and Southern Africa: implications for Food System Transformation. *Journal oflnternational Development*, 27, 628–646.

Wanwimolruk, S., Phopin, K., Boonpangrak, S. & Prachayasittikul, V. (2016). Food safety in Thailand 4: comparison of pesticide residues found in three commonly consumed vegetables purchased from local markets and supermarkets in Thailand. PeerJ 4, e2432.

WHO.(2015). Promoting Fruit and Vegetable Consumption around the World. World Health Organization, Geneva.

WHO/FAO.(2003). Diet, Nutrition and the Prevention of Chronic Diseases. Report of a Joint FAO/WHO Expert Consultation. WHO Technical Report Series 916. World Health Organization, Geneva.

World Vegetable Center.(2016). The World Vegetable Center Approach to Household Gardening for Nutrition. World Vegetable Center, Shanhua, Taiwan.

World Vegetable Center. (2017). Healthier lives, more resilient livelihoods: World Vegetable Center Strategy 2017–2025 17–823 World Vegetable Center; Shanhua, Taiwan.

Yang, R.Y. & Keding, G.B. (2009). Nutritional contributions of important African indigenous vegetables. In: Shackleton, C.M., Pasquini, M.W., Drescher, A.W. (Eds.), African Indigenous Vegetables in Urban Agriculture. Earthscan, London & Sterling, VA, pp. 105–143.

# 19

# Bioactive Compounds in Jamun (*Syzygium cumini* L.) Ensuring Nutritional Security

Pravallikasree Rayanoothala[1*], Manaswini Mahapatra[1], Suchismita Balabantaray[1] and Siddhartha Shankar Sharma[1]

[1] Department of Agriculture and Allied sciences, C.V Raman Global University, Bhubaneswar, India

**ABSTRACT**

The phenolic chemicals found in jambolan, which are bioactive, may have significant positive effects on health. There are a number of phenolic chemicals contained in jambolan, the most prominent of which are phenolic acids, and tannins. The primary products it provides are timber and fruit. The fruit has been linked to a variety of health benefits, including those for diabetes, hyperlipidemia, ulcers, oxidative stress, allergies, arthritis, infections, infertility, fever, plaque, radiation, neuropsychopharmacology, nephropathy, and diarrhoea. The skin of the jambolan fruit is rich in anthocyanins, It has been asserted that the jambolan fruit contains a variety of other chemicals. The fruit skin and pulp, as well as the leaves, are all rich in flavonoids, and the seeds of the jambolan plant are claimed to contain gallic acid, ellagic acid, antioxidant effects have all been attributed to the phenolic chemicals found in jambolan. This section discusses the medicinal, nutritional, and physiological benefits of jamun and its many bioactive constituents. Jamun seeds include the alkaloid jambosine and the glycoside jambolin or antimellin.

*Keywords*: Jamun, antioxidants, nutritional security, bioactive compounds

## Introduction

The term "bioactive phytochemicals" refers to a group of substances present in foods that are not considered nutrients but have been shown to have positive health effects when consumed in small amounts (lowering the prevalence of chronic diseases). Researchers have taken an interest in phenolic compounds because of the antioxidant benefits they may provide (Singh *et al.*, 2016). Many studies have shown the vital role that phenolic chemicals play in improving human health, disproving this long-held belief. As a result of this shift in thinking, scientists and academics in the domains of food technology and allied disciplines have been increasingly curious about the characterization and quantification of phenolic

* Corresponding author.

chemicals found in a wide range of foods. The jambolan tree, or *Syzygium cumini* Skeels., is a huge evergreen tree that is high in phenolic compounds and is found across the tropics and subtropics. Other names for this fruit include jamun, jambul, black plum, and Indian blackberry (Tavares *et al.,* 2016). The plant was transported to Southern Africa from its native range in India and Southeast Asia so that humans may enjoy its tasty fruits (Oliveira *et al.,* 2016). As well as its native territory of Eastern Africa and the all places where Jambolan has been cultivated. Florida isn't the only U.S. state where you can find jambolan. This plant has a long history of medicinal and culinary use in India due to its edible fruits, seeds, leaves, and bark (Syama *et al.,* 2017). The phytochemical components of these plant sections have the ability to exert biological effects (Ayyanar and Subash-Babu 2012). The main phenolic compounds found in the jambolan plant are phenolic acids, flavonoids, and tannins. These chemicals have earned a reputation as effective free radical scavengers. The jambolan fruit is rich in anthocyanins, a type of flavonoid with potent antioxidant qualities (Lestario *et al.,* 2017).

Anthocyanins, which are water soluble, add natural colour to foods and other ingredients that contain a lot of liquid (Veigas *et al.,* 2007). Jambolan's secondary components include ellagic acid, kaempferol, condensed tannins, and hydrolyzable tannins, These bioactive chemicals provide plants their pharmacological relevance due to their wide range of health-promoting properties (Afify *et al.,* 2011)., anti-hypergly cemic Anti - inflammatory, anti - allergic, anti - cancer, antibacterial, chemopreventive, and antioxidant activities are all attributed to jambolan (Afify *et al.,* 2011).

High levels of phenolic chemicals can be found in jambolan. Bioactive secondary phytochemicals called phenolic compounds are produced mostly by the shikimic acid or phenylpropanoid pathways in all higher plants. As a result of their protective roles, they are found in high numbers in the outer layers of plant tissues and in seeds. The number of phenolic hydroxyl groups and structural components joining benzene rings can be used to classify these chemicals (Singh *et al.,* 2016). Gallic acid and ellagic acid are two examples of hydroxybenzoic acid-derived phenolic acids; hydroxycinnamic acid is another. Flavonoids are phenolic compounds with a C6-C3-C6 structure, which consists of fifteen carbon atoms and two aromatic rings connected by a three carbon bridge (a heterocyclic ring). Anthocyanins, isoflavones, & flavones are some of the chemicals present. Tannins are high-molecular-weight, water-soluble phenolic chemicals with a bitter and astringent taste (usually from 500 to 3000). Color (particularly anthocyanins, a flavonoid family), flavour, and food preservation are all provided by phenolic compounds found in foods. The Folin-Ciocalteu reagent method is the gold standard for measuring total phenolic content; it involves the formation of a blue complex from the reduction of phosphomolybdic or phosphor-tungstic acid in an alkaline solution. Moreover, phenolic substances can be confirmed using mass spectrometry. Typically, reversed phase C18 columns are used in HPLC analysis. In most cases, polar solvents make up half of the solvent system in a binary solvent system. The phenolic components in fresh fruit samples, such jambolan, need to be removed. These fruits are extremely perishable, so they are typically preserved through freeze drying or another way. The extraction process can have a major effect on the concentration of phenolic chemicals in the final product. There are a number of methods proposed in the literature, but many of them require a lot of manual work and are hard to duplicate (Aqil *et al.,* 2014). Several methods have been reported to be quite effective in extracting jambolan from fruits and seeds, yielding a substantial amount of phenolic chemicals Aqil *et al.* (2012) used Diaion HP-20 resin and Amberlite XAD-761 column chromatography to enrich jambolan pulp and seed extracts. Acidified 75% ethanol was used in the extraction process, along with HP-20 and XAD-761 resins, and 2N HCl was used to hydrolyze the mixture.

**Table 1 :** Bioactive compunds in jambolan plant

| **Jambolan plant parts** | **Total flavonoid content** | **Main compounds identified** | **Total phenolic content (mg GAE/100 g)** | **References** |
|---|---|---|---|---|
| Fruit pulp extract | 13 500 mg QE/ 100 g FW | -- | 2359 FW | Luximon- Ramma *et al.* (2003) |
| Fruit skin (7 days after drying) | - | - | 9600 | Banerjee *et al.* (2005) |
| Fruit pulp | 7 mg/100 g | Cyanidin, petunidin, malvidin | 390 | Benherlal & Arumughan (2007) |
| Fruit C3RE/g – | – | | 995 DW | Reynertson *et al.* |
| Jambolan fruit (peel and pulp) extract | – | – | 185 | Maria do Socorro *et al.* (2010) |
| Fruit (fully ripe) pulp extract | — | | 208.3 | Brand~ao *et al.* (2011) |
| Fruit (pulp and peel) extract | 91.2 mg GAE/100 g | Delphinidin glucosides, Cyanidin glucosides, Malvidin glucosides, Petunidin glucosides, Galloylglucose ester, Myricetin derivatives | 148.3 | Faria *et al.* (2011) |
| Fruit pulp | 231.5 mg QE/100 g | – | 281.1 FW | Singh *et al.* (2015) |

| Fruit pulp FW | 25.29 mg/100 g | Gallic acid, chlorogenic acid, ferulic acid, rutin, myricetin, quercetin | 206.9 FW | Branco *et al.* (2016) |
|---|---|---|---|---|
| Kernel extract Fruit (freeze–dried) extract | 3200 mg/100 g – | 771 mg/100 g DW | 37 000 | Brito *et al.* (2007) |
| Fruit peel extract | – | – | 560 | Veigas *et al.* (2007) |
| Jambolan fruit (peel and pulp) extract | – | – | 185 | Maria do Socorro *et al.* (2010) |

The extract has a rather high concentration of anthocyanins (0.54%) after being processed in this way. For their part, Veigas *et al.* (2007) used a different resin, Amberlite XAD-7, to extract anthocyanins from jambolan pulp. Jambolan juice has a high concentration of phenolic chemicals, but research into this area is scant. Recent research by Tavares *et al.* (2017) has demonstrated that the anthocyanins present in jambolan juice degrade more noticeably than the flavonols do, allowing for easier extraction of hydrolysable tannins. Nevertheless, hydrolyzable tannins and flavonols were more sensitive to oxidation &heating duration, and increasing the dehydration temperature reduced anthocyanin content. They found that beneficial components like anthocyanins are significantly destroyed at temperatures above 70 °C in jambolan juice treatment.

## Tannins

Hydrolyzed tannins (tannins that, when hydrolyzed, give gallic or ellagic acids) and condensed tannins (made by the condensation of flavans) require complex analysis to determine their structure. Hydrolyzable tannins increase the sourness of jambolan fruit. Hydrolyzable tannins (ellagitannins and gallotannins) as well as condensed tannins (proanthocyanidins) were found in the jambolan fruit's peel and pulp (Tavares *et al.,* 2016). Hydrolyzable tannins in jambolan fruit are ellagitannins, composed of glucose in their centre and gallic and ellagic acid units on either side, as reported by Zhang and Lin (2009). Hydrolyzable tannins were identified in jambolan fruit extract by Gordon *et al.* (2011), and they included 12 gallotannins, 1 hexahydroxydiphenoyl (HHDP)-gallotannin, and 1 trisgalloyldiglucose. Some of the components of hydrolyzable tannins are gallic acid, nonahydroxytriphenolyl (NHTP), hydroxyhexyl diphenol (HHDP), trisgalloyl, or valoneic acid (Gordon *et al.,* 2011; Tavares *et al.,* 2016).

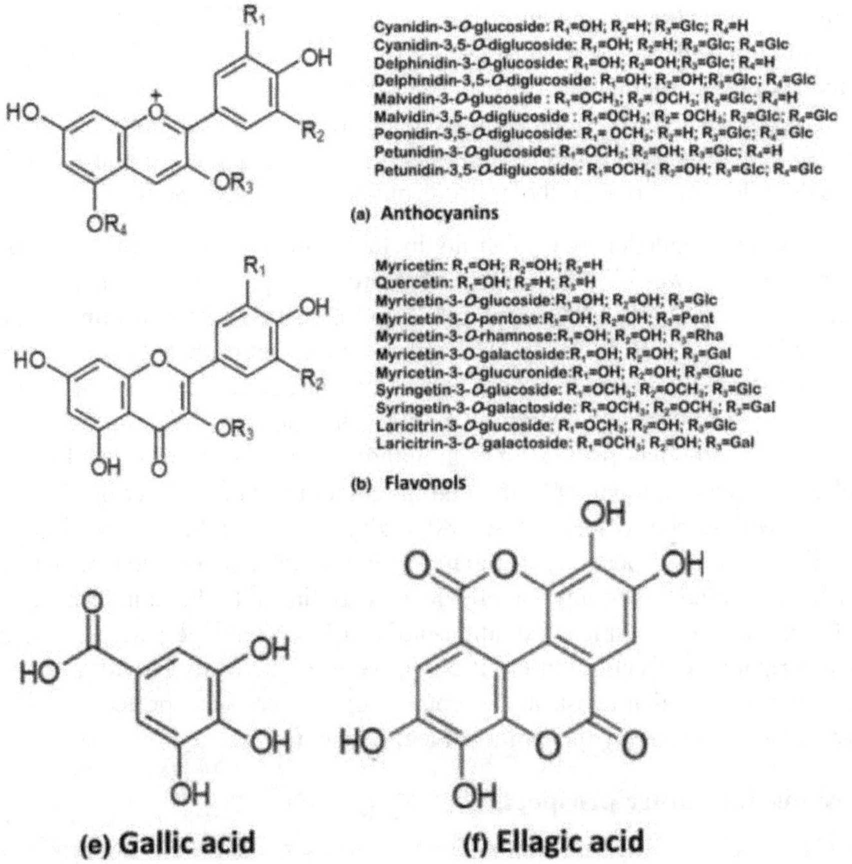


**Figure 1 :** Structures of phenolic compounds (anthocyanins, flavanols, gallic acid, ellagic acid) identified in jambolana (Singh *et al.*, 2018)

## Quantity of phenolic compounds

The phenolic content of jambolan plant sections is shown in Table 1 and Figure 1. Pulp from the jambolan tree has a TPC concentration of 1.15 percent, while seed powder has a TPC content of 2.69%. (Aqil *et al.*, 2012). Jambolan fruit's phenolic content increased in immature stages and reduced as the fruit ripened and matured (Brandrao *et al.*, 2011).

The TFC of various jambolan plant components is shown in Table 1. The highest levels of TFC were found in the skin, followed by the pulp and the seed (Ali *et al.*, 2015). There have been claims that methanol is superior to methylene chloride for flavonoid extraction. There were reported values of 622 and 204 mg QE g 1 DW for TFC in methanolic and methylene chloride extracts of jambolan leaf, respectively (Mohamed *et al.*, 2013). The total anthocyanin concentration (TAC) of jambolan plant sections is shown in Table 1. Jambolan fruit has different levels of anthocyanins at different times during its growth. The total alkaloid content per 100 grammes of fresh jambolan fruit is 79 milligrammes. The group that Brito belongs to (2007). The total anthocyanin content (TAC) in unripe jambolan fruits is fairly low, but it increases dramatically as the fruit ripens and matures. TAC levels are quite low in unripe jambolan fruits but rise sharply as the fruit ripens.

Capacity to inhibit oxidation Several fruits include anthocyanins and flavonoids, which are more powerful antioxidants than regular phenols. By acting as scavengers or deactivators, these compounds stop free radicals from forming in the first place (Singh *et al.,* 2016, 2017). Jambolan's antioxidant properties come from the high concentration of phenolic chemicals it contains. Because it contains more bioactive components, fruit peel has higher antioxidant activity than fruit pulp and fruit seeds. Ripe jambolan fruit has a high anthocyanin concentration, making it an excellent source of antioxidants and natural colourants (Lestario *et al.,* 2017). Pretreatment with jambolan seed extract (80 mg/kg1 body weight) reduced illness and mortality in mice exposed to c-radiation. Free radical scavenging bioactive components including flavonoids and ellagic acid are linked to the radioprotective effect of jambolan seed extract. Radiation-induced DNA damage was prevented in human peripheral cells cultured in vitro that were subjected to 3 Gy of gamma radiation, and intestinal mucosa and crypts in mice were also protected from radiation-induced damage by the jambolan leaf extract (Jagetia *et al.,* 2008).

## Conclusions and future prospects

Jambolan's phenolic content and antioxidant properties make it a useful ingredient in the development of nutritionally sound meals. Yet, a complete understanding of their bioavailability is needed before their health-promoting benefits can be thoroughly investigated. Many unanswered questions remain, and the protective effects of these drugs have largely been shown through in vitro and animal model studies. Further study can be conducted in a number of directions. To properly understand the effects of the phenolic chemicals in jambolan, we need more clinical trials and epidemiological studies. To lose as few chemicals as feasible during jambolan fruit preparation, more research is required. There is no established market for jambolan and its derivatives in developing countries, and the substance has been underutilised in more developed nations. Promotion of this plant for its health benefits and pharmaceutical recognition will benefit from the findings of phytochemical research and clinical studies.

## Acknowledgments

We thank all the resources helped us to learn and write the chapter on bioactive compounds in jamun.

## References

Afify, A.E.M.M., Fayed, S.A., Shalaby, E.A. & El-Shemy, H.A. (2011). Syzygium cumini (pomposia) active principles exhibit potent anticancer and antioxidant activities. African Journal of Pharmacy and Pharmacology, 5, 948–956.

Ali, T.M., Abbasi, K.S., Ali, A. & Hussain, A. (2015). Some compositional and biochemical attributes of jaman fruit (*Syzygium cumini* L.) from Potowar region of Pakistan. Research in Pharmacy, 3, 1–09.

Aqil, F., Gupta, A., Munagala, R. *et al.* (2012). Antioxidant and antiproliferative activities of anthocyanin/ellagitannin-enriched extracts from Syzygium cumini L. (Jamun, the Indian Blackberry). Nutrition and Cancer, 64, 428–438.

Aqil, F., Jeyabalan, J., Munagala, R., Singh, I.P. & Gupta, R.C. (2016). Prevention of hormonal breast cancer by dietary jamun. Molecular Nutrition & Food Research, 60, 1470–1481.

Aqil, F., Munagala, R., Jeyabalan, J., Joshi, T., Gupta, R.C. & Singh, I.P. (2014). The Indian Blackberry (Jamun), Antioxidant Capacity, and Cancer Protection. In Cancer (pp. 101–113).

Ayyanar, M. & Subash-Babu, P. (2012). *Syzygium cumini* (L.) Skeels: A review of its phytochemical constituents and traditional uses. Asian Pacific Journal of Tropical Biomedicine, 2, 240–246.

Baliga, M.S., Bhat, H.P., Baliga, B.R.V., Wilson, R. &Palatty, P.L. (2011). Phytochemistry, traditional uses and pharmacology of *Eugenia jambolana* Lam. (black plum): a review. Food Research International, 44, 1776–1789.

Balwinder Singh, Jatinder Pal Singh, Amritpal Kaur &Narpinder Singh (2018). Insights into the phenolic compounds present in jambolan (Syzygium cumini) along with their health-promoting effects, International Journal of Food Science and Technology, doi:10.1111/ijfs.13841

Banerjee, A., Dasgupta, N. & De, B. (2005). In vitro study of antioxidant activity of *Syzygiumcumini* fruit. Food Chemistry, 90, 727–733.

Barh, D. & Viswanathan, G. (2008). *Syzygium cumini* inhibits growth and induces apoptosis in cervical cancer cell lines: a primary study. Ecancermedicalscience, 2, 83.

Benherlal, P.S. &Arumughan, C. (2007). Chemical composition and in vitro antioxidant studies on *Syzygium cumini* fruit. Journal of the Science of Food and Agriculture, 87, 2560–2569.

Branco, I.G., Moraes, I.C.F., Argandona, E.J.S. ~ *et al.* (2016). Influence of pasteurization on antioxidant and in vitro anti-proliferative effects of jambolan (*Syzygium cumini* (L.) Skeels) fruit pulp. Industrial Crops and Products, 89, 225–230.

Brand~ao, T.S.D.O., Sena, A.R.D., Teshima, E., David, J.M. & Assis, S.A. (2011). Changes in enzymes, phenolic compounds, tannins, and vitamin C in various stages of jambolan (*Syzygium cumini* Lamark) development. Food Science and Technology (Campinas), 31, 849–855.

Brito, E.S., De Araujo, M.C.P., Alves, R.E., Carkeet, C., Clevidence, B.A. & Novotny, J.A. (2007). Anthocyanins present in selected tropical fruits: acerola, jambol~ao, jussara, and guajiru. Journal of Agricultural and Food Chemistry, 55, 9389–9394

Faria, A.F., Marques, M.C. &Mercadante, A.Z. (2011). Identification of bioactive compounds from jambol~ao (Syzygium cumini) and antioxidant capacity evaluation in different pH conditions. Food Chemistry, 126, 1571–1578.

Gordon, A., Jungfer, E., da Silva, B.A., Maia, J.G.S. & Marx, F. (2011). Phenolic constituents and antioxidant capacity of four underutilized fruits from the Amazon region. Journal of Agricultural and Food Chemistry, 59, 7688–7699.

Grover, J.K., Vats, V. &Rathi, S.S. (2000). Anti-hyperglycemic effect of Eugenia jambolana and Tinosporacordifolia in experimental diabetes and their effects on key metabolic enzymes involved in carbohydrate metabolism. Journal of Ethnopharmacology, 73, 461–470.

Jagetia, G.C., Shetty, P.C. & Vidyasagar, M.S. (2008). Treatment of mice with leaf extract of jamun (*Syzygium cumini* L. Skeels) protects against the radiation-induced damage in the intestinal mucosa of mice exposed to different doses of c-radiation. Pharmacology, 1, 169–195.

Lestario, L.N., Howard, L.R., Brownmiller, C., Stebbins, N.B., Liyanage, R. & Lay, J.O. (2017). Changes in polyphenolics during maturation of Java plum (*Syzygium cumini* Lam.). Food Research International, 100, 385–391.

Maria do Socorro, M.R., Alves, R.E., de Brito, E.S., Perez-Jimenez, J., Saura-Calixto, F. & Mancini-Filho, J. (2010). Bioactive compounds and antioxidant capacities of 18 non-traditional tropical fruits from Brazil. Food Chemistry, 121, 996–1002.

Mohamed, A.A., Ali, S.I. & El-Baz, F.K. (2013). Antioxidant and antibacterial activities of crude extracts and essential oils of *Syzygium cumini* leaves. PLoS ONE, 8, 1–8.

Oliveira, E.R., Caliari, M., Soares J unior, M.S., Boas, V. & de Bar- ros, E.V. (2016). Bioactive composition and sensory evaluation of blended jambolan (*Syzygium cumini*) and sugarcane alcoholic fermented beverages. Journal of the Institute of Brewing, 122, 719–728.

Parmar, J., Sharma, P., Verma, P. & Goyal, P.K. (2010). Chemopreventive action of *Syzygium cumini* on DMBA-induced skin papillomagenesis

Reynertson, K.A., Yang, H., Jiang, B., Basile, M.J. & Kennelly, E.J. (2008). Quantitative analysis of antiradical phenolic constituents from fourteen edible Myrtaceae fruits. Food Chemistry, 109, 883–890.

Singh, J.P., Kaur, A., Shevkani, K. & Singh, N. (2015). Influence of jambolan (*Syzygiumcumini*) and xanthan gum incorporation on the physicochemical, antioxidant and sensory properties of glutenfree eggless rice muffins. International Journal of Food Science & Technology, 50, 1190–1197.

Tavares, I.M.d.C., Lago-Vanzela, E.S., Rebello, L.P.G. *et al.* (2016). Comprehensive study of the phenolic composition of the edible parts of jambolan fruit (*Syzygium cumini* (L.) Skeels). Food Research International, 82, 1–13.

Tavares, I.M.d.C., Nogueira, T.Y.K., Mauro, M.A. *et al.* (2017). Dehydration of jambolan [*Syzygium cumini* (L.)] juice during foam mat drying: quantitative and qualitative changes of the phenolic compounds. Food Research International, 102, 32–42.

Veigas, J.M., Narayan, M.S., Laxman, P.M. &Neelwarne, B. (2007). Chemical nature, stability and bioefficacies of anthocyanins from fruit peel of *Syzygium cumini* Skeels. Food Chemistry, 105, 619– 627.

# 20

# Meet the Incredible, the Unsung Heroes of Crops in Alleviating Iron Deficiency Anemia

Sushree Sangita Choudhury[1*], Hemlata Singh[2] and Jyostnarani Pradhan[2]

[1] Department of Food & Nutrition, Collegeof Community Science, Dr. Rajendra Prasad Central Agricultural University, Samastipur, Bihar-848125

[2] Department of Botany, Plant Physiology & Biochemistry, Dr. Rajendra Prasad Central Agricultural University, Samstipur, Bihar-848125

**ABSTRACT**

Iron deficiency anemia (IDA) is the most familiar kind of nutritional anemia which affects people globally. Supplementation, fortification and dietary intervention are the three initiatives for alleviating IDA. Dietary intervention is preferable to others in terms of long-term acceptability, cost-effectiveness, compliance, risk of iron overabundance, and a valuable impact on iron consumption. As a result, it is critical that locally accessible, affordable but high-nutritional-value materials should be employed as a catalyst to enhance the nutritive value. Millets are generally cultivated for their small edible seeds. These non-glutinous crops are enriched with many health-promoting constituents like proteins, carbohydrates, dietary fibers, fats, minerals, and phytochemicals. Generally, food utilization of millets has been confined to only conventional consumers and very few Indians are acquiring the knowledge of their health benefits and nutritional value. Therefore, different processing of millets using contemporary as well as traditional methods for the preparation of value-added food products would diversify their utilization of the diet. A review of the literature suggests that millets are excellent sources of iron for combating iron deficiency anemia. Therefore, the present chapter aims to provide updated comprehensive information on different types of iron-rich value-added products developed from millets and their pharmacological properties in order to open a new perspective for future functional food and pharmacological research.

*Keywords*: Food, IDA, Millets, Value-added products

## Introduction

Anemia is a state of hematological abnormalities that includes depletion in oxygen-carrying capacity or a deduction in the proportion of healthy red blood cells in the body. Iron deficiency anemia (IDA) is the most familiar kind of nutritional anemia

* Corresponding author.

which affects people globally. Being an important element in the living system, iron plays a significant role in many biological functions like energy production, cell proliferation, and respiration. IDA is the terminal point of lack of iron in the body. The individuals were categorized as normal, mild, moderate, or severely anemic relying on their hemoglobin levels (Table 1).

**Table 1 :** Classification of different levels of anemia

| Level of hemoglobin(g/dl) | Severityof anemiaas per concentration of hemoglobin |
|---|---|
| ≥12 | Non-anemic |
| 11-11.9 | Mild |
| 8-10.9 | Moderate |
| <8 | Severe |

*Source: WHO (2011)*

According to WHO (2019), globally 29.9 percent of women aged 15-49 years and 39.8 percent of children aged 6-59 months suffered from anemia. Among them, 57.0 percent of women aged 15-49 years and 67.1 percent of children aged 6-59 months in India were anemic (NFHS-5, 2019).

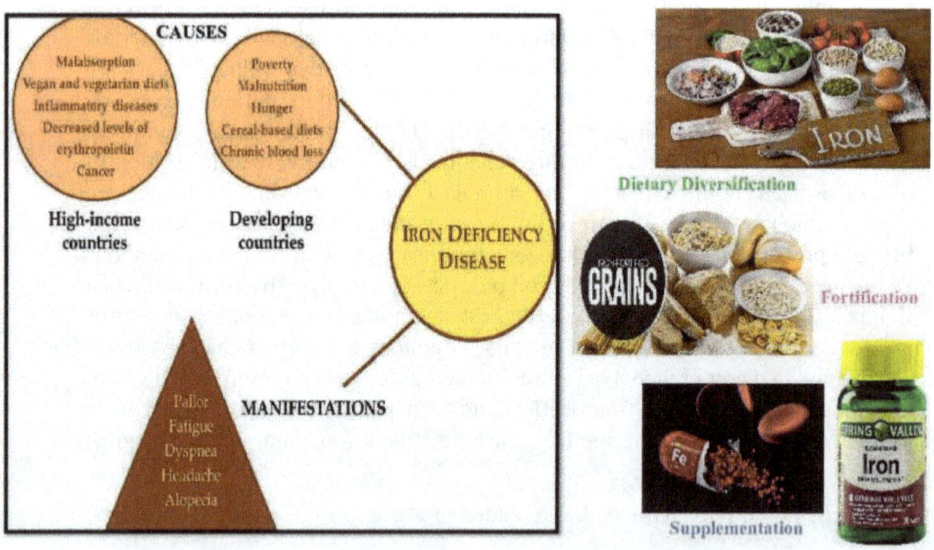


***Source:*** Liberal *et al. (2020)*

**Figure 1 :** Etiologies, manifestations and treatments for IDA

Deficient intake, inadequate and impaired absorption, greater demand, perinatal and postnatal wastage of blood, unusual intracellular transport, scanty presentation to erythroid precursors, etc. are some etiologies of IDA (Lanzkowsky, 2016). IDA is a chronic condition that often goes undiagnosed because it is asymptomatic. Patients are usually affected between the ages of 6 months and 3 years, or between the ages of 11 and 17 years due to expeditious growth and enlarging blood volume at these ages. There are ordinarily no symptoms of mild anemia. Pallor, anorexia, irritability, fatigue, and pica (a strange craving for inedible such as sand, dirt and clay) may occur in severe deficiency. Before the anemia corrects itself, iron treatment reverses these symptoms in a brief period of time.

Supplementation, fortification, and dietary diversification are the three initiatives for alleviating IDA. Dietary intervention is preferable to others in terms of long-term acceptability, cost-effectiveness, compliance, risk of iron overabundance, and a valuable impact on iron consumption.As a result, it is critical that locally accessible, affordable but high-nutritional-value materials should be employed as a catalyst to enhance the nutritive value.

India represents itself as a "Golden land of agriculture," where our diligent farmers grow varieties of nutrient-rich crops including millets, which are generally cultivated for their small edible seeds. The millet consists of major millets such as Sorghum, Pearl millet, and a group of six minor millets which comprise of Finger millet, Kodo millet, Foxtail millet, Proso millet, Little millet and Barnyard millet. Millets mainly grow in semi-arid regions due to their short growing period and higher productivity even under extreme environmental conditions and are considered smart crops. They are considered as the 6$^{th}$ cereal crops in reference to world's agricultural production and very important from food security point at regional and farm level. Therefore, more than one-third of the world's population uses millets in their diet (Ambati and Sucharitha 2019).

The world productivity of millets is estimated to be 89.17 Million Metric Tonnes (MMT) from an area of 74.00 Million hectares (Mha) (FAO Statistics, 2020). Sorghum and Pearl millet are considered as the most prominent millet crops, accounting for more than 90% of global millets cultivation, followed by Finger millet, Proso millet, Barnyard millet,Foxtail millet, Little millet and Kodo millet. India is the world's largest and leading producer of millet. Millets are grown over an area of 12.45 Mha in India, yielding 15.53 Million Tonnes (MT) at a productivity of 1247 kg/hectares. Bajra represents more than half of the country's millet acreage with a roughly equivalent share of production (7.05Mha). It is worth noting that India is the world's most significant producer of Barnyard millet (99.9%), Finger millet (53.3%), Kodo millet (100%), Little millet (100%) and Pearl millet (44.5%), yielding around 12.46 MMT from an area of 8.87 Mha (Associated Chambers of Commerce and Industry of India 2021).

**Caryopsis (grain)**

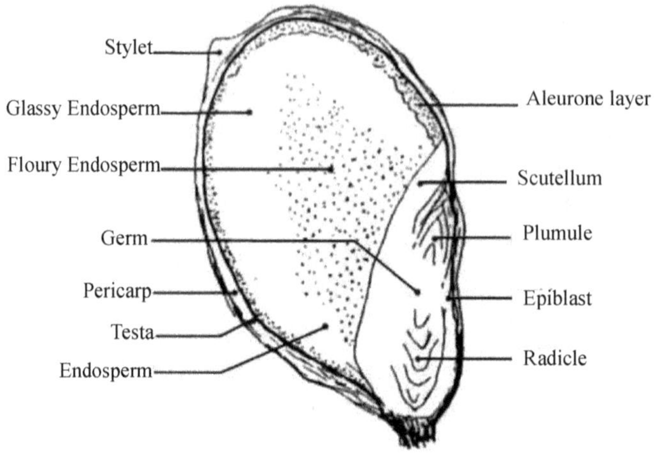


**Figure 2 :** General structure of millet grain

Millets possess a striking role in the conventional diets of many regions all over the country. Millets are acknowledged as "*coarse cereals*" but considering their nutrient composition they are now regarded as "*nutricereals*" (Saini *et al.*, 2021). These non-glutinous millets are rich in nutrients and known as "*Non-acid forming foods*" (Sarita and Singh, 2016). They are augmented with nutrients and serve as agood source of many health-promoting constituents like good quality proteins, carbohydrates, dietary fibres, fats, minerals, antioxidants and phytochemicals (Bhat *et al.*, 2018). In millets, pearl millet, sorghum, finger millet and foxtail millet are generally considered as good sources of iron which will be beneficial to control iron deficiency anemia. This was in line with many previous studies. Priya and Kowsalya (2015) formulated convenience food mixes by using pearl millet, finger millet, sorghum with green gram, bengal gram and groundnut which resulted in micronutrient-rich mixes that serve as a sustainable solution to solve the problem of hidden hunger. Kaur *et al.* (2016) evaluated that wheat flour was replaced with up to 30 percent ragi flour and 30 percent soybean flour in sukhdi which aids in enhancing the intake of protein, crude fibre, and iron and can prevent anemia which was widely prevalent amongst various age groups. Marak *et al.* (2019) indicated that the addition of foxtail millet flour with wheat flour enhanced the nutritional quality of cookies.

## Nutritional composition of different millets

Pearl millet (*Pennisetum glaucum* (L.) R.Br.) is superior in ash (2.1%), protein quality (14.0%), fiber (2.0%), and fat (5.7%) content when compared to other major cultivated cereal crops such as wheat and rice (Kavitha and Parimalavalli, 2014). It is a good source of calcium, iron (8.8mg/100g) as well as zinc (Yadav *et al.* 2014). This iron-rich millet being packed with polyphenol which possesses Antioxidant Activity (AOA) and also contains phytate (647mg/100g), tannin (0.010%) as catechin equivalent (Osman, 2011). Being a great source of energy (349 kcal), carbohydrate (72.6%), protein (10.4%), fiber (1.6%) including micronutrients Sorghum (*Sorghum bicolor* L. Moench) is a vital source of trace minerals, particularly iron and zinc. This grain possesses 1.3 to 3.3% of ash with Fe content ranging between 5.54–7.65 mg/100 g in raw sorghum. Sorghum's chemical composition and the presence of anti-nutritional factors like phytate determine its nutritional quality. Likewise, Finger millet (*Eleusine coracana* Gaertn.) possesses carbohydrate (81.5%),dietary fibre (18% to 20%), crude fibre (4.3%), starch (65% to 75%), protein (9.8%), fat (1% to 1.7%) and mineral (2.7%) which is comparable with other millets and cereals like wheat and rice (Saleh *et al.*2013). It is packed with rich sources of zinc (2.53mg/100g), iron (3.9mg/100g), and polyphenols. Certain anti-nutritional factors like tannins (0.04-3.47%) and phytates (0.48%) are also adorned this millet (IFCT, 2017 and Rathore *et al.* 2019). Similarly, the Foxtail millet (*Setariaitalica* P. Beauv.) is a good source of starch, protein, dietary fibers, fats, vitamins and minerals. The moisture, total ash, crude protein, crude fat, crude fibre and carbohydrate of foxtail millet are 9.35 percent, 3.10 percent, 10.29 percent, 3.06 percent, 4.25 percent and 69.95 percent respectively. An adequate amount of zinc (4.1mg/100g) is present in foxtail millet with fair source of iron (2.7mg/100g). This millet also contains a significant amount of total phenolic content i.e. (33.17mg (GAE)/100g) with tannin (2.80mg/100g) and phytate content (0.341mol/kg) (Sharma *et al.*, 2015).

**Table 2 :** Nutritional value of millets and their comparison to rice and wheat

| Millets | Protein (g) | Total Fat (g) | Total Dietary Fibre (g) | Carbohydrates (g) | Energy (KJ) | Calcium (mg) | Iron (mg) |
|---|---|---|---|---|---|---|---|
| Pearl millet | 10.96 | 5.43 | 11.49 | 61.78 | 1456.00 | 27.35 | 6.42 |
| Sorghum | 9.97 | 1.73 | 10.22 | 67.68 | 1398.00 | 27.60 | 3.95 |
| Finger millet | 7.16 | 1.92 | 11.18 | 66.82 | 1342.00 | 364.00 | 4.62 |
| Little millet | 8.92 | 2.55 | 6.39 | 65.55 | 1449.00 | 16.06 | 1.26 |
| Kodo millet | 8.92 | 2.55 | 6.39 | 66.19 | 1388.00 | 15.27 | 2.34 |
| Foxtail millet | 12.30 | 4.30 | 8.00 | 60.09 | 331.00 | 31.00 | 2.80 |
| Barnyard millet | 6.20 | 2.20 | 10.10 | 65.55 | 307.00 | 24.00 | 1.40 |
| Proso millet | 12.50 | 1.10 | 2.20 | 70.04 | 341.00 | 14.00 | 0.80 |
| Whole wheat | 10.59 | 1.47 | 11.23 | 64.72 | 1347.00 | 39.36 | 3.97 |
| Raw milled rice | 7.94 | 0.52 | 2.81 | 78.24 | 1491.00 | 7.49 | 0.002 |

*Source:* Indian Food Composition Tables, NIN – 2017 and Nutritive value of Indian foods, NIN – 2007

Despite all the nutritional qualities present in millets, certain anti-nutritional factors like phytates and tannins are also present in them which are minimized by different processing methods like germination, fermentation, popping, malting etc. Some investigators like Ranasalva and Visvanathan (2014) revealed that bread produced from cooked fermented pearl millet flour substituting refined wheat flour enhanced digestibility and also reduced antinutritional compounds. Another study conducted by Sharma *et al.* (2015) indicated that optimized germinated foxtail millet flour contained higher dietary fibre, protein, iron, sodium, magnesium, calcium and lower anti-nutritional factors like tannin and phytate. Kumari *et al.*(2019) developed a crunchy nutritious bar by using popped pearl millet which was popped by a high temperature and short time method at 230 ± 5 °C . The result indicated the positive effect of popping on the nutritional enhancement of grain. Shingote *et al.* (2021) analyzed the effect of malting on the nutritional composition of finger millet. The result showed a positive impact.

Millets are nutritionally superior as these grains possess a high amount of proteins, micronutrients, flavonoids and polyphenols thus they were used to combat micronutrient malnutrition through the biofortification of staple crops (Singh *et al.*, 2019). Millets have significant nutraceutical and therapeutical properties like anti-diabetic, anti-hyperlipidemic, anti-allergic, anti-carcinogenic, anti-inflammatory, anti-aging, nephroprotective etc. It also helps in healing the wound, building up the nervous system and enhancing haemoglobin level (Chauhan and Sarita, 2018). Neglected crops like millets were able to manage premature aging, diabetes, and obesity by being a significant source of nutraceuticals. Hence, they were able to provide solutions for security issues of both health and food because of their functional properties also their capability to withstandcritical weather conditions (Banerjee and Maitra 2020).

Generally, food utilization of millets has been confined to only conventional consumers and very few Indians are acquiring the knowledge of their health benefits and nutritional value. Therefore, different processing of millets using contemporary as well as traditional methods for the preparation of value-added food products would diversify their utilization of the diet. Hence, iron-rich value-added millet-based products are useful to provide most of the daily dietary iron requirements of adolescent girls which will be beneficial to control iron deficiency anemia. To promote these millets, nutritionists are trying their best to increase their consumption by supplying feeding trials among all groups of people specifically who are at the bay of anemia. Awareness among the people aids in creating a positive outlook towards this millet.

Some relevant reviews of the literature suggest that millets are excellent sources of iron for combating iron deficiency anemia. Macharia-Mutie *et al.* (2013) revealed that supplementation of 80g maize-based porridge by incorporating amaranth flour (56g amaranth flour: 24g maize flour) for 80 days had improved iron intake completeness while declining iron deficiency of preschool children aged 12-23 months in rural Kenya. Srivastava and Kumari (2019) developed supplementary food for adolescent girls (10- 18 years) by using ingredients like 60g quality protein maize, 22.5g green gram, 10.5g ragi, 10g gingelly seed, 5g amaranth leaves and 60g jaggery. After supplementation, there was an augmentation in haemoglobin levels by 1.04g/dl which indicated the positive impact of this food supplementation on the health of adolescent girls. A systematic review and meta-analysis were carried out by Anitha *et al.* (2021) on the bioavailability of iron in millet-based (Finger millet, Pearl millet, Teff, and Sorghum or a mixture of millets) products. Their findings indicated an elevation of hemoglobin level from moderate anemic to non-anemic level. Overall, they concluded that millets were a magnificent source of iron with economic potential for reducing iron deficiency anemia. Arunjyothi and Jahan (2021) assessed the impact of the intervention of finger millet ladoos on anaemic adolescent girls from different Telangana zones. They provided two finger millet ladoos of each 65gm daily for a period of 12 weeks. Further, they concluded that post-intervention analysis revealed improvement in Hb levels among adolescent girls with moderately to mildly anemic conditions.

The present chapter aims to provide updated comprehensive information on different types of iron-rich value-added food products developed from millets and their pharmacological properties in order to open a new perspective for future functional food and pharmacological research.

## Different products prepared from different millets

Akoth *et al.* (2012) compared the effectiveness of the most preferred two breakfast cereals products in the market in opposition to instant breakfast cereal products prepared from optimized flours of white sorghum, red sorghum, and pearl millet; they also used pigeon peas for legume complementation. The results revealed that white sorghum held the badge of most acceptable breakfast cereal product followed by pearl millet and red sorghum breakfast cereal with high nutritive values like the market products.

Singh *et al.* (2014) developed and standardized iron-rich ladoo made from pearl millet and concluded that a food-based initiative employing pearl millet continued to improve the Hb status of adolescent girls on par with elemental Fe supplementation.

A study of Selvi (2015) reported that haemoglobin concentration was improved by 1.26 g/dl after supplementation of two multigrain cookies (150 g) and 25 g of RTE crispy snack in daily diet among 100 adolescent girls (16 - 19 years) for 90 days.

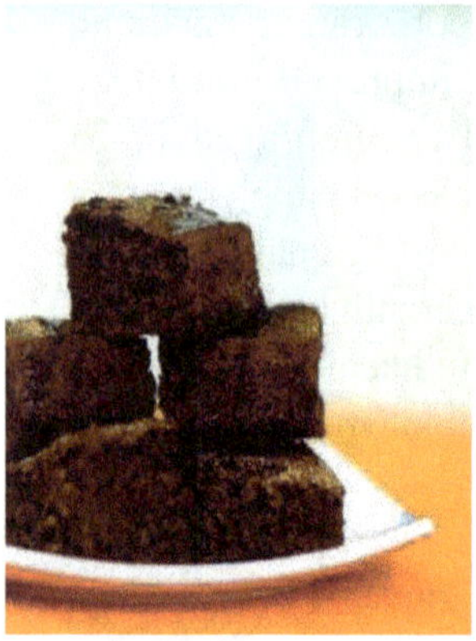

Sorghum Chocolate Brownie

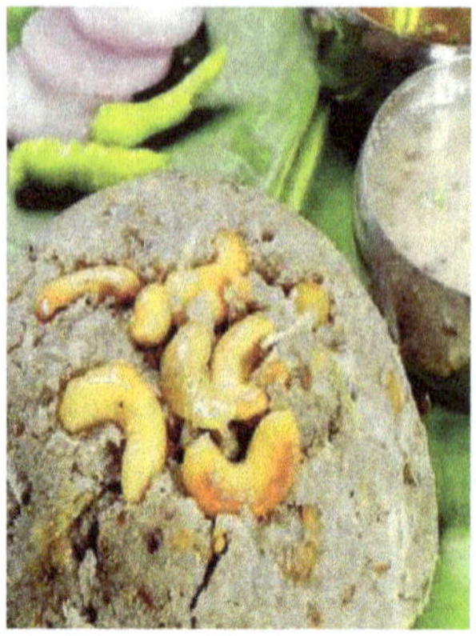

Pearl Millet Upma

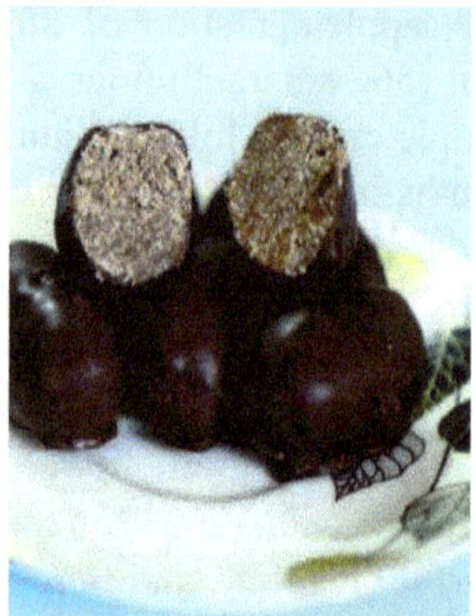

Finger Millet Bounty Bars

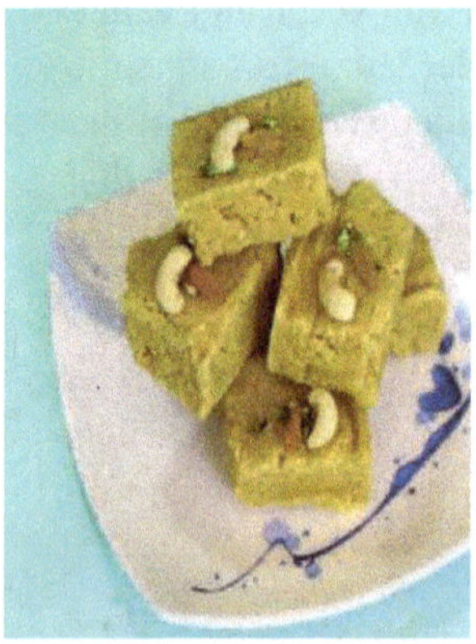

Sorghum Mysore Pak

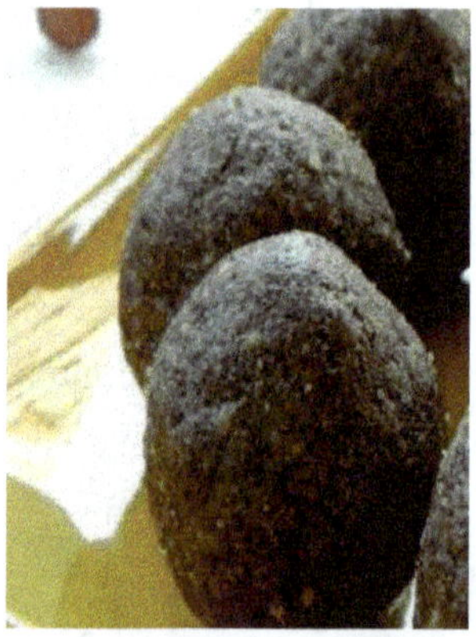

Finger Millet Ladoo

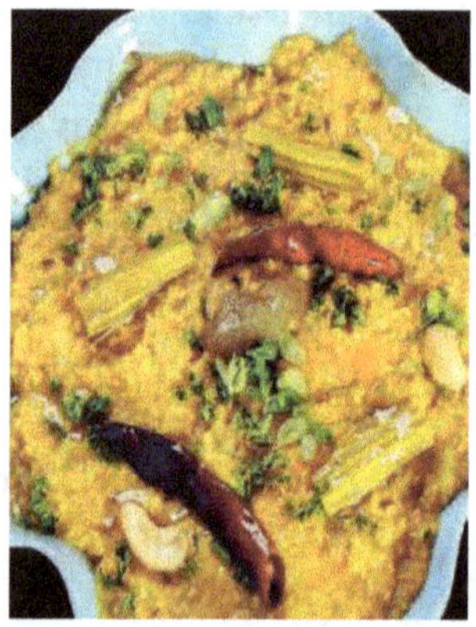

Foxtail Millet Bisi belle bath

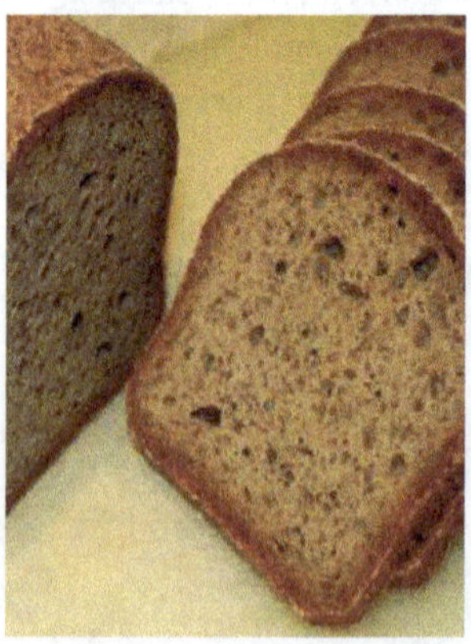

Foxtail Millet Bread

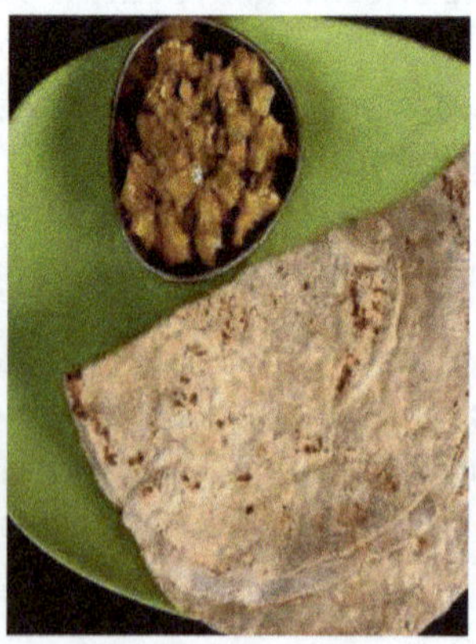

Pearl Millet Roti

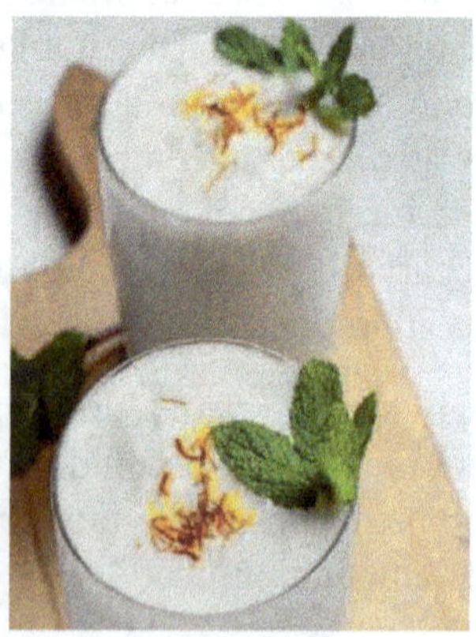

Sorghum Lassi

**Figure 3 :** Different millet-based products

Vanishree *et al.* (2016) developed a novel health drink by incorporating sprouted and dried pearl millet flour, finger millet flour, malted soya flour, milk powder, sugar powder, popped and milled amaranth seed powder in various combinations. Subjective evaluations of fortified samples indicated that 50 percent pearl millet incorporation followed by 60 percent with respective other ingredients was the most acceptable sample to combat nutritional anaemia.

Infante *et al.* (2017) evaluated the acceptability and iron bioavailability of bio-fortified sweet potato carotenoids in supplemented sorghum cookies. As a result, sorghum cookies served as functional food supplements to preclude or regulate anaemia caused by iron deficiency.

The subjective findings of Yadav and Dubey (2017) revealed that ladoo prepared by using 28.34g pearl millet, 15g turnip leaves, 28.33g gram flour, 28.33g flaxseed, 50g jaggery and 50g ghee scored highest in all aspects of hedonic scale and was useful to eradicate micro-nutrient deficiencies in adolescent girls.

A study of Sheela *et al.* (2018) revealed that millet milk extracted from selected millets (Foxtail millet, Little millet, Kodo millet, Proso millet and Barnyard millet) was a good source of nutrition composition with great implications to be used in the food industry sector primarily for formulating processed foods, functional foods, fermented foods and health mixes.

Vahini (2018) developed millet-based bar by using millet flakes (Foxtail, Barnyard millet flakes, Oats, Ragi flakes, Puffed rice in a ratio of 30:30:15:15:10) with other ingredients and at last interpreted that millet bar was well-accepted and provided necessary quantities of balanced nutrition for adolescent girls.

According to Anitha *et al.* (2019), all millet-based recipes had high acceptability, with the highest scores proceeding to the following three items: finger millet idli, little-pearl millet bisi belle bath, and pearl-little millet upma; millets also had significant potential to supplement rice in adolescent school feeding programmes for increased nutrient outcomes of children.

Jandu and Kawatra (2019) originated pearl millet-based bakery products (kulcha) which act as an alternative to wheat-based bakery products; also beneficial for human health to eradicate nutrient deficiencies.

Agrahar-Murugkar (2020) evaluated that the incorporation of malted finger-millet flour accompanied with refined wheat flour was used to improve the bio-accessibility of mineral especially iron and zinc in breads and biscuits which give rise to enhance mineral status of the population.

Bafna *et al.* (2020) developed a nutri-rich bhakri instant mix by using finger millet flour, pearl millet flour, wheat flour, flaxseeds, dry fenugreek leaves and found it good for better health and nutritional security.

Barbhai *et al.* (2021) discerned that buns prepared with 20% foxtail millet and muffins developed with 30% kodo millet enhanced bran-rich fractions accompanied by a significant increase in iron, zinc, calcium, dietary fibre, antioxidant capacity and phytonutrient constituent.

Belwal and Sujatha (2021) compared traditional recipes made of cereals with foxtail millet breakfast recipes. The results revealed that foxtail millet was easily incorporated in the local and common recipes.

Kulkarni *et al.* (2021) prepared cookies by substituting whole wheat flour with pearl millet flour (60%) which was highly accepted and potentially superior in terms of a nutritional point of view.

Mounika and Sireesha (2021) revealed that multi-millet bread which was formulated with pearl millet, sorghum, whole wheat flour, baker's yeast, sugar and butter in the ratio of 40:20:20:3:15:5 was highly accepted and packed with the goodness of fibre, iron, protein.

## Conclusion

In light ofsome relevant investigation outcomes, it can be deduced that consumption of various millet-based diets with special emphasis to pearl millet, sorghum, finger millet and foxtail millet by using different processing method in regular mealsby different age groups, especially vulnerable populationswill benefit to ameliorate iron deficiency anemia as millets are good sources of organic iron in contrast to other cereals.

## References

Agrahar-Murugkar, D. (2020). Food to food fortification of breads and biscuits with herbs, spices, millets and oilseeds on bio-accessibility of calcium, iron and zinc and impact of proteins, fat and phenolics. *LWT-Food Science and Technology*. **130**: 109703.doi: https://doi.org/10.1016/j.lwt.2020.109703.

Akoth, O. C., Oduor, S., Mwasareu, M. A., Ochieng, J. K., and Mathooko, F. M. (2012). Development of instant breakfast cereals from optimized flour of pearl millet red and white sorghum. *Journal of Applied Biosciences*. **51:** 3559-3566.

Ambati, K., and Sucharitha, K. V. (2019). Millets- review on nutritional profiles and health benefits. *International Journal of Recent Science Research*. **10** (7): 33943-33948.

Anitha, S., Kane-Potaka, J., Botha, R., Givens, D. I., Sulaiman, N. L. B., Upadhyay, S., and Bhandari, R. K. (2021). Millets can have a major impact on improving iron status, hemoglobin level and in reducing iron deficiency anemia–A systematic review and meta-analysis. *Frontiers in Nutrition*. **8**. doi: 10.3389/fnut.2021.725529.

Anitha, S., Kane-Potaka, J., Tsusaka, T. W., Tripathi, D., Upadhyay, S., Kavishwar, A., Jalagam, A., Sharma, N., and Nedumaran, S. (2019). Acceptance and impact of millet-based mid-day meal on the nutritional status of adolescent school going children in a peri urban region of Karnataka state in India. *Nutrients*. **11**(9): 2077. doi:10.3390/nu11092077

Arunjyothi, R., and Jahan, A. (2021). Effect of nutritional intervention in ameliorating anemia among adolescent girls of rural Telangana state. *The Pharma Innovation*. **10**(2): 185-188. doi: 10.11648/j.ijnfs.20130206.14

Associated Chambers of Commerce and Industry of India. Knowledge paper on millets 2021 status and way forward. 2021. https://www.assocham.org/ uploads / files/ Report_Millets2021_FINAL.pdf

Bafna, J., Kalpana, B., and Ramya, K. G. (2020). Development of nutri-rich bhakri (snack) instant mix. *Journal of Pharmacognosy and Phytochemistry*. **9**(3): 28-31.

Banerjee, P., and Maitra, S. (2020). The role of small millets as functional food to combat malnutrition in developing countries. *Indian Journal of Natural Sciences*. **10**(60): 20412- 20417.

Barbhai, M. D., Hymavathi, T. V., Kuna, A., Mulinti, S., and Voliveru, S. R. (2021). Quality assessment of nutri-cereal bran rich fraction enriched buns and muffins. *Journal of Food Science and Technology*. **59**(6): 2231-2242. doi: https://doi.org/10.1007/s13197-021-05236-9

Belwal, E., and Sujatha, M. (2021). Development of foxtail millet incorporated breakfast recipes and their comparison with traditional recipes made of cereals. *International Journalof Home Science*. 7(3): 147-151. doi:https://doi.org/10.22271/23957476.2021.v7.i3b.1196

Bhat, B. V., Rao, D. B., and Tonapi, V. A. (2018). The story of millets, Karnataka state department of agriculture in association with ICAR. Indian Institute of Millet Research, Hyderabad, India.

Chauhan, E.S. and Sarita (2018). Exploration of gluten-free baked food products incorporated by germinated finger (*Eleusine coracana*) and pearl (*Pennisetum glaucum*) millet: A therapeutic approach. *International Journal of Health Sciences and Research.* **8**(3): 232-242.

FAO Statistics. (2020). Statistical year book world food and agriculture, 2020. https://www.fao.org

Gopalan, C., Rama Sastri, B. V., & Balasubramanian, S. C. (2007). Nutritive value of Indian foods, Hyderabad, India

Infante, R. A., Natal, D. I. G., de Castro Moreira, M. E., Bastiani, M. I. D., Chagas, C. G. O., Nutti, M. R., and Martino, H. S. D. (2017). Enriched sorghum cookies with biofortified sweet potato carotenoids have good acceptance and high iron bioavailability. *Journal of Functional Foods*. **38**: 89-99. doi: http://dx.doi.org/10.1016/j.jff.2017.08.044

Jandu, R., and Kawatra, A. (2019). Nutritional composition of kulcha prepared from three varieties of pearl millet by incorporating soyabean flour. *The Pharma Innovation Journal*. **8**(6):52-54.

Kaur, J., Kanbi, V. H., and Chaudhary, M. K. (2016). Development and evaluation of soybean and finger millet incorporated sukhdi: An Indian snack. *International Journal of Farm Sciences*. **6**(4):6-13.

Kavitha, S., and Parimalavalli, R. (2014). Effect of processing methods on proximate composition of cereal and legume flours. *Journal of Human Nutrition and Food Science*. **2**(4):1051.

Kulkarni, D. B., Sakhale, B. K., and Chavan, R. F. (2021). Studies on development of low gluten cookies from pearl millet and wheat flour. *Food Research*. **5**(4): 114-119. doi:https://doi.org/10.26656/fr.2017.5(4).028

Kumari, R., Singh, K., Kumar, A., Singh, R. R., and Bhatia, N. (2019). Evaluation of nutrient content in crunchy bar developed from popped pearl millet *(Pennisetum glaucum)*. *Journal of AgriSearch*. **6**(Special Issue):150-152.

Lanzkowsky, P. (2016). Iron-deficiency anemia. In Lanzkowsky's Manual of Pediatric Hematology and Oncology.*Academic Press*. 69-83.

Liberal, Â., Pinela, J., Vívar-Quintana, A. M., Ferreira, I. C., and Barros, L. (2020). Fighting iron-deficiency anemia: innovations in food fortificants and biofortification strategies. *Foods*. **9**(12): 1871.

Longvah, T., Ananthan, R., Bhaskarachary, K., and Venkaiah, K. (2017). *Indian Food Composition Tables*, National Institute of Nutrition, Hyderabad, India.

Macharia-Mutie, C. W., Omusundi, A. M., Mwai, J. M., Mwangi, A. M., and Brouwer, I. D. (2013). Simulation of the effect of maize porridge fortified with grain amaranth or micronutrient powder containing NaFeEDTA on iron intake and status in Kenyan children. *Public Health Nutrition*. **16**(9): 1605-1613. doi:10.1017/S1368980012005174

Marak, N. R., Malemnganbi, C. C., Marak, C. R., and Mishra, L. K. (2019). Functional and antioxidant properties of cookies incorporated with foxtail millet and ginger powder. *Journal of Food Science and Technology*. **56**(11): 5087-5096. doi: https://doi.org/10.1007/s13197-019-03981-6

Mounika, M. D., and Sireesha, G. (2021) Development of multi millet bread with pearl millet and sorghum millet. *Wesleyan Journal of Research*. **14**(80): 90-100.

NFHS-5.(2019-21).Factsheet-NFHS-5.http://rchiips.org/nfhs/factsheet_NFHS-5.sht ml

Osman, M. A. (2011). Effect of traditional fermentation process on the nutrient and antinutrient contents of pearl millet during preparation of Lohoh. *Journal of the Saudi Society of Agricultural Sciences*. **10**(1): 1-6. doi: 10.1016/ j.jssas.2010.06.001

Priya, S.S., and Kowsalya, S. (2015). Formulation and evaluation and convenience food mixes from malted millets. *International Journal of Scientific Research*. **4**(11):409-411.

Ranasalva, N., and Visvanathan, R. (2014). Development of cookies and bread from cooked and fermented pearl millet flour. *African Journal of Food Science*.**8**(6): 330-336.

Rathore, T., Singh, R., Kamble, D. B., Upadhyay, A., and Thangalakshmi, S. (2019). Review on finger millet: Processing and value addition. *The Pharma Innovation Journal*.**8**(4): 283- 329.

Saini, S., Saxena, S., Samtiya, M., Puniya, M., and Dhewa, T. (2021). Potential of underutilized millets as nutri-cereal: An overview. *Journal of Food Science and Technology*. **58**(12): 4465-4477. doi: https://doi.org/10.1007/s13197-021-04985-x

Saleh, A. S., Zhang, Q., Chen, J., and Shen, Q. (2013). Millet grains: Nutritional quality, processing and potential health benefits. *Comprehensive Reviews in Food Science and Food Safety.* **12**(3): 281-295.

Sarita, E. S., and Singh, E. (2016). Potential of millets: Nutrients composition and health benefits. *Journal of Scientific and Innovative Research.* **5**(2): 46-50.

Selvi, M. T. (2015). Effect of nutri dense pack on academic performance and imparting changeability on snacking pattern of adolescents (Project Report). PSG College of Arts and Science, Coimbatore.

Sharma, S., Saxena, D. C., and Riar, C. S. (2015). Antioxidant activity, total phenolics, flavonoids and antinutritional characteristics of germinated foxtail millet (*Setariaitalica*). *Cogent Food and Agriculture.* **1**(1):1081728. doi: http://dx.doi.org/10.1080/23311932.2015.1081728

Sheela, P., Kanchana, S., Maheswari, T. U., and Hemalatha, G. (2018). Optimization of parameters for the extraction of millet milk for product development. *Research Journal of Agricultural Sciences.* **9**(6): 1345-1349.

Shingote, A. B., Sadawarte, S. K., Gaikwad, K. K., Gajmal, D. B., and Pawar, V. S. (2021) Effect of pretreatments on nutritional composition of sorghum, green gram and ragi. *Biological Forum – An International Journal.* **13**(1): 500-505.

Singh, R. B., Khan, S., Chauhan, A. K., Singh, M., Jaglan, P., Yadav, P., Takahashi, T., and Juneja, L. R. (2019). Millets as functional food, a gift from Asia to Western World. *The Role of Functional Food Security in Global Health.* 457-468. doi: https://doi.org/10.1016/B978-0-12-813148-0.00027-X

Singh, T. S., Goyal, M., and Sheth, M. (2014). Intervention trials with pearl millet-based iron rich ladoo and iron folic acid (IFA) tablets on hemoglobin status of adolescent females in Bikaner city. *Studies on Ethno-Medicine.* **8**(1): 77-82.

Srivastava, S., and Kumari, P. (2019). Impact of nutritional supplementation of quality protein maize based supplementary foods on nutritional status of adolescent girls. *Journal of Pharmacognosy and Phytochemistry.* (05) (Special Issue):417-419.

Vahini, R. V. (2018). Nutritional and microbiological assessment of nutrient enriched millet bar for adolescent female athletes. *International Journal of Engineering and Scientific Research.* **8**(1): 204-208.

Vanishree, S., Kammar, M.R., and Nidoni, U. (2016). Development and evaluation of pearl millet based novel health drink. *Advances in Life Sciences.* **5**(13): 5483-5486.

WHO. (2011). 'Haemoglobin concentrations for the diagnosis of anaemia and assessment of severity'. https://apps.who.int/iris/handle/10665/85839

WHO. (2019). Anemia in women and children. URL: https://www.who.int/data /gho/data/themes/topics/ anaemia_in _women _and_ children

Yadav, D. N., Sharma, M., Chikara, N., Anand, T., and Bansal, S. (2014). Quality characteristics of vegetable blended wheat pearl millet composite pasta. *Agricultural Research.* **3**(3): 263-270.

Yadav, K., and Dubey, R. P. (2017). Management of micronutrient deficiencies in adolescent girls: An interventional approach. *Plant Archives.* **17**(2): 973-976.

21

# Importance of Millets for Enhancement of Calcium Content and Thickness in Eggshell of Granivorous Birds

Renu Bala[1]* and Kamalpreet Kaur[2]

[1]Department of Biology, S. D. College, Barnala-148101, Punjab, India

[2]Department of Biology, S. D. College, Barnala-148101, Punjab, India

**ABSTRACT**

The distribution of food and types of the seeds available in a particular region are important aspects that affect suitability of the habitats for granivorous bird species. The intensification of agriculture and changes in agricultural practiceshaveled to the decline of granivorous birds.Pigeons and Ring Dove feed on the ground and are mainly grain-eater. Their food consists mainly of rice grains, millets, maize and other cereal grains pecked from the ground.The thickness of eggshell of eggs depends on the diet source, habitat quality (e.g. availability of the calcium) and the environment (e.g. presence of persistent biological contaminants). Calcium and eggshell thickness ofgranivorous birds are declining. The present study showed that White Pigeon under study were fed by trainers on artificial feed and they have been found to be with the highest calcium content (83%), followed by Blue-Rock Pigeon (70.20%) and Ring Dove (67.07%). This is considerably($p \leq 0.05$) higher in white pigeons than in Blue Rock Pigeons and Ring Doves.Eggs from White Pigeon had the thickest eggshell followed by eggs from Blue-Rock Pigeon and Ring Dove which had the lowest eggshell thickness. The reduction in thickness and calcium content in eggshells of selected birds may be attributed to monoculture of rice and wheat in the study area of Punjab, related agro-chemical pollution in habitats where bird species live and may result in failure of development of their chicks and hence reproduction.Accoding to Ministry of Agriculture and Farmer Welfare, Government of India (2022), millet production is not dependent on the use of agro-chemicals. Hence, present study suggests that cultivation of millets will be helpful in protecting birds, ecosystem, general environment and health of people by reducing/negligible use of agro-chemicals.

*Keywords*: Blue-Rock Pigeon, calcium, eggshell, Ring Dove, White Pigeon, Thickness

* Corresponding author.

## Introduction

Over the past 30 years, the range and population of many bird species linked with lowland farms have decreased, raising serious conservation concerns (Krebs *et al.,* 1999, Donald *et al.,* 2001). These decreases have been caused by agricultural intensification and modifications to farming methods throughout this time (Chamberlain *et al.,* 2000). One potential reason for the fall in the amount and accessibility of seed food is a reduction in the survival rate of seed-eating birds (Peach *et al.* 1999, Wilson *et al.,* 1999, Siriwardena *et al.,* 2001). The amount of grain and weed seed food on farms throughout the winter has also decreased because to more effective harvesting, storage, and seed cleaning techniques as well as aggressive herbicide regimes (Brickle and Harper 2000; Moorcroft *et al.,* 2002).

2023 will be recognised as the International Year of Millets, according to a resolution passed by the The United Nations General Assembly (UNGA). This highlights the value of millets and how they contribute to increased food security. Millets include pearl millet (major millet) (*Cenchrus americanus*), finger millet (*Eleusine coracana*), kodo millet (*Paspalum scrobiculatum*), foxtail millet (*Setar iaitalica*), proso millet (*Panicum miliaceum*), barnyard millet (*Echinochloa esculenta*), little millet (*Panicum sumatrense*), teff (*Eragrostist ef*), guinea millet (*Brachiaria deflexa*), fonio (*Digitaria exilis*), browntop millet (*Urochloa ramosa*) and Job's tears (*Coix lacryma-jobi*) (Rao *et al.,* 2021). Millets, a kind of grain from the Poaceae grass family, are among the earliest crops still grown today. As millet grains are so high in essential elements including calcium, dietary fibre, polyphenols, and protein, they are regarded as special crops (Devi *et al.,* 2014). For many nations in Asia and Africa, they serve as a staple food supply. The majority of millet produced is mostly utilised for human consumption, with a smaller amount also being used as animal and bird feed and to make beer (*Obiana,* 2020). In recent years, there has been an increase in the use of millet grains in animal feed. According to Baurhoo *et al.* (2011), broilers' development, bone calcium content, and feed efficiency have all significantly improved after maize was replaced in their diets with pearl millet.

Blue-Rock Pigeon (*Columba livia*) lives in a variety of habitats, including cracks in structures, openings in water pipes, tiny dumping grounds in waterways, bare-rock cliffs, home gardens, and house vents in both rural and urban environments. Due to their domestic origin and biological makeup, the majority of pigeons are classified as "granivorous" and are strongly related to human settlements. Due to the abundance of leftover food in both rural and urban areas, as well as grain storage structures, the Blue-Rock pigeon population has expanded over the past few decades. White pigeons (Albino) are being raised as pets in the study area.

Pigeons are powerful flyers with good homing instincts (Batool *et al.* 2019). Dhanda and Dhindsa (1993) noted that Ring Dove (*Streptopelia capicola*) had been building open nests in branches of trees.

The food type that birds consume is ecologically, economically and fundamentally important. Food availability has a vital role in diet of species of bird. Birds can have certain flexibility in the choice of food (Molokwu *et al.*, 2011, Camin *et al.*, 2015). Generalist birds are those that use a variety of food-gathering techniques or consume a wide range of foods, while specialists are those who focus their energy and attention on a particular type of food or use a single method of food acquisition (Gill, 1995).

Blue Rock Pigeon and Ring Dove feed on the ground and mainly grain-eater, while quite frequently they are invading diverse niches of food. The pigeon food consists mainly of rice grains, millet, maize and other cereals pecked from the ground. This bird species feeds also on banyan figs and other fruits like berry and occasionally eggs and larvae of insects (Bhattacharya, 1994). In addition to grains of wheat, jowar, paddy, millet and other pulses and cereals, mustard seeds, linseeds and several weeds are very frequently fed. Rana (1991) concluded that depending on the food availability, the ring dove frequently changes its habit of food; the bird feeds also on insects in the monsoon. Foraging in pigeon is done as a flock in a circular formation of which 10% of birds are feeding and 80% stay at periphery. Other 10% don't feed and move back and forth around the source of food (Murton *et al.*, 1972).

The research in birds has been mainly focused on egg shell thinning, as the large number of birds are not able to successfully reproduce mostly in the parts of the northern hemisphere since 1950 mainly due to pollutants continuously persisting in the environment, monoculture of rice and wheat and lack of millets(Wegner *et al.*, 2005, Jagannath *et al.*, 2008).An eggshell is a mineralized superficial cover of the egg in all birds which consists of the inner and outer shell membranes, the true egg shell and the cuticle. It is hard in some, and soft in other birds. The eggshell is a protein medium lined with mineral crystals, generally of a calcium complex like 95-97 percent of crystals of calcium carbonate. Softer eggs are less mineralized as compared to harder eggs (Eruvbetine, 2003).

The unity of eggshells, being composed of calcium carbonate, is vital for successful reproduction in birds (Gill, 2007). No doubt agriculture fields offers an extremely predictable and concentrated food source for birds (Gabbe *et al.*, 2002; Goetz *et al.*, 2007). The agricultural activities have led to the reshuffling of many bird species with an appropriate reduction in the abundance of bird species (Malhi, 2008). Blue-Rock Pigeon, White Pigeon, and Ring Dove are very commonly found birds in the study area which is agriculture land with added chemicals. Thus, the present study “Importance of Millets for enhancement of calcium content and thickness in eggshell of granivorousbirds”has been carried out in order to add to literature that habitat influences the eggshells of birds.

## Materials and Methods

### *Experimental design*

The present study was conducted from March 2022 to June 2022 at Biology Lab-I, S. D. College, Barnala, Punjab (India). Three birds, Blue-Rock Pigeon, White Pigeon, and Ring Dove, were chosen based on their feeding guild. Four eggs of each selected bird were collected from four nests (one from each clutch) after all eggs were laid and brought to the laboratory for egg parameter evaluation. Calcium content and thickness of eggshells were estimated.

### Eggshell thickness

For the measurement, three little egg shell pieces were used. They underwent air drying. During the measurements, vaterite-coated areas were avoided. The thickness might vary greatly according to the vaterite. Each eggshell has three measurements on each of its three sections. For the egg’s mean measurement, the three measures (in centimetres) were averaged (Dirksen and Boudewijn, 2001; Reis *et al.,* 2019).

### Eggshell composition

The inner membrane of the egg was removed after collecting the entire egg shell. After being crushed, it was put into a 250 ml beaker. It was then mixed with 50 ml of 3M HCl. The liquid was filtered (using filter paper) and allowed to dry over night after some time, when the bubbling ceased and the foam dissipated. Instead of calcium carbonate, the residual material was eggshell (mass of unreacted eggshell). The mass and percent content of calcium carbonate were then determined using the technique described by Butcher & Miles, 2000.

### *Full equation of reaction*

$$CaCO_3\ (s) + 2HCl\ (aq) \longrightarrow CaCl_2\ (aq) + CO_2\ (g) + H_2O\ (l)$$

### *Calculations*

Mass of unreacted eggshell = mass of filter paper and unreacted eggshell – the mass of filter paper.

Mass of $CaCO_3$ in eggshell = mass of eggshell – the mass of unreacted eggshell

$$CaCO_3 \text{ in eggshell} = \frac{\text{Mass of } CaCO_3}{\text{Mass of eggshell}}$$

$$\% \, CaCO_3 \text{ in eggshell} = \frac{\text{Mass of } CaCO_3}{\text{Mass of eggshell}} \times 100$$

## Statistical analysis

Eggshell calcium content and thickness in eggs of selected birds were compared by using one-way ANOVA (computer software SPSS16).

## Results and Discussion

In the present study, it has been observed that White Pigeon has the highest concentration of $CaCO_3$ i.e. 0.83±0.01 gm (83%), followed by the Blue-Rock Pigeon i.e. 0.69±0.02 gm (69.44%) and Ringneck Dove i.e. 0.67±0.01 gm (67.07±1.79%) which has the lowest value of $CaCO_3$ (Table 1, Fig 1).

According to our experimental analysis, the eggshell thickness was thickest in eggs of White Pigeon (0.18±0.01 mm) followed by eggs of Blue-Rock Pigeon and Ring Dove i.e. 0.14±0.01 mm and 0.11±0.04 mm respectively.

Moreover, amongst granivorous birds, the calcium content is significantly ($p \leq 0.05$) more in white pigeon when compared to Blue Rock Pigeon and Ring Dove.

**Table 1:** Calcium content (grams and percentage) and thickness in eggshells of Granivorous birds

| S. No. | Parameters → / Birds ↓ | Calcium carbonate content (gm) | Percentage of Calcium (%) | Eggshell Thickness (mm) |
|---|---|---|---|---|
| 1 | Blue Rock Pigeon | $0.69 \pm 0.02^{b}$ | $69.44 \pm 2.39^{b}$ | $0.14 \pm 0.02^{a}$ |
| 2 | White Pigeon | $0.83 \pm 0.01^{c}$ | $82.50 \pm 0.71^{c}$ | $0.18 \pm 0.01^{a}$ |
| 3 | Ring Dove | $0.67 \pm 0.01^{b}$ | $67.07 \pm 1.79^{b}$ | $0.11 \pm 0.04^{a}$ |

The Values are mean ± S.E.

Values with different superscripts in a column reveal significant ($p \leq 0.05$) difference

This may be due to the reason that the White Pigeons, being domesticated receive additional, regular nourishment by their caretaker while other two birds feed on food contaminated with chemicals in the fields etc. Various studies have been carried out by different authors in different areas. Jabbal and Khera (2016) have reported that in Blue-Rock pigeons average eggshell thickness varied from 0.15 mm to 0.20 mm, and calcium content of eggshell varied from 77.56 % to 91.10% in eggs collected from different locations of district Ludhiana. Shwetha *et al.* (2018) found that the content of calcium was higher in the eggshell of lapwing *i.e.* 96.46% and hybrid hen *i.e.*, 95.28% followed by pigeon *i.e.*, 68.06% in eggs collected from different locations of Karnataka.

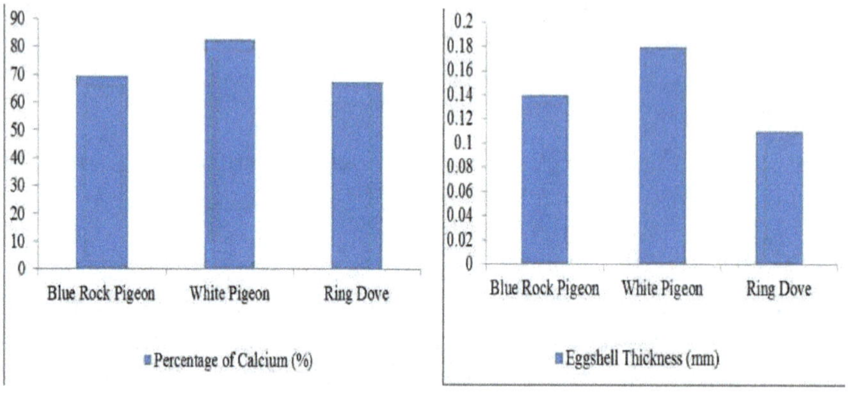


**Figure 1 :** Calcium content percentage and thickness in eggshells of selected birds

In the present study, the eggshell thickness range of the egg of pigeon (*Columba livia*) is in conformity with the range of eggshell thickness given by Sidel (1993) (0.15 mm to 0.20 mm with the mean eggshell thickness of 0.175 mm). Hence, different habitat quality (e.g. availability of calcium), different feeding habits and different environmental conditions (e.g. presence of persistent biological contaminants) in which the bird species live seems to be the reasons for differences in thickness and calcium content in the eggshell of selected birds in the present study.

Numerous authors have reported that variations in the thickness of the shell among clutches are caused by differences in the stages of incubation, differences related to clutch size, genetic and physiological differences between females, differences in diet among females within and between local populations, differences in gene pools between local populations, differences in environmental conditions, and other unknown factors (Romanoff and Romanoff 1949; Kaur and Khera 2017). Basesd on feeding habits of the Indian birds, very clear differences in the persistent toxic substances loads were observed as granivores< Omnivores<insectivores<coastal piscivores<midland piscivores and scavengers (Fybe *et al.,* 1991).

Many authors (Fernie *et al.,* 2009; Wilkin *et al.,* 2009) have reported that the development of the embryo also leads to thinning of the eggshell in many avian species as the embryos use calcium and minerals present in the eggshell for the development of the brain, skeleton, and muscles (Castilla *et al.* 2007; Karlsson and Lilja 2008). This may be due to the reason given by Gosler *et al.,* (2005) that the eggshell thinning can be compensated by a thicker layer of eggshell pigment deposition. Increased thickness of the membranes of the eggshell as reported by others (Felsenstein, 2008; Jagannath *et al.,* 2008; Ketta and Tumova 2016) has not been found the reason in present study. Cereal grain should continue to be a key component in situations where seed is being provided for farmland birds by growing seed-bearing crops, either on setaside land or under agri-environment schemes (Stoate *et al.,* 2004). This should be done using whatever variety is grown most easily and produces the most seed based on local climate and soil conditions.

## Conclusion

Birds require high amounts of calcium and eggshell thickness for egg production and the proper development of young chicks. Without it, young birds may not be healthy, and damaged eggshells may result in clutch abandonment because the hatchlings fail to hatch or malformed or even die. From the current study, it can be concluded that the eggshell thickness and calcium content in the eggs of various bird species change depending on habitat specific diet and trophic level specific feeding and foraging activities in particular environment. Because millets utilise fewer agrochemicals (Ministry of Agriculture and Farmer Welfare, Government of India 2022), birds that consume them may be able to produce eggs with thicker shells, which helps to increase the survival rate of hatchlings. As a result, more agricultural land must be used for millet cultivation.

## References

Batool, F., Khan, H.A., Saif-ur-Rehman, M. (2020). Feeding ecology of Blue Rock Pigeon (*Columba livia*) in the three districts of Punjab. Pakistan. Brazilian Journal of Biology, 80(4), 881-890.*https://doi.org/10.1590/1519-6984.225451*

Baurhoo, NB., Baurhoo, A.F. and Mustafa, Z.X. (2011).Comparison of corn-based and Canadian pearl millet-based diets on performance, digestibility, villus morphology, and digestive microbial populations in broiler chickens.Poultry Science, 90, 579–86.

Bhattacharyya, B. N. (1994). Diversity of feeding adaptations in certain columbid birds: A functional morphological approach. Journal of Biosciences, 19, 415-27.

Brickle, N.W. and Harper, D.G.C. (2000).Habitat use by Corn Buntings Miliariacalandra in winter and summer. In: Aebischer NJ, Evans AD, Grice PV and Vickery JA (eds) Ecology and Conservation of Lowland Farmland Birds. British Ornithologists' Union, Tring.

Butcher, G.D., Miles, R.D. (2000). Concepts of Egg shell Quality. Inquiry-Based Experiments in Chemistry,Oxford, New York. Pp 159-165.

Camin, S.R, Cueto, V.R., de Casenave, J.L. and Marone, L. (2015).Exploring food preferences and the limits of feeding flexibility of seed-eating desert birds.Emu Austral Ornithology, 115(3), 261-69.

Castilla, A.M., Herrel, A., Diaz, G. and Francesch, A. (2007). Developmental stage affects eggshell breaking strength in two ground-nesting birds: the partridge (*Alectorisrufa*) and the quail (*Coturnix japonica*). Journal of Experimental Zoology, 307, 471-477. *https://doi.org/10.1002/jez.400*

Chamberlain, D.E., Fuller, R.J., Bunce, J.C., Duckworth, J.C. and Shrubb, M. (2000). Change in the abundance of farmland birds in relation to the timing of agricultural intensification in England and Wales. Journal of Applied Ecology, 37, 771–788.

Devi, P.R., Vijayabharathi, R., Sathyabama, S., Malleshi, N.G. and Priyadarisini, V.B. (2014). Health benefts of fnger millet (*Eleusine coracana* L.) polyphenols and dietary fbre: a review. Journal of Food Science and Technology, 6, 1021–40. https://doi.org/10.1007/s13197-011-0584-9.

Dhanda, S.K. and Dhindsa, M.S. (1993). Eviction of Ring Dove, *Streptopeliadecaocto*, from a nest box by Common Myna, *Acridotheres tristis*.Pavo: Indian Journal of Ornithology, 31, 35-38.

Dirksen, S. and Boudewijn, T. (2001).Egg shell thickness measurements of Cormorant eggs: methods and some backgrounds.*www.cormorants.freehostia.com*

Donald, P.F., Green, R.E. and Heath, M.F. (2001).Agricultural intensification and the collapse of Europe's farmland bird populations.Proceedings of the Royal Society of London Series B, 268, 25–29.

Eruvbetine, D. (2003). Canine nutrition and health.Kensington Pharmaceuticals, Lagos,Nigeria.

Felsenstein, J. (2008). Comparative methods with sampling error and within-species variation: contrasts revisited and revised. The American Naturalist, 171, 713–725. *https://doi.org/10.1086/587525*

Fernie, K.J., Shutt, L., Letcher, R.J., Ritchie, I.J. and Bird, D.M. (2009). Environmentally relevant concentrations of DE-71 and HBCD alter eggshell thickness and reproductive success of American kestrels. Environmental Science & Technology, 43, 2124-30.

Fybe, R.W., Banasch, U., Benevides, V., Benevides, N.H., LusCombe, A. and Sanchez, J. (1991). Organochlorine residues in potential prey of peregrine falcons, *Flaco peregrines* in Latin America. Nat Field, 104, 211–228.

Gibbs, D., Barnes, E. and Cox, J. (2001). Pigeons and Doves: A Guide to the Pigeons and Doves of the World. The Auk, 118(4), 1117-1118.*http://dx.doi.org/10.1642/0004-8038(2001)118[1117:]2.0.CO;2*

Gill, (1995).Ornithology. Pp. 1-766. W H Freeman and Company, New York, USA.

Gill, F.B. (2007).Ornithology (3 rded). Freeman W H and Company, New York.

Goetz, S. Steinberg, D., Dubayah, R. and Blair, B. (2007).Laser remote sensing of canopy habitat heterogeneity as a predictor of bird species richness in an eastern temperate forest, USA .Remote Sensing of Environment,108, 254-263.*http://dx.doi.org/10.1016/j.rse.2006.11.016*

Gosler, A.G., Higham, J.P. and Reynolds, J. (2005). Why are birds' eggs speckled? EcolLett, 8, 1105–13.

Jabbal, G.K. and Khera, K.S. (2016). Morphometric analysis of eggs collected from Moga, PAU and Industrial Area of Ludhiana. Indian Journal of Applied Research, 6(1), 418-420.

Jagannath, A., Shore, R.F., Walker, L.A., Ferns, P.N. and Gosler, A.G. (2008). Eggshell pigmentation indicates pesticide contamination. Journal of Applied Ecology, 45, 133-40.

Karlsson, O. and Lilja, C. (2008).Eggshell structure, mode of development and growth rate in birds. Journal of Zoology, 111, 494–502.*https://doi.org/10.1016/j.zool.2007.11.005*

Kaur, M. and Khera, K.S. (2017).Egg parameters of the Red Wattled Lapwing (*Vanellusindicus*) in agricultural ecosystem of Punjab. Journal of Applied and Natural Science, 9(3), 1419-1421. *http://dx.doi.org/10.31018/jans.v9i3.1377*

Ketta, M. and Tumova, E. (2016).Eggshell structure, measurements, and quality-affecting factors in laying hens: a review. Czech Journal of Animal Science, 61(7), 299–309. *https://doi.org/10.17221/46/2015-CJAS*

Krebs, J.R., Wilson, J.D., Bradbury, R.B. and Siriwardena, G.M. (1999).The second silent spring? Nature, 400, 611–612.

Malhi, C.S. (2008). Successful breeding of five beneficial birds species in wooden boxes (Artificial nest boxes and earthen pots). Journal of Environment and Ecology, 26, 915-924.

Molokwu, M.N., Nilsson, J.A. and Olsson, O. (2011). Diet selection in birds: trade-off between energetic content and digestibility of seeds. Behavioral Ecology, 22(3), 639-47.

Moorcroft, D., Whittingham, M.J., Bradbury, R.B. and Wilson, J.D. (2002). The selection of stubble fields by wintering granivorous birds reflects vegetation cover and food abundance. Journal of Applied Ecology, 39, 535–547.

Murton, R.K., Coombs, C.F.B., and Thearle, R.J.P. (1972). Ecological studies of the Feral Pigeon Columba livia var. II. flock behaviour and social organization. Journal of Applied Ecology, 9(3), 875-89.

Obiana, A.B. (2020). Overview: importance of millets in Africa 2003. Published online at http://www.afripro.org.uk/papers/Paper02Obil

Peach, W.J., Siriwardena, G.M. and Gregory, R.D. (1999).Longterm changes in over-winter survival rates explain the decline of reed buntings Emberizaschoeniclus in Britain. Journal of Applied Ecology, 36, 798–811.

Rana, B.D. (1991). Ecology of the Indian Ring Dove in an arid environment.IntSymp on Environmental and Hormonal approaches to Ornithology.Pp 560.GarhwalUniversity Srinagar, Uttar Pradesh (Abstr).

Rao, B.D., Dinesh, T.M. andNune, S.D. (2021).Policy analysis and strategies. In: Millets and pseudo cereals. Woodhead Publishing. https://doi. org/10.1016/B978-0-12-820089-6.00011-2.

Reis, T.L., Quintero, J.C.P., Moraes, J.E., Pizzolante, C.C. and Calixto, L.F.L. (2019). Correlation among the main parameters of eggshellquality analysis of Hen And Quail eggs. Boletim de Indústria Animal, 76, 1-6.*https://doi.org/10.17523/bia.2019.v76.e1456*

Robinson, R.A. and Sutherland, W.J. (2002). Post war changes in arable farming and biodiversity in Great Britain. Journal of Applied Ecology, 39, 157–176.

Romanoff, A.L. and Romanoff, A. (1949).*The Avian Egg.* John Wiley and Sons Company, New York. Pp. 1-918.

Shwetha, A., Dhananjaya, Shravana, K.S.M. and Ananda (2018).Comparative study on calcium content in egg shells of different birds. International Journal of Zoology Studies, 3(4), 31-33.

Siriwardena, G.M., Baillie, S.R., Crick, H.Q.P. and Wilson, J.D. (2001). Variation in the survival rates of some British passerines with respect to their population trends on farmland. Bird Study, 45, 276–292.

Stoate, C., Henderson, I.G. and Parish, D.M.B. (2004). Development of an agri-environment scheme option: seed-bearing crops for farmland birds. Ibis, 146(2), 203–209.

Wegner, P., Kleinstauber, G., Baum, F. and Schilling, F. (2005).Long-term investigation of the degree of exposure of German peregrine falcons (*Falco peregrinus*) to damaging chemicals from the environment. Journal of Ornithology, 146, 34–54.

Wilkin, T.A., Gosler, A.G., Garant, D., Reynolds, S.J. and Sheldon, B.C. (2009). Calcium effects on life-history traits in a wild population of the great tit (*Parus major*): analysis of long-term data at severalspatial scales. Oecologia, 159, 463-472.*http://dx.doi.org/10.1007/s00442-008-1222-8*

Wilson, J.D., Morris, A.J., Arroyo, B.E., Clark, S.C. and Bradbury, R.B. (1999).A review of the abundance and diversity of invertebrate and plant foods of granivorous birds in northern Europe in relation to agricultural change.Agriculture, Ecosystem & Environment, 75, 13–30.

22

# Climate Change Resilient through Modern Farming in Vegetable Cultivation

Suprava Biswal[1*], Ambika Prasad Mishra[2]

[1] Department of Vegetable and Spice Crops, Uttar Banga Krishi Viswavidyalaya, Pundibari – 736165, India

[2] Department of Soil Science and Agricultural Chemistry, Faculty of Agriculture, Sri Sri University, Cuttack 754006, India

**ABSTRACT**

Vegetables are the high valued crops for human kind as it is rich source of important vitamins and minerals especially, micronutrients and phytochemicals promote good health which helps in reduction of mal nutrition.It is also primarily responsible for the positive health effects due to contains generous amount of numerous antioxidant substances, carotenoids and phenolics. Farmers are favored for their economics due to the short period of cultivation.But due to world's biggest threat that is climate change, which has made vegetable cultivation vulnerable to extreme weather occurrences including high temperatures, unpredictable rainfall that causes flooding, and drought situations.Vegetables are very perishable in nature due to high water content *i.e.,* 90%. Therefore, high temperature makes the cell damage and vulnerable for carry out all physiological and biological process inside the cell. Shedding down of flower bud and small fruit of solanaceous, cucurbitaceous and other types of vegetables also occur under high temperature stress. Not only drought, high temperature causes the cell damage but also erratic rainfall pattern results flood condition also dangerous for crop growth and development. In flooded condition, tomato plants produced ethylene hormone which is detrimental for fruit quality due to absence of oxygen.Increases in carbon dioxide, nitrous oxide, methane, and other harmful gases as a result of human activity are the primary cause of climate change. The majority of carbon dioxide is produced by burning of fossil fuels with emission of harmful industrial gases, methane is produced by raising livestock, and nitrous oxide is produced by using inorganic fertilizer. According to FAO, worlds vegetable production is get lowered around 18.68% due to adverse climatic effect.As a result, by 2050, an estimated 175 million more people could have zinc deficiency and 122 million more could have protein deficiency. People in poverty, who rely primarily on plant sources for sustenance, will be most affected by these effects.Therefore, to mitigate climate change problem crop prototype or idiotype will be helpful in a

* Corresponding author.

significant manner.Climate change is not only responsible for abiotic stresses but also it is responsible for spreading of biotic stress. So, incorporation of new crop prototype or new cultivar in a farming system which are resistant to biotic and abiotic stresses along with rich in high nutrition content. Climate change is not only a potential for the future; it is a reality that we are all already experiencing. Therefore, in modern farming systems modified and new innovation technology regarding water, soil and food security can be helpful to cope up in the climate change issue.

*Keywords*: vegetable, phytochemical, antioxidant, mal nutrition, resistance, climate change

## Introduction

'Vegetable cultivation' is a Latin term that stands for "pot herb culture," and it refers to the production of vegetables in which all parts can be consumed as cooked, raw, half cooked, or whole. Vegetables are an important food source in the human diet because they are high in bioactive compounds, dietary fiber, vitamins, minerals, and other phytochemical substances such as flavonoids, bioactive peptides, and phenolic compounds. It also contains a variety of antioxidant chemicals that aid in the removal of free radicals from the human body's metabolism process, and these are recognized as vitamin-A, vitamin-C, and vitamin-E.Because vegetable crops include a high concentration of numerous body-building materials, they serve to reduce the risk of chronic diseases such as diabetes, various types of cancer, heart disease, and obesity.According to ICMR, New Delhi recommended around 285gm-300gm of vegetables should be consumed by every individual in their daily diet period. However, the availability of vegetables is 145gm/person, which is insufficient to meet their daily dietary requirements.With growing awareness of the health benefits of vegetable crops, demand in both the domestic and foreign markets is rising. Furthermore, the growing population necessitates the cultivation of a fundamental dietary vegetable crop. As a result, a steady supply of vegetables throughout the year is required. However, in today's world, 'climate change' is the most serious threat to crop development and other living components in the ecosystem. As a result, farmers have recently been faced with the difficulty of producing abundant, safe, and nutritious vegetables for a growing global population while dealing with climate change issues and various types of biotic stress. According to IPCC (2018), worlds vegetable production is get lowered around 18.68% due to adverse climatic effect. As a result, by 2050, an estimated 175 million more people could have zinc deficiency and 122 million more could have protein deficiency. People in poverty, who rely primarily on plant sources for sustenance, will be most affected by these effects.Many issues related to climate change can be overcome by implementing current technology work in the field and improving crop prototypes. So, during climate change, the primary goal should be the development of various biofortified cultivars using gene modification or genetic engineering technology, raising cultivars resistant to all types of biotic and abiotic stresses, growing green-house crops, protected cultivation, and organic farming, crop residue management and so on.

## Reason behind the climate change

Climate change is the most significant challenge for global farmers. The fundamental source of climate change is caused by both natural and human-induced factors. Since the beginning of the industrial revolution, humans have been the primary cause of climate change due to the conversion of natural resources through the use of more and more fossil fuels. The emergence of various industries throughout the Industrial Revolution was the primary source of the creation of carbon dioxide gases, nitrous oxide, methane gas, ChloroFluro Carbon gas (CFC), and so on. According to the IPCC, carbon dioxide levels have risen from 350ppm to 410ppm in the last 20 years. All of these gases are referred to as green-house gases andtermed as the green-house effect.The increase in those gases generates a 1.5°C rise in temperature in the current climate, up from 1°C in the previous 20 years. As a result, numerous natural forest lands or ecosystems have been turned into agricultural land, industrial land, new building construction, and other uses. Furthermore, the world's growing population necessitates more food for existence. Meeting the food requirement for growing population expansion can be a difficult task for farmers. As a result, farmers are used to incorporating inorganic fertilizer, mostly nitrogenous based fertilizer, ammoniacal based fertilizer, insecticides, and pesticides to increase crop growth rate and output. However, it eventually degrades soil quality and causes soil erosion by the lower down of organic matter. So, the modern farming practices can be a useful for resolving the issue of climate change.

## Effect of climate change on vegetable production

Climate change can have significant effects on vegetable cultivation in several ways:

### 1. *Changes in temperature*

Temperature plays a crucial role in vegetable cultivation, as it affects the growth and development of the plants, their yield, and the quality of the produce. Here are some effects of temperature changes on vegetable cultivation:

(a) **Germination:** Temperature has a significant impact on the germination of seeds. Most vegetable seeds germinate best in temperatures between 15°C to 30°C. If the temperature is too low, the seeds may not germinate, and if it's too high, they may become dormant.

(b) **Growth and development:** Different vegetables have specific temperature requirements for optimal growth and development. For example, warm-season vegetables like tomatoes and peppers require higher temperatures between 18°C to 30°C to grow, while cool-season vegetables like spinach and broccoli grow best in temperatures between 10°C to 20°C.

(c) **Flowering and fruiting:** Temperature also influences the flowering and fruiting of vegetable plants. For example, some vegetables like eggplant and okra require warm temperatures to produce fruit, while others like lettuce and spinach can bolt and produce seed prematurely if exposed to high temperatures.

(d) **Yield and quality:** Extreme temperature changes can have negative impacts on the yield and quality of vegetable crops. High temperatures can cause the plants to wilt, reduce yield, and affect the quality of the produce. Low temperatures can also damage the plants and reduce yield.

(e) **Pests and diseases:** Temperature changes can also impact the susceptibility of vegetable plants to pests and diseases. High temperatures can increase pest and disease pressure, while low temperatures can slow down the growth of the plants, making them more vulnerable to pests and diseases.

Every crop requires optimum temperature for their growth and development. Both the high and low temperature affect the physiological process of the crop. High temperature (26°C) causes lower flower trusses results low fruit set as well as low yield in tomato along with uneven ripening or blotchy ripening occurred at fruit maturation time of tomato. Low temperature (14°C) takes more days for flowering to fruit set due to lower pollen activity and germination results poor fruit set (Adams *et al.,* 2001).The main reason behind the pollen desiccation at high temperature is increase of hexose: sucrose ratio up to three times more as compared to normal ratio due to activity of soluble acid invertase and sucrose synthase in matured anther of tomato. The gene expression for particular hexose: sucrose ratio, m-RNA coding for particular cell wall bound acid invertase results decrease in sucrose synthase and increase in acid invertase in matured anther of tomato (Pressman *et al.,* 2006). High and low temperature not only affect the fruit growth but also affect the leaf growth. At low temperature (15°C) the number of leaves has increased but at high temperature, reduction of leaf primordia growth occurs due to high competition for assimilates which conserved before at photosynthesis time in the early growth stages of tomato (Hussey, 1963). High temperature (33°C) causes low fruit set with low seed set and low fruit weight (Thuy and Kenji, 2015) whereas at low temperature (18°C) causes flower malformation results development of parthenocarpic fruit in capsicum crop (Karma *et al.,* 2018). Rising temperatures can also cause heat stress in vegetables, which can reduce yield and quality. For example, high temperatures can cause lettuce to bolt, resulting in bitter-tasting leaves. On the other hand, low temperature can delay crop growth, reduce yields, and increase the risk of frost damage.Rising temperature is also responsible for harmful insect, pest and disease incidence. Bacterial spot, anthracnose, bacterial wilt and phytophthora infestation is maximum at high temperature in capsicum crop (Karma *et al.,* 2018). Reduction of head and curd quality of cabbage and cauliflower due to high temperature prevails throughout the crop growth period encourages fungal disease caused by various strains of *Alternaria spp.* Disease incidence was severe at 22-26°C temperature and 800-850 ppm of $CO_2$ concentration in cabbage cauliflower crop (Siciliano *et al.* 2016). The high temperature at 32.5 or 35°C, was suitable for diamond back moth attack (*Plutella xylostella*) which is a devastating pest of cole crops (Golizadeh *et al.,* 2007).

## 2. *Effect of drought on vegetable cultivation*

Drought can have a significant impact on vegetable cultivation in several ways. Here are some effects of drought on vegetable cultivation:

(a) **Reduced yield:** Drought can cause a significant reduction in vegetable yield due to the lack of water, which can stress the plants and affect their growth and development. This can lead to smaller fruits or vegetables or a lower number of crops overall.

(b) **Delayed germination:** Drought conditions can delay the germination of vegetable seeds, which can affect the growth and development of the plant. This can cause the plant to be weaker and more susceptible to diseases and pests.

(c) **Stunted growth:** Drought can stunt the growth of vegetable plants, causing them to be shorter and smaller than usual. This can also affect the quality of the produce, as smaller plants may not produce as many fruits or vegetables or may produce smaller-sized fruits or vegetables.

(d) **Reduced nutritional value:** Drought can also reduce the nutritional value of vegetables, as water stress can affect the plant's ability to absorb nutrients from the soil. This can lead to a reduction in the vitamins and minerals present in the vegetables, which can have an impact on the health benefits they provide.

(e) **Increased susceptibility to pests and diseases:** Drought-stressed plants are more susceptible to pests and diseases, as they are weaker and more vulnerable. This can lead to a higher rate of plant disease and pest infestations, which can further reduce the vegetable yield.

Water is a key element for carry out all the metabolic process of the plant. If the water is not available to the plant system through irrigation or through rain, physiological process like photosynthesis process will be hamperedand plant will die eventually. Due to unavailability of water to the root system accumulation of salt occurred in to the root zone area due to osmotic effect which is the ultimately reason of more water stress condition of the plant.Reduction of relative water content inside the plant system, relative growth rate and increase of proline content along with abscisic acid in tomato plant under drought condition (Khan *et al.,* 2015). Ors*et al.* (2021) proved that combination effect of drought along with salt stress was detrimental for tomato growth and development as compared to individual stress effect. Those combination stress effect mostly damage the physiological and photosynthesis process of the plant. Other process was also affected due to stress like stomatal conductance, chlorophyll value and plant dry weight. They had also observed that electrolyte leakage of the leaves was highest under stress condition like reduction of nitrogen, phosphorous, potassium, iron, calcium and zinc nutrient but increase of sodium, boron and chloride content of the tomato seedlings. Decrease in tomato fruit weight can be correlated with salt content of the soil, which mostly seen in arid and sub arid region. But quality of the fruit like total soluble solid, color index and total soluble sugar content was highest under salt stress affected fruit crop of tomato (Yang *et al.,* 2019). As like tomato, chile ancho pepper was also affected by drought situation results reduction of leaf water content, stomatal conductance, whole plant transpiration, tissue relative water content, plant biomass and leaf transpiration surface area which ultimately affects the growth and development of the crop (Davies *et al.,* 2002). In some of the crop drought stress situation can be identified by looking at small leaf size and lower root to shoot ratio *i.e.,* in pepper plant (Phimchan *et al.,* 2012).

### 3. *Effect of flood conditions on vegetable cultivation*

It can have both positive and negative effects on vegetable cultivation. Here are some of the ways in which floods can impact vegetable crops:

#### *Positive effects*

(a) **Increased soil fertility:** Floods can deposit nutrient-rich sediment on fields, which can improve soil fertility and provide a boost to crops.

(b) **Water availability:** Floods can help alleviate water shortages and provide a reliable water source for vegetable crops.

(c) **Control of pests and diseases:** Flooding can help control certain pests and diseases that can damage crops.

#### *Negative effects*

(a) **Soil erosion:** Floods can cause erosion and soil loss, which can harm the growth of crops and reduce yields.

(b) **Waterlogging:** Prolonged flooding can cause waterlogging, which can suffocate plant roots and cause damage or even death to vegetable crops.

(c) **Loss of yield:** Flooding can cause significant crop losses due to water damage, soil erosion, and other factors.

(d) **Contamination:** Floodwaters can carry pollutants, chemicals, and other contaminants, which can affect the quality and safety of vegetable crops.

In a flooding situation all the soil pores *i.e.,* macro and micro pores filled with water. Due to waterlogged condition plant roots are unable to draw nutrients and other elements from the soil. Soil aeration is also hampered due to absence of oxygen. Therefore, death of the root occurs and ultimately it damages the plant system. Growth parameters like plant height, stem base diameter, number of leaves, size of the leaves, number of fruits per plant and dead plant % was maximum in waterlogged condition up to 12 days of tomato crop cultivar Pusa Ruby (Tareq *et al.*, 2020). Every crop has their own recovery system to cope up with any type of stress. During flooding condition of the tomato crop, usually water potential increases up to certain point and water deficit occurs inside the plant system. Under that water deficit condition, proline accumulation occurred which helps in development of adventitious root. Adventitious root again helped in resumed the plant growth system and allow to stand under waterlogged condition (Aloni and Rosenshtein, 1982). In waterlogged condition, taproot system of the plant converted into the adventitious root system. There are 2 types of plant hormone produced in the plant system during waterlogged condition i.e., ethylene and abscisic acid (Bouzroud *et al.,* 2018). Spreading of diseases is also high in waterlogged condition. Fruit rot of chili is caused by *Phytophthora capsici* soil organism spread through soil during waterlogged condition from infected plant to noninfected plant of chili (Sanogo, 2006). Overall, the impact of floods on vegetable cultivation can vary depending on the severity and duration of the flood, as well as the type of vegetable crop and the management practices used by farmers. In some cases, floods can even lead to improvements in crop yields, but in most cases, the negative impacts tend to outweigh the positive ones.

### 4. *Changes in soil quality*

Climate change can have significant impacts on soil quality, which in turn can affect vegetable cultivation. Some of the potential effects of climate change on soil quality include:

(a) **Soil erosion:** Climate change can lead to more extreme weather events, such as heavy rainfall and flooding, which can cause soil erosion. This can result in the loss of valuable topsoil, which is essential for vegetable cultivation.

(b) **Soil compaction:** Increased drought and heat can lead to soil compaction, making it difficult for vegetable roots to grow and access nutrients.

(c) **Soil nutrient depletion:** Rising temperatures and changing rainfall patterns can affect the nutrient content of soil, making it more difficult for vegetables to grow. This can result in lower crop yields and decreased quality of produce.

(d) **Soil acidity and soil salinity:** Climate change can also lead to changes in soil pH levels, which can affect the growth and development of vegetables.

(e) **Soil moisture content:** Changes in rainfall patterns can lead to either too much or too little moisture in the soil, which can affect the growth and development of vegetables.

To mitigate the impacts of climate change on soil quality, farmers can adopt sustainable soil management practices, such as reducing tillage, using cover crops, and practicing crop rotation. Additionally, they can use soil amendments, such as organic matter and fertilizer, to maintain soil health and fertility.

## Modern farming tools used to avoid climate change

There are several modern farming tools and techniques that can help mitigate the impact of climate change on vegetable cultivation. Here are a few examples:

1. *Precision agriculture*

Precision agriculture has several benefits for vegetable cultivation in the context of climate change:

(a) **Adaptation to changing weather patterns:** Climate change has led to more frequent and severe weather events such as droughts, floods, and heatwaves. Precision agriculture technologies, such as soil moisture sensors and weather monitoring systems, can help farmers adapt to these changing weather patterns by providing real-time data on soil moisture and weather conditions. This allows farmers to adjust irrigation and fertilization schedules to optimize crop growth and minimize water and nutrient losses.

(b) **Reduction of greenhouse gas emissions:** Agriculture is a significant contributor to greenhouse gas emissions, which contribute to climate change. Precision agriculture technologies can help reduce these emissions by optimizing fertilizer and pesticide application rates, reducing fuel consumption through optimized tractor routes, and reducing soil disturbance through minimum tillage techniques.

(c) **Conservation of natural resources**: Climate change can lead to the depletion of natural resources such as water and soil fertility, making it difficult for farmers to grow crops. Precision agriculture technologies can help conserve these resources by optimizing water use through drip irrigation, reducing soil erosion through cover cropping, and minimizing fertilizer use through precision nutrient management.

(d) **Improved crop resilience:** Climate change can increase the incidence and severity of pests and diseases, which can negatively impact crop yields. Precision agriculture technologies can help improve crop resilience by providing early detection of pest and disease outbreaks, enabling farmers to take quick action to prevent crop losses.

Precision farming is a site-specific farming technology where main objective are lower cost of production, higher crop productivity with minimizes the change climate impact on today's farming system. Rosa *et al.* (2000) used delta data precision farming system to evaluate processing tomato yield with plant parameters. They proved that site specific application of water and nutrient management helped in higher yield without hampering the soil quality. Schillaci *et al.* (2012) concluded that implementation of a machine vision algorithm in a precision farming system helped to carry out different farming activities like application of all inputs with desired quantity at specific site and harvesting of the tomato crop based on visual image collected from different places through artificial intelligence technology system.Amala and Syriac (2016) standardized the fertigation level for tomato crop growth and development under precision farming system *i.e.,* 125% recommended dose of nitrogen and potassium applied at 4 days interval. It is also help to detect various type of diseases through artificial intelligence. Durmus *et al.* (2017) used robotic system to identified and took close picture of tomato diseased leaves by using sensors. In this case human error was minimized results higher productivity of tomato crop. Naresh *et al.* (2011) cultivated cabbage as well as other types of vegetable-based farming system by using of conservation agricultural practices through laser-assisted precision land levelling technology. In this technology, crop stand occurred in a better way along with achieving all input use efficiency results crop productivity was increased 10% along with savings of water was 22% at western UP, Lucknow. Deshmukh *et al.* (2009) proved that site specific nutrient management helped to achieve yield of chili crop @ 30q/ha. with highest B:C ratio was 2.58. Shanmugam *et al.* (2015) applied biointensive pest management practices through precision farming to minimized the infestation of major pest of brinjal i.e., brinjal shoot and fruit borer (*Leucinodes orbonalis*). They recorded the lower damage of shoot (9.06%, 9.46%) and fruit (16.53%, 15.06%) of brinjal crop during kharif and rabi season which was earlier for shoot (11.40%, 11.46%) and fruit (16.93%, 17.20%) during kharif and rabi season under conventional farming practices.To avoid abnormal size in grafted seedlings of cucurbits used of automatic seedlings feeding device i.e., robotic system in precision farming was helped to get uniform grafted seedlings (Ohkoshi *et al.,* 2016). Another and important part of precision agriculture is application of nanofertilizers and nanopesticides. Chhipa (2017) studied the importance of nano-fertilizers (nitrogen, phosphorous, potassium, iron, manganese, zinc, copper, molybdenum and carbon nanotubes) observed as site directed application with required quantity and nanopesticides (Cu, ZnO, $SiO_2$, Ag and nanoformulations) was highly efficient to manage a broad-spectrum pest population.

Overall, precision agriculture has the potential to help vegetable farmers adapt to the challenges of climate change by providing real-time data and insights that allow them to optimize their farming practices and conserve natural resources. By using precision agriculture, farmers can reduce their environmental impact, improve crop yields, and ensure the long-term sustainability of their farming operations.

### 2. *Drip irrigation*

Drip irrigation is a type of irrigation system where water is applied directly to the soil near the root zone of the plant through a series of tubes or emitters. This method of irrigation can help in vegetable cultivation in areas affected by climate change in several ways:

(a) **Water conservation:** Drip irrigation can help conserve water by delivering water directly to the plant's root zone, reducing the amount of water lost to evaporation or runoff. This is especially important in areas affected by drought or where water resources are scarce.

(b) **Improved plant growth:** Drip irrigation can help improve plant growth by providing a consistent supply of water and nutrients to the plant's root zone. This can help plants grow faster and produce higher yields, which is important for vegetable cultivation.

(c) **Reduced soil erosion:** Drip irrigation can help reduce soil erosion by applying water slowly and evenly to the soil, reducing the amount of water runoff that can wash away topsoil and nutrients.

(d) **Increased efficiency:** Drip irrigation can be more efficient than traditional irrigation methods, such as sprinklers or flood irrigation. This is because drip irrigation delivers water directly to the plant's root zone, reducing the amount of water lost to evaporation or runoff.

Sub-surface drip irrigation system can give good outcome as compared to surface drip irrigation system. Kumar *et al.,* (2022) proved that the highest yield and maximum number of fruits per plant was achieved in sub surface drip irrigation system with using of mulch at salinity soil condition of brinjal variety Navkiran. Combination of 2 or more factor has more importance for improving crop growth and development than individual factor. Biswas *et al.,* (2015) showed that combine effect of drip irrigation and mulching on tomato gave higher economic return with higher yield and high water-use efficiency. Polythene mulch with drip irrigation of 50% water supplied were observed as best for crop yield, highest productivity and highest net returns as compared to paddy straw mulch with 100% water supplied through drip irrigation. Singandhupe *et al.* (2003) compared furrow irrigation with drip irrigation through fertigation system. They revealed that fertigation through drip irrigation gave higher yield with high water use efficiency and uptake of nutrients was more in drip irrigation system. Selvaperumal and Muthuchamy (2018) also concluded that drip fertigation (80% RDF) and black plastic mulch (thickness of 50 pm) gave maximum yield, number of fruits and net return of the chili crop. Similarly, study was carried out by Pandey *et al.*, (2013) where combination of drip irrigation, plant spacing (at 30cm) and nitrogen fertigation level helped to obtained early higher fruit yield, net income and minimizes of pest, diseases infestation of the crop. Blaine *et al.* (2006) observed that processing tomato yield was increased at saline ground water condition at depth of less than 1 meter. Because during salinity condition water is not available to plant system for carry out all the metabolism process. Therefore, they concluded that supply of water through drip irrigated processing tomato should be similar with the evapotranspiration loss of seasonal crop because lower water supply indicates lower yield under salinity condition of the soil. The key characteristic of processing tomato is total soluble solids concentration and many researchers proved that drip irrigation caused the reduction of soluble solids concentration. Johnstone *et al.* (2005) carried out a field experiment to see how late-season irrigation affects tomato quality. Generally, when there is a drought, the fruit size and crop weight are dramatically reduced. They discovered that if water shortage exists, it has no effect on the total soluble solids concentration and brix of processing tomato at the turning stage of maturity time, but water should be applied at the crop's early growth stages using drip irrigation system in drought-stressed areas. Singh *et al.* (2017) cultivated vegetable like cauliflower, chili and higher yielding factor observed at 80% irrigation level of pan evaporation with fertigation level of 75% recommended dose of fertilizer. Drip irrigation can also be helpful in reduction of diseases. Singh and Pandey (2014) noticed that reduction of harmful disease of chili i.e., anthracnose of chili caused by fungal organism *Colletotrichum sps.* occurred through drip irrigation system. There were only 4% infestation occurred when drippers placed at 60 cm apart as compared to closed dripper and flood irrigation system. Drip irrigation system was also helped in achieving of maximum chili yield as well as net income of the crop. Not only anthracnose in chili is get suppressed through drip irrigation but also *Phytophthora* root rot disease of chili can be suppressed through drip irrigation. Xie *et al.* (1999) applied irrigation on daily drip basis, 3 days interval drip system and alternate row furrow irrigation on chile plants *i.e., Capsicum annum* New Mexico '6-4'. They observed that highest yield as well as *Phytophthora* root rot infestation was low in daily drip and 3 days interval drip system.

Overall, drip irrigation can be an effective tool for vegetable cultivation in areas affected by climate change, helping to conserve water, improve plant growth, reduce soil erosion, and increase efficiency.

3. *Protected cultivation*

It refers to the practice of growing crops under a controlled environment, such as in greenhouses or polytunnels, to protect them from external factors like extreme weather, pests, and diseases. This method of cultivation has several benefits when it comes to vegetable cultivation in the context of climate change:

(a) **Protection from extreme weather events:** Protected cultivation provides a stable environment for vegetable crops, shielding them from extreme weather events such as droughts, floods, and heatwaves. This helps ensure a more consistent yield and reduces the risk of crop failure due to unpredictable weather patterns.

(b) **Reduced water use:** By controlling the environment inside the greenhouse or polytunnel, protected cultivation reduces the amount of water needed to grow vegetables. This is especially important in areas where water scarcity is a concern.

(c) **Protection from pests and diseases:** Protected cultivation can also help reduce the spread of pests and diseases that can be exacerbated by climate change. By providing a closed environment, pests and diseases are less likely to enter, reducing the need for chemical treatments.

(d) **Extended growing season:** Protected cultivation can also extend the growing season for vegetable crops, allowing farmers to grow crops for longer periods of time. This can help meet demand for fresh produce during times when traditional outdoor cultivation may be limited due to weather conditions.

Shamshiri (2017) recorded optimum temperature and optimum relative humidity at early growth stages, vegetative growth stages and flowering to fruit development stages for tropical green-house planted with tomato and that valued should be lies between 0 and 1. They showed that optimum maximum (0.92) and minimum temperature (0.42) was observed at vegetative growth stages while optimum relative humidity (0.62, 1) was observed at early growth stages of the protected tomato grown crop. They also examined that at various light conditions (night, sun and cloud) specific growth stages were hampered and after critical observation they found out during night hours of early growth stages period, highest optimum temperature and relative humidity occurred while increasing of light conditions did not affect the optimum temperature during vegetative growth stages of the tomato. Now adays, increasing of temperature is a biggest threat for flower and fruit setting of the crop. Harel *et al.* (2014) conducted an experiment to observe the effect of increased temperature during summer month of the Mediterranean region inside the protected structure of the pollen viability, flower development and fruit setting in the tomato crop. They found out decreasing of 1-1.5°C temperature inside the protected structure as compared to outside temperature with 50-70% RH which helped in pollen viability resulted good fruit settings of the tomato crop. Relative humidity was maintained through fogging system. Therefore, flower and fruit drop can be managed during hotter months of the growing period through protected structure equipped with useful instrument. Cheema *et al.*, (2004) cultivated tomato cultivar Avinash-2, CLN 2026D and Naveen inside the net house. They revealed that only 3-9% damage occurred by attack of *Spodoptera litura* whereas, aphid and *Helicoverpa armigera* attack was totally absent results higher fruit yield in tomato. Santosh *et al.* (2017) evaluated that value of water-use efficiency varied with use of different protected structure. They recorded that low crop evapotranspiration value showed in shadow hall (1.2-2.9 mm/day) followed by shade net house (1.4-3.7 mm/day) and polyhouse (1.3-3.2 mm/day) whereas, in open field condition value was 2-4.9 mm/day. Minimum water used only for crop growth and development under different protected structure like polyhouse (35.6%), shade net house (35.2%) and shadow hall (25.5%). Pandey *et al.* (2020) proved that protected cultivation was responsible for higher production of cole crops as compared to open field condition in the hilly areas. Protected cultivation in hilly area gave the new way for income generation to the small and marginal scale farmer.

Overall, protected cultivation offers a way to adapt to the impacts of climate change on vegetable cultivation by providing a controlled environment that is less vulnerable to extreme weather events and other environmental stresses.

4. *Crop modelling*

Crop modelling can help in vegetable cultivation in the face of climate change by predicting how changes in temperature, precipitation, and other climatic factors will impact the growth and development of different crops. Specifically, crop modelling can help in the following ways:

(a) **Selecting suitable crop varieties:** By simulating the impact of different climatic conditions on crop growth and yield, crop models can help identify crop varieties that are better adapted to the changing climate. For example, if the model predicts that temperatures will rise in a particular region, farmers can choose crop varieties that can tolerate higher temperatures.

(b) **Optimizing crop management:** Crop models can also help farmers optimize their crop management practices, such as planting dates, irrigation schedules, and fertilizer applications. By simulating the impact of different management strategies on crop growth and yield, farmers can identify the best practices for their specific conditions.

(c) **Assessing risk:** Crop models can also help assess the risk of crop failure due to climate change. By simulating the impact of extreme weather events, such as droughts and floods, on crop growth and yield, farmers can take proactive measures to reduce their risk of crop loss.

Mostly tolerant genotypes are preferred over susceptible for farming under various environmental stress condition. Tolerant genotypes (SRC-517, BARI Morich-2) showed as higher accumulation of proline content and total antioxidant capacity under waterlogged condition. But reduction of leaf area, photosynthetic compound and relative water content were observed in susceptible genotypes (AHM-206, RI-1(6) of chili crop. TSS (total soluble solid) content also reduced in waterlogged condition but after stress TSS content increased in tolerant genotypes of chili crop (Molla *et al.,* 2022). Tolerant genotypes have certain character for resistant to diseases. Fruit rot in chili caused by *Phytophthora capsici* is spreading through soil under waterlogged condition from infected plant to noninfected plant. But tolerant genotypes Criollo de Morelos 334and New Mexico 6-4) had peculiar feature where saturated and unsaturated soil condition did not create any disease symptoms to the chili crop (Sanogo, 2006). Thakur *et al.* (2019) developed chili leaf curl virus resistant hybrid by using of genetic male sterility breeding method. They crossed MS-341 (male sterile susceptible line) with S-343 (resistant donor line) for development of chili hybrid resistant to leaf curl virus. They observed, in the subsequent generation number of resistant genotypes was more as compared to susceptible genotypes that implies leaf curl disease resistant bearing line i.e., S-343 controlled by dominant gene. Therefore, it can be used in improving other susceptible genotypes of chili to lower down the leaf curl viral diseases.Phimchan *et al.* (2012) took three different pungency level of capsaicinoids content i.e., low, medium and high group of chili crop. They concluded that yield did not compromise in high capsaicinoids group cultivar whereas yield reduction was observed in low pungency group cultivar. But medium pungency group of cultivars did not show any symptoms under drought stress condition.

Vegetable grafting is becoming increasingly important in climate-resilient farming. Rivero *et al.* (2003) grown grafted and non-grafted tomato plants tolerant to high temperature (35°C). During growing period, they recorded highest PAL (phenylalanine Ammonium-Lyases) activity, phenol, o-diphenols concentration, decreased of dry matter content and decreased of polyphenol oxidase activity at highest temperature. Grafted plants had less phenolase activity as compared to non-grafted tomato plants because usually phenol act as defense mechanism against any stresses therefore, they observed as less produced phenol resulted less photosynthetic product used under high temperature condition. Usually, tomato has temperature stress at 35°C temperature whereas, watermelon has 15°Cstress temperature (Rivero *et al.,* 2001). Grafting of tomato plants on the brinjal root stock can help to reduce the issues of flooding and other soil borne diseases. Some eggplant rootstock *i.e.,* AVRDC recommended eggplant accessions EG195 and EG203 can be used as against soil borne diseases like bacterial wilt, root knot nematode, flooding and *Fusarium* wilt of tomato (Black *et al.,* 2003). Some tomato accessions are also available to avoid problem of Fusarium wilt, bacterial wilt and flooding condition of the tomato *i.e.,* AVRDC recommended line Hawaii 796 (Black *et al.,* 2003).

Climate change difficulties can also be mitigated via genome editing technologies, allowing for optimal growth and development. Zhang *et al.* (2020) grown thermotolerance transgenic tomato plants to observe the effect on crop growth under high temperature condition. Transformation of 2 enzymes named as betaine aldehyde dehydrogenase (BADH) and choline oxidase (COD) are responsible for synthesis of glycinebetaine (GB). Glycinebetaine mainly responsible for accumulation of reactive oxygen species (ROS) during stress period of the plant. In ROS, $H_2O_2$, $O_2^{\cdot-}$ and malondialdehyde were mostly observed in transgenic plant. They showed that glycinebetaine concentration in the water deficit plant was 1.9 µmol/gm to 3.4 µmol/gm of fresh weight of leaves whereas, this value was negligible in the water tolerance plants. Again, they found out that accumulation of heat shock protein 70 was more in transgenic plants. Wang *et al.* (2020) identified tomato low temperature stress resistance gene expression *i.e.,* SIMYB102. Low temperature stress resistance mostly found in reproductive part of the plant as compared to vegetative part example, it observed more in fruits than roots of the tomato plant. Accumulation of protein under stress condition is more and that was associated with over expressions of low temperature stress resistance gene SIMYB102. They also concluded that not only one gene was responsible for low temperature stress resistance but also other gene were there for responsible in low temperature stress resistance like SICBF1, SICBF3, SIDREB1, SIDEB2, and SIICE1 whereas, upregulated genes were SIP5CS and SIAPX2. Ezin *et al.* (2012) recorded 2 flooding tolerance genotypes i.e., CLN2498E and CA4 whereas, LA1579 genotype in tomato crop was sensitive to flooding. They also observed some key characteristic in susceptible genotype like up regulated gene action in alcohol dehydrogenase activity was four times higher and sucrose synthase decreased as the flooding days increased from 0 to 8 days.Despite this, tolerant genotypes did not produce a high yield due to flower and fruit dropping during the crop's reproductive stage. Wu *et al.* (2020) were introduced few recessive mutant genotypes for flood tolerance in grafting tomato. They observed development of adventitious root system in the stem with some chlorotic leaves in submergence tomato mutant genotypes. That mutation was mapped into the phytochromobilin synthase gene AUREA, where only one amino acid was responsible for conversion of asparagine to tyrosine compound. It can be a novel technology for improvement of crop genotype against flooding condition. Usman *et al.* (2017) were transferred heat shock protein gene from AVPP0702 (*Capsicum annum*) to susceptible genotypes of chili through marker assisted back cross breeding. They developed back cross breeding population from 3 generations and using of SSR polymorphic heat shock protein-linked markers (Hsp70-u2 and Agi42). They also recorded highest fruit yield characteristic in the improved genotypes and up regulation of heat shock protein activity observed when high temperature occurred. Sahitya *et al.* (2019) altered some aquaporin gene expressions to avoid the problem of drought situation in chili crop. They confirmed that presence of total 12 aquaporin upregulated gene action in drought tolerant genotype of chili *i.e.,* KCa-4884 whereas, downregulated aquaporin gene expression was observed in susceptible genotypes G-4. They also concluded that photosynthetic rate and relative water content were highest whereas, stomatal conductance was low in tolerant genotypes of chili.

Overall, crop modelling can provide valuable insights into how climate change will impact vegetable cultivation, and help farmers adapt their practices to ensure sustainable and productive crop production in the face of a changing climate.

5. *Organic farming*

Organic farming can have several benefits in vegetable cultivation when it comes to climate change. Here are a few examples:

(a) **Reduced greenhouse gas emissions:** Organic farming practices typically rely on natural fertilizers such as compost and manure instead of synthetic fertilizers, which require significant amounts of fossil fuels to produce. As a result, organic farming can reduce greenhouse gas emissions and help mitigate climate change.

(b) **Improved soil health:** Organic farming practices prioritize soil health, which can increase the soil's ability to store carbon. Organic farmers may use techniques such as crop rotation, cover cropping, and reduced tillage to improve soil health, leading to increased soil organic matter and improved water-holding capacity.

(c) **Reduced pesticide use:** Organic farmers use natural pest management methods such as crop rotation, companion planting, and natural predators to control pests and diseases. This can reduce the need for synthetic pesticides, which can have harmful impacts on the environment and contribute to climate change.

(d) **Water conservation:** Organic farming practices can also help conserve water, which is especially important in areas experiencing drought due to climate change. Practices such as mulching, cover cropping, and reduced tillage can help retain moisture in the soil, reducing the need for irrigation.

To the maximum extent possible organic farming rely upon application of types of manure, green manures, organic biostimulants, biodynamics compost, recycling of crop residue, crop rotation, mulching, inter cropping, cover cropping, biofertilizer based manure etc. To obtain better soil productivity as well as helps to improvement of crop growth, yield and quality factors. Application of various doses bulky organic manure like farmyard manure, vermicompost and poultry manure observed highest growth parameter in vegetable crops. Similar findings were recorded by Pandey *et al.* (2006) in pea crop and Adhikari *et al.* (2016) in capsicum. Organic bulky manure (vermicompost and poultry manure) is not only used in open field condition but also it can supply better nutrient sources under poly house condition by Dixit *et al.* (2018) in the cultivar GS-600 indeterminate type tomato. There are other types of bulky organic manure also helps to enhanced the crop growth, yield and quality parameter such as leaf manure, neem cake, night soil, vermicompost but among them use of vermicompost enhanced the crop quality such as capsaicin, vitamin-C, vitamin-A content as well as increased soil physio-chemical properties like cation exchange capacity, organic carbon, water holding capacity, other micro-macro nutrients- Ca, Mg, Na, Fe, Mn, Zn, Cu etc. Similar findings were observed by Kumar *et al.* (2016) in chilli crop. Utilization of concentrated organic manure (sesame meal, alfalfa meal) and mines product like peat, vermiculite mix has many benefits for enhancing the crop growth as well as soil microbial activity at different crop growth stages in tomato crop by Jack *et al.* (2011).

Enriched manure or biofertilizer enriched manure has many benefits due to availability of nutrients to the root system of the crop. Inoculation of biofertilizer like Phosphorous solubilizing bacteria (PSB), *Azotobacter sp.*, *Azospirillum sp.*, *Rhizobium sp.* used for legume crops helps to enhancement of fruit quality such as antioxidant property, vitamin-A, C etc. fruit length, fruit girth, number of fruits per plant and higher yield. Similar findings were recorded by Gopinath and Mina (2011) and Khurshid *et al.* (2021). Yadav *et al.* (2019) carried out a field trail to examine the combine effect of organic manure (farmyard manure, vermicompost) with biofertilizers (*Rhizobium*, phosphorous-solubilizing bacteria) on growth, yield parameters of cowpea legume crop. They found higher plant height, branches per plant, leaf area, leaf area index, root growth, higher nodule number and higher yield were highest at application of farmyard manure + vermicompost + *Rhizobium* + phosphorous-solubilizing bacteria. Nanobased biofertilizer is a recent advance in modern organic farming. Nano means small size that is about 1-100 nm helps improvement of nutrient use efficiency. Use of nanosilver and nitroxin biofertilizer recorded highest tuber diameter, number of tubers per each plant, average weight of each tuber and tuber yield observed by Davod *et al.* (2011). Biodynamic compost is another type of nutrient management in modern organic farming which preparation based on available of farm material instead of outside material. Application of biodynamic compost aid boosts the crop quality like crude fiber, crude ash, dry matter, anti-oxidant compounds like total phenolics, total anthocyanin, total leucoanthocyanins in coloured potatoes by Jariene *et al.*

(2015) and accumulation of starch content, accumulation of Magnesium, Pottasium nutrient etc. by Vaitkeviciene *et al.* (2016). Biodynamic compost can also use as spray during at different crop growth stages to improvement of dry matter content, nitrate content, crude fiber, dry matter accumulation etc. by Bacchus (2010) in head lettuce crop and also improvement of soil properties like average soil CO2 flux, total nitrogen, phosphorous, potassium content in addition to improvement of enzyme activity like urease and saccharase by Jukneviciene *et al.* (2019).

Green manuring is one of the nutrient sources for organic farming which helps to fixation of atmospheric nitrogen by the action of nitrogen fixing bacteria. It helps to improvement of crop quality like vitamin-C content, highest lettuce yield by Caliskan *et al.* (2014). There are lot of green manuring plants helps improvement of fruit quality, yield, titratable acidity, total soluble solids, dry weight of fruit and soil parameters like electrical conductivity, pH, available nitrogen, phosphorous, potassium etc. by incorporation of winter green manuring crop like pea, Italian rye grass, vetch etc., similar findings recorded by Tuzel *et al.* (2013) in green house organic cucumber production and incorporation of summer green manuring such as soyabean, maize, cowpea resulted highest head lettuce yield recorded by Duyar *et al.* (2009).

Thereafter spraying of biostimulants like panchagavya, jeevamruth, vermiwash has many benefits for enhancing the crop growth and quality along with improvement of soil physio-chemical properties. Similar findings were reported by Chandrakala (2008) in chilli crop. All those biostimulants has boosting effect on soil properties such as pH, electric conductivity, N, P, K, organic carbon, quantity of phytohormones like indole acetic acid, gibberlic acid, kinetin, abscisic acid and enhanced the activity of microbial population like Actinomycetes, *Rhizobium*, *Azospirillum* which is helped to increase shoot biomass, shoot length, root length, high leaf yield in spinach plant. Ramesh *et al.* (2018) conducted field trail by taking three different liquid organic supplements (jeevamrut, beejamrut, vermiwash) at the concentration of 3 % and 5 % applied three different growth times on 20, 40 and 60 days after sowing of maize seeds. They found foliar spray of jeevamrut at 5% recorded higher growth, yield attributing traits such as plant height, dry matter production, leaf area index, cob diameter, cob length, test weight, number of grains per cob, grain and stover yield. Application of both foliar biostimulant with bulky organic manure confirmed higher root girth, root length, root weight, yield/plot in beet root crop at soil application of vermicompost at 5 t/ha and consortium of biofertilizers at 2 kg/ha, combined with foliar application of effective microorganism at 1:1000 dilution/ha, panchagavya at 3% and humic acid at 2% by Devi *et al.* (2016). In a study conducted by Chongre *et al.* (2019) to optimize the effect of organic manures and liquid manures (jeevamrut + farmyard manure, sanjivak + farmyard manure, panchagavya + farmyard manure, cow urine + farmyard manure, vermiwash +

cow urine + farmyard manure, vermiwash + farmyard manure, vermicompost + farmyard manure, control) on growth, yield of summer green gram. They concluded application of both farmyard manure at 12 kg as basal doses along with panchagavya at 8 kg as foliar spray after 30 and 45 days after sowing were found as higher growth, yield characters like plant height, leaf area index, dry matter, number of pods per plant, pod length, number of seeds per pod, test weight, maximum grain yield and stover yield. In another study, Ansari and Sukhraj (2010) were conducted field experiment at Guyana by applying four different components (control, cattle dung, vermicompost, vermiwash, vermicompost + vermiwash) to examine the result of growth, yield of okra crop. They were observed higher fat and protein content found in vermicompost + vermiwash treated crop along with this particular treatment causes increasing the soil physical, chemical and soil micronutrient properties of soil.

There is other nutrient management strategy available in organic farming like cover cropping system. In a study conducted by Naira and Ngouajiob (2012) recorded highest microbial populations and functional diversity on incorporation of organic amendments along with crop residue of cover crops that is rye or a mixture of rye-vetch. All the major nutrients that is N, P, K, Ca, Mg in soil positively correlated with microbial population by incorporation of crop residue of rye-vetch mixture for improvement of tomato production.

## 6. *IPM and IDM*

Climate change can have significant impacts on agricultural production, including vegetable cultivation. Changes in temperature, precipitation patterns, and extreme weather events can all affect the incidence and severity of pests and diseases. Integrated Pest Management (IPM) and Integrated Disease Management (IDM) are two approaches that can help vegetable growers manage these challenges in the context of climate change.

(a) Integrated Pest Management (IPM) is a pest management strategy that focuses on preventing pest problems before they occur, using a combination of cultural, biological, and chemical control methods. This approach involves monitoring pests and their natural enemies, setting action thresholds, and implementing control measures only when necessary.IPM can help vegetable growers adapt to changes in pest populations and reduce their reliance on synthetic pesticides. For example, using crop rotation and cover crops can help prevent soil-borne diseases and pests, while natural enemies such as predators and parasitoids can help control insect pests.

(b) Integrated Disease Management (IDM) is a similar approach to IPM, but focuses specifically on managing plant diseases. IDM involves a combination of cultural, biological, and chemical control methods to prevent, diagnose, and manage diseases. This approach includes strategies such as crop rotation, resistant cultivars, sanitation, and biological control.

7. *INM*

Integrated nutrient management is a holistic approach to plant nutrition that involves the use of various sources of nutrients to improve soil fertility and plant growth. INM focuses on the efficient use of organic and inorganic fertilizers, and the integration of different crop management practices to improve soil health, crop productivity, and sustainability.In vegetable cultivation, INM involves the use of both organic and inorganic fertilizers, along with various crop management practices, such as crop rotation, intercropping, and use of cover crops. Here are some of the key components of INM in vegetable cultivation:

(a) **Soil analysis:** Before planting, soil analysis should be conducted to determine the nutrient content of the soil and the appropriate fertilizer requirement for the crops.

(b) **Organic fertilizers:** Organic fertilizers, such as compost, manure, and crop residues, can be used to improve soil fertility, increase water-holding capacity, and add essential nutrients.

(c) **Inorganic fertilizers:** Inorganic fertilizers, such as nitrogen, phosphorus, and potassium, are also essential for crop growth and can be used in combination with organic fertilizers to meet the nutrient requirement of crops.

(d) **Crop rotation:** Crop rotation can help improve soil fertility and reduce disease and pest problems. Rotation with legumes, such as peas and beans, can fix nitrogen in the soil, which can be beneficial for subsequent vegetable crops.

(e) **Intercropping:** Intercropping involves growing two or more crops together, which can help reduce soil erosion, improve soil health, and increase overall productivity.

(f) **Cover crops:** Cover crops, such as clover or rye, can be planted in between vegetable crops to improve soil health, prevent erosion, and suppress weeds.

(g) **Use of biofertilizers:** Biofertilizers, such as *Rhizobium*, mycorrhizae, and *Azotobacter*, can be used to enhance nutrient uptake, improve soil health, and reduce the need for chemical fertilizers.

8. *IWM*

Integrated Weed Management (IWM) is a holistic approach to weed management that combines multiple weed control methods to achieve sustainable, long-term control of weeds. In vegetable cultivation, IWM aims to minimize weed competition while reducing the use of herbicides and promoting the use of other cultural and physical weed control practices.Here are some strategies that can be incorporated in an IWM program for vegetable cultivation:

(a) **Crop rotation:** Crop rotation is an effective way to manage weeds by disrupting their life cycle. This practice involves alternating vegetable crops with non-vegetable crops, such as cover crops or grains, to break the weed cycle and reduce the population of weeds that are specific to certain crops.

(b) **Mulching:** Mulching with organic materials such as straw, leaves, or grass clippings can help to suppress weed growth by blocking sunlight from reaching the soil surface. This also helps to conserve soil moisture and regulate soil temperature, which can benefit the vegetable crop.

(c) **Hand weeding:** Hand weeding is a labor-intensive but effective way to remove weeds, especially in small-scale vegetable gardens. It involves pulling or cutting the weeds out by hand, which helps to prevent weed seed dispersal and reduce competition for resources.

(d) **Cultural control:** Cultural practices such as planting at the correct density, optimizing irrigation and fertilization practices, and using appropriate tillage methods can help to create an environment that is less favorable for weed growth.

(e) **Biological control:** Biological control involves using natural enemies of weeds, such as insects or pathogens, to suppress weed growth. This strategy is not commonly used in vegetable cultivation but can be effective in some situations.

(f) **Chemical control:** While minimizing the use of herbicides is an important goal of IWM, herbicides can still be used as part of an integrated approach to weed management. Selective herbicides that target specific weeds and leave the vegetable crop unharmed can be used judiciously to control weeds and reduce weed competition.

Overall, modern farming tools and techniques can help reduce the carbon footprint of vegetable cultivation and make it more resilient to the impacts of climate change.

## Conclusion

Climate change is a pressing global issue that has led to increasing concerns about food security and sustainable agricultural practices. Modern farming techniques, such as precision agriculture and smart farming, have the potential to increase the resilience of vegetable cultivation to the impacts of climate change.Precision agriculture involves the use of technology and data analysis to optimize crop yields, reduce waste, and improve resource efficiency. Smart farming, on the other hand, uses advanced sensors, internet of things (IoT) devices, and machine learning algorithms to automate various farming processes and improve productivity.

By incorporating these modern farming techniques into vegetable cultivation, farmers can better adapt to changing weather patterns, mitigate the effects of extreme weather events, and optimize resource utilization. For instance, precision agriculture can help farmers adjust irrigation schedules to account for changes in precipitation levels, while smart farming can automate pest management and soil nutrient management to reduce waste and increase productivity. In conclusion, modern farming techniques have the potential to increase the resilience of vegetable cultivation to the impacts of climate change. By adopting these practices, farmers can improve their yields, reduce waste, and contribute to sustainable agricultural practices that are crucial to addressing the global food security challenges posed by climate change.

## Future Prospective

Climate change poses a significant threat to agriculture, including vegetable cultivation. However, modern farming practices can help make vegetable cultivation more resilient to the impacts of climate change.One approach is to use precision agriculture techniques, such as using sensors and data analytics to optimize irrigation, fertilization, and pest management. This can help reduce water and fertilizer usage and increase crop yields, making vegetable cultivation more efficient and sustainable. Another approach is to use crop varieties that are more resistant to the impacts of climate change, such as heat stress and drought. Breeding programs can develop vegetable varieties that are more resilient to changing weather patterns and can thrive in warmer and drier conditions.In addition, modern farming practices can help reduce greenhouse gas emissions from agriculture, which contributes to climate change. Practices such as reducing tillage, using cover crops, and integrating livestock into cropping systems can help sequester carbon in the soil and reduce the need for synthetic fertilizers. Overall, modern farming practices can help make vegetable cultivation more resilient to the impacts of climate change while also reducing greenhouse gas emissions. By adopting these practices, farmers can help ensure a sustainable and secure food supply in the face of a changing climate.

## References

A. K. Pandey, A. K. Singh, A. Kumar, S. K. Singh (2013) Effect of Drip Irrigation, Spacing and Nitrogen Fertigation onProductivity of Chilli (*Capsicum annuum* L.). Environment & Ecology 31 (1) : 139—142.

Adhikari P, Khanal A and Subedi R (2016) Effect of different sources of organic manure on growth and yield of sweet pepper. Adv Plants Agric Res 3(5).

Ajeet Singh,S.k. Sharma and Rahul Chopra (2017)Effect of drip fertigation scheduling on yield and economics of cauliflower (Brassicaoleracea var.botrytis) and chilli (*Capsicum annuum* L.). Annals of Plant and Soil Research 19(2):137 - 142 (2017).

Ali Golizadeh, Karim Kamali, Yaghoub Fathipour, Habib Abbasipour (2007) Temperature-dependent development of diamondback moth, *Plutellaxylostella* (Lepidoptera: Plutellidae) on two brassicaceous host plants. Insect Science 14(4):309-316.

Anil Kumar Singh and Ajit Kumar Pandey (2014) Dynamics of Anthracnose Disease of Chilli in Responses to Water and Nitrogen Management under Drip and Flood Irrigation. Vol. 1 No. 3 (2014): Journal of AgriSearchpp 151-156.

Ansari A A and Sukhraj K. 2010. Effect of vermiwash and vermicompost on soil parameters and productivity of okra (*Abelmoschus esculentus*) in Guyana. African Journal of Agricultural Research 5 (14): 1794-8.

Bacchus G L (2010) An evaluation of the influence of biodynamic practices including foliar- applied silica spray on nutrient quality of organic and conventionally fertilised lettuce (*Lactuca sativa* L.). Journal of Organic Systems 5(1).

Benj' AloniandGilaRosenshtein (1982) Effect of flooding on tomato cultivars: The relationship between proline accumulation and other morphological andphysiological changes. PHYSIOL. PLANT. 56: 513-517.

Blaine R. Hanson, Robert B. Hutmacher& Donald M. May (2006) Drip Irrigation of Tomato and Cotton Under Shallow Saline Ground Water Conditions. Irrigation and Drainage Systems volume 20, pages155–175 (2006) (springer).

Caliskan S, Yetisir H and Karanlik S (2014) Combined use of green manure and farmyard manure allows better nutrition of organic lettuce. Not Bot Horti Agrobo 42(1):248-54.

Chandrakala M. 2008. Effect of FYM and fermented liquid manures on yield and quality of chilli (Capsicum annuum L.). (M.Sc. Thesis) University of Agricultural Sciences, Dharwad, Karnataka, India.

Chongre S, Mondal R, Biswas S, Munshi A, Mondal R and Pramanick M. 2019. Effect of liquid manure on growth and yield of summer green gram (Vigna radiata L. Wilczek). Current Journal of Applied Science& Technology 38 (6): 1-7.

D.S. Cheema, P. Kaur, S. Kaur (2004) Off-Season Cultivation of Tomato Under Net House Conditions. ISHS Acta Horticulturae 659: VII International Symposium on Protected Cultivation in Mild Winter Climates: Production, Pest Management and Global CompetitionDOI: 10.17660/ActaHortic.2004.659.21

Danny Harel,HadarFadida,AlikSlepoy,Shelly Gantz andKobi Shilo (2014) The Effect of Mean Daily Temperature and Relative Humidity on Pollen, Fruit Set and Yield of Tomato Grown in Commercial Protected Cultivation. Journals of Agronomy 2014, 4(1), 167-177.

Davod T, Reza Z, Ali V A and Mehrdad C (2011) Effects of nanosilver and nitroxin biofertilizer on yield and yield components of potato minitubers. Int. J. Agric. Biol. 13: 986–90.

Deshmukh, A. K. ; Shashidhara, G. B. ; Bidari, B. I. (2009) Effect of site specific nutrient management (SSNM) through targeted yield approach on yield and nutrient uptake of chilli (Capsicum annuum L.).Asian Journal of Soil Science 2009 Vol.4 No.2 pp.287-289 ref.3.

Devi T I, Haripriya K and Rajeswari R. 2016. Effect of organic nutrients and biostimulants on yield characters of beetroot (Beta vulgaris L.). Plant Archives 16 (1): 399-402.

Dixit P S, Prasad V M, Kasera S and Singh S (2018) Effect of various organic inputs on growth and its attributes of tomato (Solanum lycopersicum L.) cv. GS-600 under polyhouse condition. International Journal of Chemical Studies 6(6): 2537-9.

Duyar H, Tuzel Y, Kilic O G and Anac D (2009) The effects of green manuring on organic head lettuce production in greenhouse. Acta Hort. 807.

E. Pressman,D. Harel,E. Zamski,R. Shaked,L. Althan,K. Rosenfeld (2006) The effect of high temperatures on the expression and activity of sucrose-cleaving enzymes during tomato (Lycopersicon esculentum) anther development. The Journal of Horticultural Science and Biotechnology Volume 81, 2006 - Issue 3 pp 341-348.

F.T Davies Jr. a, V Olalde-Portugal b, L Aguilera-Gomez b, M.J Alvarado b, R.C Ferrera-Cerrato c, T.W Boutton d (2002) Alleviation of drought stress of Chile ancho pepper (Capsicum annuum L. cv. San Luis) with arbuscular mycorrhiza indigenous to Mexico. Scientia HorticulturaeVolume 92, Issues 3–4, 14 February 2002, Pages 347-359.

G. Hussey (1963) Growth and Development in the Young Tomato: I. The Effect of Temperature and Light Intensity on Growth ff the Shoot Apex and Leaf Primord IA. Journal of Experimental Botany, Volume 14, Issue 2, May 1963, Pages 316–325.

Gopinath K A and Mina B L. 2011. Effect of organic manures on agronomic and economic performance of garden pea (Pisum sativum) and on soil properties. Indian Journal of Agricultural Sciences 81 (3): 236–9.

HalilDurmus, EceOlcayGunes and MurvetKirci (2017) Disease detection on the leaves of the tomato plants by using deep learning. 2017 6th International Conference on Agro-Geoinformatics.

Hament Thakur, S.K. Jindal, Abhishek Sharma, M.S. Dhaliwal (2019) A monogenic dominant resistance for leaf curl virus disease in chilli pepper (Capsicum annuum L.). Crop ProtectionVolume 116, February 2019, Pages 115-120. (elsevier).

Hemraj Chhipa (2017) Nanofertilizers and nanopesticides for agriculture. Springer Environmental Chemistry Letters volume 15, pages15–22 (2017).

Hui Yang, Taisheng Du, Xiaomin Mao, Risheng Ding, Manoj K. Shukla (2019) A comprehensive method of evaluating the impact of drought and salt stress on tomato growth and fruit quality based on EPIC growth model. Agricultural Water ManagementVolume 213, 1 March 2019, Pages 116-127.

J. Amala and E. K. Syriac (2016) Standardization of fertigation schedule for tomato(Solanum lycopersicum L) under open precision farming. Journal of Crop and Weed, 12(2):82-85.

Jack A L H, Rangarajan A, Culman S W, Nguan T S and Thies J E (2011) Choice of organic amendments in tomato transplants has lasting effects on bacterial rhizosphere communities and crop performance in the field. Applied Soil Ecology.

Jariene E, Vaitkeviciene N, Danilcenko H, Gajewski M, Chupakhina G, Fedurajev P and Ingold R (2015) Influence of biodynamic preparations on the quality indices and antioxidant compounds content in the tubers of coloured potatoes (Solanum tuberosum L.). Not Bot Horti Agrobo 43(2): 392-7.

JinhuiXie, Elsa S. Cardenas, Theodore W. Sammis, Marisa M. Wall, Donald L. Lindsey, Leigh W. Murray (1999) Effects of irrigation method on chile pepper yield and Phytophthora root rot incidence. Agricultural Water ManagementVolume 42, Issue 2, November 1999, Pages 127-142 (elsevier)

Jukneviciene E, Danilcenko H, Jariene E and Fritz J (2019) The effect of horn-manure preparation on enzyme activity and nutrient contents in soil as well as great pumpkin yield. Open Agriculture 4:452-9.

Junqing Wu, Jie Cheng, Chunmiao Xu, Shilian Qi, Wenru Sun, Shuang Wu (2020) AUREA maintains the balance between chlorophyll synthesis and adventitious root formation in tomato. Horticulture Research, Volume 7, 2020, 166, 1-11.

Karma Bhutia L, Khanna VK*, TombisanaMeetei NG and Nangsol Bhutia D (2018) Effects of Climate Change on Growth and Development of Chilli. Agrotechnology 2018, 7:2 1-4.

Kaswan Pankaj Kumar*, Choudhary Gulab, Singh A.K., Choudhary Ashok, Kumar Ramesh, DidalBhuwnesh (2022) Performance of brinjal to water quality under drip irrigation system. Journal of Eco-friendly Agriculture Year : 2022, Volume : 17, Issue : 2First page : ( 290) Last page : ( 292).

Khurshid A, Mushtaq F, Narayan S, Mufti S, Rasool R, Wani I M, Maqbool S, Ashraf M T, Jan U, Nazir H and Ahmed N (2021) Effect of various organic manures and bio- fertilizers on growth and yield of chilli (Capsicum annum L.) under temperate conditions of Kashmir. Int J CurrMicrobiol App Sci 10(01): 3469-74.

Kumar V, Shankar R and Singh P K (2016) Effect of vermicompost, cow dung and different organic manure combination on growth and yield of chilli crop (Capsicum annuum L) in India. International Journal of Advances in Agricultural Science and Technology 3(3):14-9.

L.L.Black, D.L. Wu, J.F. Wang, T. Kalb, D.Abbass and J.H.Chen (2003) Grafting tomatoes for production in the hot-wet season. International Cooperators' Guide, AVRDC pub #03-551.

Magaji G. Usman, Mohd Y. Rafii, Mohammad Y. Martini, Oladosu A. Yusuff, Mohd R. Ismail &Gous Miah (2017) Introgression of heat shock protein (Hsp70 and sHsp) genes into the Malaysian elite chilli variety Kulai (Capsicum annuum L.) through the application of marker-assisted backcrossing (MAB). Cell Stress and Chaperones volume 23, pages223–234. (Springer)

MD. Rezwan Molla1,2,4; MD. Motiar Rohman2,*; MD. Robyul Islam1,2; Mirza Hasanuzzaman3,*; Lutful Hassan (2022) Screening and evaluation of chilli (Capsicum annuum L.) genotypesfor waterlogging tolerance at seedling stage. BIOCELL 1-15.

Md. Zablul Tareq1, Mohammad Saiful Alam Sarker1, Muhammad Delwar Hossain Sarker1,Md. Moniruzzaman1, Abu Sayeed Md. Hasibuzzaman2 and Syed Nazrul Islam (2020) Waterlogging stress adversely affects growth and development of Tomato. Asian Journal of Crop, Soil Science and Plant Nutrition. Vol. 02, Issue 01: 44-50.

Naira A and Ngouajiob M (2012) Soil microbial biomass, functional microbial diversity, and nematode community structure as affected by cover crops and compost in an organic vegetable production system. Applied Soil Ecology 58:45– 55.

Naresh R. K., Singh B., Singh Y. P., Kumar Ashok, Singh H. L., Prakash Satya (2011) Precision farming for enhancing productivity and sustainab-ility of vegetable system in western Uttar Pradesh. Annals of HorticultureYear : 2011, Volume : 4, Issue : 1First page : ( 10) Last page : ( 19).

Ohkoshi, T. ; Kobayashi, K. ; Shigematsu, K. ; Nakayama, N. ; Yoshinaga, K. (2016) Development of automatic seedling feeding device for cucurbits grafting robot (Part 2) - Practicality evaluation of automatic stock feeder.Journal of the Japanese Society of Agricultural Machinery and Food Engineers 2016 Vol.78 No.3 pp.232-240 ref.16.

P.R. Johnstone, T.K. Hartz, M. LeStrange, J.J. Nunez, andE.M. Miyao (2005) Managing Fruit Soluble Solids withLate-season Deficit Irrigation inDrip-irrigated Processing TomatoProduction. H ORT S CIENCE 40(6):1857–1861. 2005.

Pandey A K, Gopinath K A, Chatiacharya P, Hooda K S, Sushil S N, Kundu S, Kumar G S and Gupta H S. 2006. Effect of source and rate of organic manures on yield attributes, pod yield and economics of organic garden pea (Pisum sativum sub sp. hortense) in North-West Himalaya. Indian Journal of Agricultural Sciences 76 (4): 230-4.

Pandey Vandna*, Ranjan Ritesh, Pandey Harish, Rawal Jyoti, Bala Madhu (2020) Performance of different cole crops in different growing environmental conditions under mid hills of Uttarakhand. Progressive HorticultureVolume : 52, Issue : 2First page : ( 185) Last page : ( 192).

PaongpetchPhimchan, SuchilaTechawongstien, SaksitChanthai and Paul W. Bosland (2012) Impact of Drought Stress on the Accumulation of Capsaicinoids in Capsicum Cultivars with Different Initial Capsaicinoid Levels. American Society for Horticultural Science volume 47, issue 9 pp 1204–1209.

R.B. Singandhupe, G.G.S.N. Rao, N.G. Patil, P.S. Brahmanand (2003) Fertigation studies and irrigation scheduling in drip irrigation system in tomato crop (Lycopersicon esculentum L.). European Journal of AgronomyVolume 19, Issue 2, May 2003, Pages 327-340.

Ramesh S, Sudhakar P and Elankavi S. 2018. Effect of organic foliar nutrition on growth and yield of maize (Zea mays L.). International Journal of Research Analysis Review 5 (3): 64-7.

RaminShamshiri (2017) Measuring optimality degrees of microclimate parameters in protected cultivation of tomato under tropical climate condition. MeasurementVolume 106, August 2017, Pages 236-244. (elsevier)

Rosa M Rivero, Juan M Ruiz and Luis Romero (2003) Can grafting in tomato plants strengthenresistance to thermal stress?. Journal of the Science of Food and Agriculture 83:1315–1319.

Rosa M Rivero, Juan M Ruiz, Pablo C Garcia, Luis R Lopez-Lefebre, Esteban Sanchez, Luis Romero (2001) Resistance to cold and heat stress: accumulation of phenolic compounds in tomato and watermelon plants. Plant ScienceVolume 160, Issue 2, 5 January 2001, Pages 315-321. (Elsevier)

Rosa, U. A. ; Upadhyaya, S. K. ; Koller, M. ; Josiah, M. ; Pettygrove, S. (2000) Precision farming in a tomato production system.Proceedings of the 5th International Conference on Precision Agriculture, Bloomington, Minnesota, USA, 16-19 July, 2000 2000 pp.1-15 ref.8.

S. R. Adams *, K. E. Cockshull and C. R. J. Cave (2001) Effect of Temperature on the Growth and Development of Tomato Fruits. Annals of Botany 88: 869-877, 2001.

S. Sanogo (2006) Predispositional Effect of Soil WaterSaturation on Infection of Chile Pepper by Phytophthora capsici. HORT SCIENCE 41(1):172–175.

S.K. Biswas, A.R. Akanda, M.S. Rahman, M.A. Hossain (2015) Effect of drip irrigation and mulching on yield, water-useefficiency and economics of tomato. Plant Soil Environ. Vol. 61, 2015, No. 3: 97–102.

Sanjay Patel, H.N. Jinal, N. Amaresan (2017) Isolation and characterization of drought resistance bacteria for plant growth promoting properties and their effect on chilli (Capsicum annuum) seedling under salt stress. Biocatalysis and Agricultural BiotechnologyVolume 12, October 2017, Pages 85-89.

Santosh D.T.*, Tiwari K.N., Singh Vikas Kumar (2017) Influence of different protected cultivation structures on water requirements of winter vegetables. International Journal of Agriculture, Environment and Biotechnology Year : 2017, Volume : 10, Issue : 1First page : (93) Last page : ( 103).

Sarah Bouzroud, Sandra Gouiaa ,Nan Hu ,Anne adac, Isabelle Mila, Najib Bendaou, Abdel Aziz Smouni, Mondher Bouzayen, Mohamed Zouine (2018) Auxin Response Factors (ARFs) are potential mediators of auxin action in tomato response to biotic and abiotic stress (Solanum lycopersicum). PLoS ONE 13(2): 371-380.

Schillaci G.(1), Pennisi A.(1), Franco F.(2), Longo D.(2012) Detecting tomato crops in greenhouses using a vision based method. International Conference RAGUSA SHWA 2012, September 3-6, 2012, Ragusa – Italy 252-258.

SeldaOrs a, MelekEkinci b, Ertan Yildirim b, UstunSahin a, MetinTuran c, Atilla Dursun (2021) Interactive effects of salinity and drought stress on photosynthetic characteristics and physiology of tomato (Lycopersicon esculentum L.) seedlings. South African Journal of BotanyVolume 137, March 2021, Pages 335-339.

Selvaperumal A., Muthuchamyl. (2018) Performance of Chili (Capsicum Annuum L) Under Best Management Practices. Book Engineering Interventions in Sustainable Trickle Irrigation Edition1st Edition First Published2018 ImprintApple Academic Press Pages12eBook ISBN9781315184241.

Shanmugam P. S.*, Indhumathi K., Vennila M. A., Tamilselvan N. (2015) Evaluation of biointensive pest management modules against brinjal shoot and fruit borer, LeucinodesorbonalisGuenee (Lepidoptera: Crambidae) under precision farming system. Pest Management in Horticultural EcosystemsYear : 2015, Volume : 21, Issue : 2First page : ( 154) Last page : ( 158).

Sher Hassan Khan, Arsalan Khan, UzmaLitaf, Abdul Sattar Shah, Muhammad Ali Khan, Muhammad Bilaland Muhammad Usman (2015) Effect of Drought Stress on Tomato cv. Bombino. J Food Process Technol 2015, 6:7 1-6.

Siciliano, F. Berta, P. Bosio, M.L. Gullino, A. Garibaldi (2016) Effect of different temperatures and CO2 levels on Alternaria toxins produced on cultivated rocket, cabbage and cauliflower. World Mycotoxin Journal: 10 (1)- Pages: 63 – 71.

Tianpeng Zhang, Zhimei Li, Daxing Li, Chongyang Li, Dandan Wei, Shufen Li, Yang Liu, Tony H. H. Chen &Xinghong Yang (2020) Comparative effects of glycinebetaine on the thermotolerance in codA- and BADH-transgenic tomato plants under high temperature stress. Plant Cell Reports volume 39, pages1525–1538 (Springer)

Tran Loc Thuy and Murakami Kenji (2015) Effect of High Temperature on Fruit Productivity andSeed-Set of Sweet Pepper (Capsicum annuum L.) in theField Condition. Journal of Agricultural Science and Technology A and B& Hue University Journal of Science 5 (2015) 515-520.

Tuzel Y, Duyar H, Oztekin G B, Gurbuzkilic O, Anac D, Madanlar N and Yoldas Z (2013). Effects of winter green manuring on organic cucumber production in unheated greenhouse conditions. Turkish Journal of Agriculture and Forestry.

U. Lakshmi Sahitya, M. S. R. Krishna & P. Suneetha (2019) Integrated approaches to study the drought tolerance mechanism in hot pepper (Capsicum annuum L.). Physiology and Molecular Biology of Plants volume 25, pages637–647.

Vaitkeviciene N, Jariene E, Danilcenko H, Sawicka B (2016) Effect of biodynamic preparations on the content of some mineral elements and starch in tubers of three coloured potato cultivars. J. Elem. 21(3): 927-35.

VincentEzin, Cyrille A. Vodounon, Robert de la Pena, Adam Ahanchede, and Avtar Krishan Handa (2012) Gene expression and phenotypic characterization of flooding tolerance in tomato. Journal of Evolutionary Biology Research Vol. 4 (3), pp. 59-65, December, 2012.

Wang M, Hao J, Chen X, Zhang X. 2020. SlMYB102 expression enhances low-temperature stress resistance in tomato plants. Plant Biology PeerJ 8:e10059 https://doi.org/10.7717/peerj.10059.

Yadav A K, Naleeni R and Singh D. 2019. Effect of organic manures and biofertilizers on growth and yield parameters of cowpea (Vigna unguiculata (L.) Walp.). Journal of Pharmacognosy and Phytochemistry 8 (2): 271-4.

For Product Safety Concerns and Information please contact our EU representative GPSR@taylorandfrancis.com
Taylor & Francis Verlag GmbH, Kaufingerstraße 24, 80331 München, Germany

www.ingramcontent.com/pod-product-compliance
Lightning Source LLC
LaVergne TN
LVHW082342011026
849160LV00025B/1543